Advances in Cardiomyopathies

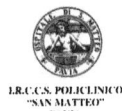
I.R.C.C.S. POLICLINICO
"SAN MATTEO"
PAVIA

Under the auspices of Policlinico San Matteo, Istituto di Ricovero e Cura a Carattere Scientifico, Pavia, Italy

Advances in Cardiomyopathies

Springer
Milano
Berlin
Heidelberg
New York
Barcelona
Budapest
Hong Kong
London
Paris
Singapore
Tokyo

F. Camerini • A. Gavazzi • R. De Maria (Eds)

Advances in Cardiomyopathies

Proceedings of the
II Florence Meeting on
Advances on Cardiomyopathies
April 24-26, 1997

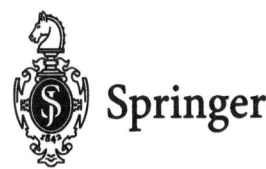 Springer

FULVIO CAMERINI
Division of Cardiology
Ospedale Maggiore
Trieste, Italy

ANTONELLO GAVAZZI
Division of Cardiology
IRCCS Policlinico S. Matteo
Pavia, Italy

RENATA DE MARIA
Institute of Clinical Phisiology, CNR
Ospedale Niguarda
Milan, Italy

© Springer-Verlag Italia, Milano 1998
Softcover reprint of the hardcover 1st edition   1998

ISBN 978-88-470-2181-5   ISBN 978-88-470-2155-6 (eBook)
DOI 10.1007/978-88-470-2155-6

Library of Congress Cataloging-in-Publication Data: Florence Meeting on Advances on Cardiomy-opathies (2nd: 1997) Advances in cardiomyopathies: proceedings of the II Florence Meeting on Advances on Cardiomyopathies, April 24-26, 1977 / F. Camerini, A. Gavazzi, R. De Maria (eds.). p. 000 cm. 17x24. Includes bibliographical references and index. ISBN 8847000092. 1. Myocardi-um-Diseases-Congresses. I. Camerini, F. II. Gavazzi, A. (Antonello), 1948-. III. De Maria, R. (Rena-ta), 1957-. IV. Title. [DNLM: 1. Myocardial Diseases congresses. WG 280 F632a 1998]. RC685.M9 F56 1997. 616.1'24-DC21. DNLM/DLC for Library of Congress 98-10658 CIP.

Typesetting: Photo Life (Milan)

Cover design: Simona Colombo

SPIN: 10661604

Preface

The Italian Study Group on Cardiomyopathies organized in Florence in April 1997, eight years after the first successful meeting, the second international symposium devoted to "Advances in Cardiomyopathies".

In these years exceptional progress has been made in the field of heart muscle diseases, in clinical research as well as in molecular biology, molecular genetics, pathophysiology and treatment. Many of these advances were presented and discussed in Florence by a distinguished team of international experts.

Hypertrophic cardiomyopathy was addressed in ten papers; in the first one Seidman reported the results obtained by the use of molecular genetic techniques which showed that hypertrophic cardiomyopathy is a heterogeneous disorder caused by different mutations of different genes and discussed the clinical role and significance of genetic testing.

Original data regarding the natural history and prognosis of symptomatic patients were obtained in the Italian multicentric study (Cecchi, Lazzeroni), while Baroldi discussed the clinico-pathologic spectrum of the disease in severely symptomatic patients treated with heart transplantation.

Sudden death in the young (Basso), the identification and management of high risk patients (Elliott), the clinical importance and the problems of detection of ischemia (Camici) were deeply discussed as well as the indications and results of different types of treatment: medical, surgical, DDD pacing (Spirito, Betocchi, Schoendube).

The sessions on dilated cardiomyopathy included many papers devoted to the study of the role of different potential etio-pathogenetic factors such as viruses (Tracy), genetic abnormalities (Towbin), organ specific autoantibodies (Caforio), beta-receptor antibodies (Waagstein), mitochondrial DNA changes (Arbustini), myocardial blood flow abnormalities (Neglia) and to their importance in clinical cardiology (Mestroni, Gavazzi).

The result of natural history of dilated cardiomyopathy obtained by the SPIC registry, which included 441 patients (De Maria) were presented, while Porcu analyzed the prognosis of a group of patients with mildly dilated cardiomyopathy.

Of high interest were the sessions devoted to treatment. Maisch discussed the role of immunosuppressive treatment in "inflammatory dilated cardiomyopathy" (myocarditis) followed by Cohn (medical treatment), Borggrefe (prevention of sudden death) and Leonen (timing of heart transplantation).

The final session was completely devoted to the treatment of heart failure with beta-blockers. The panel discussed the theoretical and experimental background (Bristow), the controlled studies (Sharpe) and the complex clinical problems (Cleland, Sinagra), indicating a useful additive role of this class of drugs in heart failure, although many problems, as for example the prevention of sudden death, are still open.

An analysis of the role of non-pharmacologic approaches (DDD pacing, cardiomyoplasty, VAD) in severely ill patients ended the meeting (Gibson, Chachques, Rinaldi).

In conclusion, the congress closed a decade of great advances in our understanding and management of cardiomyopathies.

Undoubtedly these major advances were strictly connected to the revolutionary changes in medical genetics and molecular biology, characterized by the newer techniques of gene identification and characterization as well as to careful clinical study and controlled trials in heart failure.

I think that this book is a good summary of all these complex fascinating problems.

Fulvio Camerini

Table of Contents

DILATED CARDIOMYOPATHY: Treatment

List of Contributors

A. Angelini
Istituto di Anatomia Patologica,
Università degli Studi, Padua, Italy

E. Arbustini
Istituto di Anatomia Patologica, Patologia
Cardiovascolare e Diagnostica Molecolare
IRCCS Policlinico San Matteo, Pavia, Italy

E. Ardemagni
Divisione di Cardiochirurgia, IRCCS Policlinico San Matteo, Pavia, Italy

M.K. Baig
Department of Cardiological Sciences,
St. George's Hospital Medical School,
London, UK

N. Banchieri
Istituto di Anatomia Patologica, IRCCS,
Policlinico San Matteo, Pavia, Italy

G. Baroldi
Istituto di Fisiologia Clinica CNR, Sezione
di Milano, Dipartimento Cardiotoracico
De Gasperis, Ospedale Niguarda, Milan,
Italy

M. Bartoli
Istituto di Fisiologia Clinica CNR, Pisa,
Italy

C. Basso
Istituto di Anatomia Patologica, Università
degli Studi, Padua, Italy

O. Bellini
Istituto di Anatomia Patologica, Patologia
Cardiovascolare e Diagnostica Molecolare,
IRCCS, Policlinico San Matteo, Pavia,
Italy

P. Bellone
Servizio di Cardiologia, Ospedale
Sant'Andrea, La Spezia, Italy

L. Beretta
Divisione di Cardiologia, Istituto Villa
Marelli, Milan, Italy

C. Bethge
Jüdisches Krankenhaus, Berlin, Germany

S. Betocchi
Istituto di Medicina Interna, Cardiologia e
Cardiochirurgia, Università Federico II,
Naples, Italy

M. Block
Innere Medizin, Kardiologie, Medizinische
Klinik und Poliklinik, Westfälische
Wilhelms Universität, Münster, Germany

E. Bonacina
Servizio di Anatomia Patologica, Ospedale
Niguarda, Milan, Italy

M. Borggrefe
Innere Medizin, Kardiologie, Medizinische
Klinik und Poliklinik, Westfälische
Wilhelms Universität, Münster, Germany

C. Bosman
Istituto di Anatomia Patologica, Ospedale
Pediatrico Bambin Gesù, Rome, Italy

K.R. Bowles
Department of Pediatrics (Cardiology),
Molecular and Human Genetics, Baylor
College of Medicine and Texas Children's
Hospital, Houston, USA

G. Breithardt
Innere Medizin, Kardiologie,
Medizinische Klinik und Poliklinik,
Westfälische Wilhelms Universität,
Münster, Germany

M. Bristow
Division of Cardiology, University of
Colorado, Denver, USA

C. Briguori
Istituto di Medicina Interna, Cardiologia e
Cardiochirurgia, Università Federico II,
Naples, Italy

A.L.P. Caforio
Cattedra di Cardiologia, Università degli
Studi, Padua, Italy, and Department of
Cardiological Sciences, St. George's Hospi-
tal Medical School, London, UK

F. Camerini
Divisione di Cardiologia, Ospedale
Maggiore, Trieste, Italy

P.G. Camici
MRC Cyclotron Unit and Royal Post-
graduate Medical School, Hammersmith
Hospital, London, UK

C. Campana
Divisione di Cardiologia, IRCCS,
Policlinico San Matteo, Pavia, Italy

A. Carpentier
Département de Chirurgie Cardiaque et
Vasculaire Hospital Broussais Université
de Paris "Pierre et Marie Curie", Paris,
France

G. Castelli
Servizio di Cardiologia S. Luca, Azienda
Ospedaliera Careggi, Florence, Italy

G. Catani
Istituto di Anatomia Patologica, Ospedale
S. Michele Brotzu, Cagliari, Italy

F. Cecchi
Divisione di Cardiologia S. Luca, Azienda
Ospedaliera Careggi, Florence, Italy

J.C. Chachques
Département de Chirurgie Cardiaque et
Vasculaire Hospital Broussais Université
de Paris "Pierre et Marie Curie", Paris,
France

N.M. Chapman
Department of of Pathology and
Microbiology, University of Nebraska
Medical Center, Omaha, USA

D. Chersevani
Divisione di Cardiologia, Ospedale
Maggiore, Trieste, Italy

M. Chiariello
Istituto di Medicina Interna, Cardiologia e
Cardiochirurgia, Università Federico II,
Naples, Italy

G.P. Chiriatti
Divisione di Cardiologia, Ospedale di
Pescia, Pescia, Italy

M. Ciaccheri
Servizio di Cardiologia S. Luca, Azienda
Ospedaliera Careggi, Florence, Italy

J.G.F. Cleland
Department of Medical Cardiology,
Glasgow Royal Infirmary, and Clinical
Research Institute in Heart Failure,
Glasgow, UK

J.N. Cohn
Cardiovascular Division, Department of
Medicine, University of Minnesota Medi-
cal School, Minneapolis, Minnesota, USA

E. Colombi
Divisione di Cardiologia, IRCCS,
Policlinico San Matteo, Pavia, Italy

D. Corrado
Istituto di Anatomia Patologica, Università
degli Studi, Padua, Italy

A.M. D'Armini
Divisione di Cardiochirurgia, IRCCS,
Policlinico San Matteo, Pavia, Italy

B. Dal Bello
Patologia Cardiovascolare e Diagnostica
Molecolare, Istituto di Anatomia
Patologica, IRCCS, Policlinico San Matteo,
Pavia, Italy

L. De Biase
Istituto di Chirurgia del Cuore e Grossi
Vasi, Università La Sapienza, Rome, Italy

R. De Maria
Istituto di Fisiologia Clinica CNR, Sezione
di Milano, Dipartimento Cardiotoracico De
Gasperis, Ospedale Niguarda, Milan, Italy

M. Diegoli
Istituto di Anatomia Patologica,
Patologia Cardiovascolare e Diagnostica
Molecolare, Laboratorio Ricerca Trapianti,
IRCCS, Policlinico San Matteo, Pavia,
Italy

A. Di Lenarda
Divisione di Cardiologia, Ospedale
Maggiore, Trieste, Italy

A. Dolara
Divisione di Cardiologia S. Luca,
Azienda Ospedaliera Careggi, Florence,
Italy

E. Donegani
Cattedra di Cardiochirurgia, Università di
Torino, Turin, Italy

R. Dougthy
Department of Medicine, Faculty of
Medicine and Health Sciences, University
of Auckland, Auckland, New Zealand

P.M. Elliott
Department of Cardiological Sciences,
St. George's Hospital Medical School,
London, UK

A. Falaschi
International Centre for Genetic Enginee-
ring and Biotechnology, AREA Science
Park, Trieste, Italy

R. Fasani
Istituto di Anatomia Patologica,
Patologia Cardiovascolare e Diagnostica
Molecolare, Laboratorio Ricerca Trapianti,
IRCCS, Policlinico San Matteo,
Pavia, Italy

A. Fiocchi
Divisione di Cardiochirurgia, Ospedali
Riuniti, Bergamo, Italy

G. Gagliardi
Divisione di Cardiologia, Ospedale
Pediatrico Bambin Gesù, Rome, Italy

P. Gallo
Cattedra di Anatomia Patologica Cardio-
vascolare, Dipartimento di Medicina
Sperimentale e Patologia, Università La
Sapienza, Rome, Italy

M. Gallopin
Istituto di Clinica Medica Generale e
Cardiologica, Università di Firenze,
Florence, Italy

A. Gavazzi
Divisione di Cardiologia, IRCCS, Policlinico San Matteo, Pavia, Italy

G. Gensini
Istituto di Clinica Medica Generale e
Cardiologica, Università di Firenze,
Florence, Italy

M. Giacca
International Centre for Genetic Enginee-
ring and Biotechnology, AREA Science
Park, Trieste, Italy

E. Giagnoni
Divisione di Cardiologia, Istituto Villa
Marelli, Milan, Italy

D. Gibson
Cardiac Department, Royal Brompton
Hospital, London, UK

A. Giorgetti
Istituto di Fisiologia Clinica CNR, Pisa,
Italy

M. Giraldi
Divisione di Cardiologia, IRCCS, Policlinico San Matteo, Pavia, Italy

J.H. Goldman
Department of Cardiological Sciences,
St. George's Hospital Medical School,
London, UK

J.F. Goodwin
Department of Clinical Cardiology, Royal
Postgraduate Medical School and Department of Cardiological Sciences, St. George's Hospital, London, UK

M. Grasso
Istituto di Anatomia Patologica,
Patologia Cardiovascolare e Diagnostica
Molecolare, Laboratorio Ricerca Trapianti,
IRCCS, Policlinico San Matteo, Pavia,
Italy

D. Gregori
Dipartimento di Scienze Economiche e
Statistiche, Università di Trieste, Trieste,
Italy

E. Gronda
Divisione di Cardiologia, Dipartimento
Cardiotoracico De Gasperis, Ospedale
Niguarda, Milan, Italy

A.J. Haven
Department of Cardiological Sciences,
St. George's Hospital Medical School,
London, UK

M. Herzum
Medizinische Klinik, Kardiologie,
Klinikum der Philipps Universität,
Marburg, Germany

G. Hufnagel
Medizinische Klinik, Kardiologie,
Klinikum der Philipps Universität,
Marburg, Germany

C. Inserra
Divisione di Cardiologia, IRCCS,
Policlinico San Matteo, Pavia, Italy

V. Kanjuh
Institute for Cardiovascular Diseases,
Medical Center of Serbia, Belgrade,
Yugoslavia

S. Klugmann
Divisione di Cardiologia, Ospedale
Maggiore, Trieste, Italy

U. Kühl
Medizinische Klinik II, Kardiologie,
Universitätsklinikum Benjamin Franklin,
Berlin, Germany

A. L'Abbate
Istituto di Fisiologia Clinica CNR, Pisa,
Italy

M. Laudisa
Divisione di Cardiologia, IRCCS,
Policlinico San Matteo, Pavia, Italy.

E. Lazzeroni
Divisione di Cardiologia, Azienda Ospedaliera di Parma, Parma, Italy

O. Leone
Istituto di Anatomia Patologica, Università
degli Studi, Bologna, Italy

M.F. Leonen
Department of Internal Medicine, Wayne
State University School of Medicine,
Detroit, USA

U. Livi
Istituto di Chirurgia Cardiovascolare,
Centro di Cardiochirurgia «V. Gallucci»,
Padua, Italy

F. Longaro
Divisione di Cardiologia, Ospedale
Maggiore, Trieste, Italy

M.A. Losi
Istituto di Medicina Interna, Cardiologia e
Cardiochirurgia, Università Federico II,
Naples, Italy

G. Magrini
Istituto di Anatomia Patologica,
Patologia Cardiovascolare e Diagnostica
Molecolare, IRCCS, Policlinico San
Matteo, Pavia, Italy

B. Maisch
Medizinische Klinik, Kardiologie,
Klinikum der Philipps Universität,
Marburg, Germany

R. Maksimović
Institute for Cardiovascular Diseases,
Medical Center of Serbia, Belgrade,
Yugoslavia

M. Matulic
International Centre for Genetic Engineer-
ing and Biotechnology, AREA Science
Park, Trieste, Italy

W.J. McKenna
Department of Cardiological Sciences,
St. George's Hospital Medical School,
London, UK

L. Mestroni
International Centre for Genetic Engineering and Biotechnology, AREA Science
Park, and Divisione di Cardiologia, Ospedale Maggiore, Trieste, Italy

G. Minzioni
Divisione di Cardiologia, IRCCS,
Policlinico San Matteo, Pavia, Italy

L. Miocic
International Centre for Genetic Engineer-
ing and Biothechnology, AREA Science
Park, Trieste, Italy

A. Montereggi
Divisione di Cardiologia S. Luca,
Azienda Ospedaliera Careggi, Florence,
Italy

P. Morbini
Istituto di Anatomia Patologica, Patologia
Cardiovascolare e Diagnostica Molecolare,
IRCCS, Policlinico San Matteo, Pavia,
Italy

D. Neglia
Istituto di Fisiologia Clinica CNR, Pisa
Italy

J.B. O'Connell
Department of Internal Medicine, Wayne
State University School of Medicine,
Detroit, USA

I. Olivotto
Divisione di Cardiologia S. Luca,
Azienda Ospedaliera Careggi, Florence,
Italy

R. Ortiz-Lopez
Department of Pediatrics (Cardiology),
Molecular and Human Genetics, Baylor
College of Medicine and Texas Children's
Hospital, Houston, USA

M. Ostojič
Institute for Cardiovascular Diseases,
Medical Center of Serbia, Belgrade,
Yugoslavia

F. Pagani
Divisione di Cardiochirurgia, IRCCS,
Policlinico S. Matteo, Pavia, Italy

S. Pankuweit
Medizinische Klinik, Kardiologie,
Klinikum der Philipps Universität,
Marburg, Germany

A. Parma
Servizio di Anatomia Patologica, Ospedali
Riuniti, Bergamo, Italy

O. Parodi
Istituto di Fisiologia Clinica CNR, Pisa,
Italy

M. Parolini
Istituto di Fisiologia Clinica CNR,
Sezione di Milano, Dipartimento Cardioto-
racico De Gasperis, Ospedale Niguarda,
Milan, Italy

M. Pauschinger
Medizinische Klinik II, Kardiologie,
Universitätsklinikum Benjamin Franklin,
Berlin, Germany

A. Perkan
Divisione di Cardiologia, Ospedale
Maggiore, Trieste, Italy

A. Pilotto
Istituto di Anatomia Patologica
Patologia Cardiovascolare e Diagnostica
Molecolare, Laboratorio Ricerca Trapianti,
IRCCS, Policlinico San Matteo, Pavia,
Italy

B. Pinamonti
Divisione di Cardiologia, Ospedale
Maggiore, Trieste, Italy

A. Poletti
Divisione di Cardiologia, Ospedale
Maggiore, Trieste, Italy

M. Ponzetta
Divisione di Cardiologia, IRCCS,
Policlinico San Matteo, Pavia, Italy

M. Porcu
Divisione di Cardiologia, Ospedale
S. Michele Brotzu, Cagliari, Italy

I. Portig
Medizinische Klinik, Kardiologie,
Klinikum der Philipps Universität,
Marburg, Germany

A. Pucci
Dipartimento di Scienze Biochimiche e
Oncologia Umana, I Sezione di Anatomia
Patologica, Università di Torino,
Turin, Italy

A. Raisaro
Divisione di Cardiologia, IRCCS,
Policlinico San Matteo, Pavia,
Italy

C. Rapezzi
Istituto di Malattie Cardiovascolari,
Università degli Studi, Bologna,
Italy

G. Renosto
Divisione di Cardiologia, Presidio Ospedaliero Multizonale, Treviso, Italy

M. Rinaldi
Divisione di Cardiochirurgia, IRCCS,
Policlinico San Matteo, Pavia, Italy

A. Ristič
Institute for Cardiovascular Diseases,
Medical Center of Serbia, Belgrade,
Yugoslavia

C. Rocco
Divisione di Cardiologia, Ospedale
Maggiore, Trieste, Italy

A. Sachero
Divisione di Cardiologia, Istituto Villa
Marelli, Milan, Italy

G. Sambuceti
Istituto di Fisiologia Clinica CNR, Pisa,
Italy

F.A. Schoendube
Klinik für Thorax-Herz-Gefässchirurgie,
Universitätsklinikum RWTH, Aachen,
Germany

U. Schönian
Medizinische Klinik, Kardiologie,
Klinikum der Philipps Universität,
Marburg, Germany

H.P. Schultheiss
Medizinische Klinik II, Kardiologie,
Universitätsklinikum Benjamin Franklin,
Berlin, Germany

R. Sebastiani
Divisione di Cardiologia, IRCCS,
Policlinico San Matteo, Pavia, Italy

D. Seferovič
Institute for Cardiovascular Diseases,
Medical Center of Serbia, Belgrade,
Yugoslavia

P.M. Seferovič
Institute for Cardiovascular Diseases,
Medical Center of Serbia, Belgrade,
Yugoslavia

C. Seidman
Howard Hughes Medical Institute and
Cardiovascular Division, Brigham
and Women's Hospital, Boston, USA

N. Sharpe
Department of Medicine, Faculty
of Medicine and Health Sciences,
University of Auckland, Auckland, New
Zealand

S. Simeunovič
Institute for Cardiovascular Diseases,
Medical Center of Serbia, Belgrade,
Yugoslavia

G. Sinagra
Divisione di Cardiologia, Ospedale
Maggiore, Trieste, Italy

P. Spirito
Servizio di Cardiologia, Ospedale Sant'Andrea, La Spezia, Italy

S. Stepanovič
Institute for Cardiovascular Diseases,
Medical Center of Serbia, Belgrade,
Yugoslavia

B. Swynghedauw
U127 INTERN, Hôpital Lariboisière, Paris,
France

G. Thiene
Istituto di Anatomia Patologica, Università
degli Studi, Padua, Italy

J.A. Towbin
Department of Pediatrics (Cardiology),
Molecular and Human Genetics, Baylor
College of Medicine and Texas Children's
Hospital, Houston, USA

S. Tracy
Department of Pathology and Microbio-
logy, University of Nebraska Medical
Center, Omaha, USA

J.D. Vasiljevič
Institute for Cardiovascular Diseases,
Medical Center of Serbia, Belgrade,
Yugoslavia

M. Vatta
International Centre for Genetic Enginee-
ring and Biotechnology, AREA Science
Park, Trieste, Italy

M. Viganò
Divisione di Cardiochirurgia, IRCCS,
Policlinico San Matteo, Pavia

Q. Wang
Department of Pediatric (Cardiology),
Molecular and Human Geneticc, Baylor
College of Medicine and Texas Children's
Hospital, Houston, USA

A. Wilke
Medizinische Klinik, Kardiologie,
Klinikum der Philipps Universität,
Marburg, Germany

T. Zerjal
International Centre for Genetic Enginee-
ring and Biotechnology, AREA Science
Park, Trieste, Italy

Introduction: II Florence Meeting on Advances in Cardiomyopathies

J.F. Goodwin

I am honoured and delighted to be asked by the Italian Study Group on Cardiomyopathies and Professors Baroldi, Camerini and De Vita to take part in this important meeting. Cardiomyopathies go from strength to strength in their importance. I well recall that, when involved in planning the Scientific Programme for the World Congress of Cardiology in 1970, I proposed a Session on Cardiomyopathies, a suggestion that was greeted without enthusiasm! Now large lecture theatres at major Cardiological meetings are filled to capacity when the topic is Cardiomyopathies. Fifty years ago or so, Proctor Harvey, Burch and Mattingly in the United States were studying cases of heart muscle disease of unknown cause. Brigden gave his St Cyres lecture in 1957 on "uncommon myocardial diseases". Teare described asymmetric hypertrophy of the heart, now known as hypertrophic cardiomyopathy and Brock was operating to relieve muscular sub-aortic obstruction. But what we now recognise as hypertrophic cardiomyopathy was probably first discovered by Liouville in 1869 [1].

The recognition of cardiomyopathy as an entity and cardiomyopathies as an important group of disorders with a broad classification into hypertrophic, congestive (now dilated) and restrictive forms respectively [2] was an important step forward. The term cardiomyopathy was at that time confined to cases in which no cause for myocardial disease was apparent, but now with the new definition and classification that Professor Camerini will speak about, our research over the past thirty years has come full circle and a modified classification is needed. I once described a classification as a "bridge between ignorance and knowledge"[3]. But bridges need maintenance, strengthening and modification from time to time. Any classification which is not subjected to regular critical examination tends to become a monument to past endeavours. Thanks to notable international research by authorities in their fields, we have learnt a great deal about hypertrophic and dilated cardiomyopathy and we are at least halfway across the bridge, though there are still many challenges to be met, notably the cause of hypertrophic cardiomyopathy, the relation of virus infection to dilated cardiomyopathy, the ramifications of restrictive cardiomyopathy and the challenge of effective treatment for all cardiomyopathies.

The application of molecular biology and genetics to the study of cardiomyopathies has been a major advance, which has not only shed light

on the dark places of ignorance in cardiomyopathies, but has also provided a
window from which to study myocardial function in general and the secrets
of ventricular hypertrophy and failure.

In the course of the next two days we are going to hear from the giants of
cardiomyopathy research about hypertrophic and dilated cardiomyopathies,
genetics, the role of viruses as well as immunity in dilated cardiomyopathy,
the natural history and treatment, the problems of sudden death, the role of
beta adenergic blocking agents in dilated cardiomyopathy, cardiac pacing,
ventricular assist methods, cardiomyoplasty, transplantation and management
in general. The Speakers come from many countries, notably Italy, USA,
Canada, Germany, the United Kingdom and France. I greatly appreciate the
enterprise of the Italian Study Group on Cardiomyopathies in setting up this
important meeting and I have much pleasure in handing over now to my old
friend and colleague, Professor Fulvio Camerini.

References

1. Liouville H (1869) Rétrécissement cardiaque sous aortique. Gazette Med Paris 24.61
2. Goodwin JF (1964) Cardiac function in primary myocardial disorders. Brit Med J
   1:1527-1595
3. Olsen EGJ, Goodwin JF (1993) Definition, classification and terminology. In: Goodwin
   JF, Olsen EGJ (eds) Cardiomyopathies - Realisations and expectations. Springer-Verlag,
   Heidelberg, pp 3-5

The Classification of Cardiomyopathies

G. Sinagra, L. Mestroni and F. Camerini

The 1980 Classification and Its Evolution

The term cardiomyopathy was probably used for the first time in 1957, when W. Bridgen [1] described the diseases of the myocardium of "non-coronary" etiology. Previously, a variable terminology had been used for these diseases, such as "myocardosis" ,"cardiac myopathy", "myocarditis" etc.

In following years Goodwin et al [2] suggested a classification of these diseases, but the first official approach to this issue was made by the WHO Expert Committee on Cardiomyopathies and by the WHO/ISFC Task Force, which, in 1980, published the "Report of the WHO/ISFC Task Force on the definition and classification of cardiomyopathies [3].

Cardiomyopathies were defined by the Task Force as "heart muscle diseases of unknown cause". Three main forms were recognized: 1) Dilated

Table 1. Evolution of cardiomyopathy classification (from [3,4])

WHO CLASSIFICATION	
1985	1995
DILATED CMP	DILATED CMP
HYPERTROPHIC CMP	HYPERTROPHIC CMP
RESTRICTIVE CMP	RESTRICTIVE CMP
	ARRHYTHMOGENIC RV CMP
SPECIFIC HEART MUSCLE DISEASES	SPECIFIC CARDIOMYOPATHIES
Infective	Inflammatory
Metabolic	Metabolic
General Systemic Diseases	General Systemic Diseases
Heredo Familial	Muscular Dystrophies
	Neuromuscolar Disorders
	Ischemic
	Valvular
	Hypersensitive
Sensitivity and Toxic Reactions	Sensitivity and Toxic Reactions
Peripartal CMP	Peripartal CMP
UNCLASSIFIED (Fibroelastosis, Fiedler's myocarditis)	UNCLASSIFIED (Fibroelastosis, noncompacted myocardium, mildly dilated CMP, mitochondrial involvement)

Cardiomyopathy; 2) Hypertrophic Cardiomyopathy and 3) Restrictive Cardiomyopathy, while the term "Specific Heart Muscle Disease" was applied to diseases of myocardium "of known cause or associated with disorders of other systems" [3] (Table 1). This terminology and the proposed classification were widely accepted and were found to be useful both in the clinical setting and in research.

However, more recently, new pathophysiological aspects and new forms of cardiomyopathies have been recognized and described requiring a revision of this classification. Furthermore, over time, the term "cardiomyopathy" was used inappropriately, with discrepancies between the WHO/ISFC Task Force suggestions and the commonly used scientific terminology.

In fact with the term *Cardiomyopathies,* by definition idiopathic forms, were named also specific forms, such as "Diabetic Cardiomyopathy", "Cardiomyopathy of Duchenne Disease", "Alcoholic Cardiomyopathy", "Ischemic Cardiomyopathy" and "Adriamycin Cardiomyopathy". Consequently, to distinguish the *true* cardiomyopathies from *specific* forms, the redundant prefix "idiopathic" was frequently used. For these reasons, the task force of the WHO/ISFC reported new guidelines for the definition and classification of cardiomyopathies in 1995 [4].

Dilated Cardiomyopathy

The most frequent form of cardiomyopathy is *dilated cardiomyopathy.* The reported incidence ranges from 0.73 patients/100.000 individuals/year [5] to 6.95/100.000/year [6] and prevalence from 8.3 patients/100.000 individuals [7] to 36.5/100.000 [8].

Dilated cardiomyopathy was considered a heart muscle disease of unknown etiology characterized by impaired systolic function of the left or both ventricles usually associated with cardiac enlargement.

To explain the chronic and progressive myocardial damage, three main etiopathogenesis were proposed: 1) a chronic viral infection of the myocardium with consequent cell damage; 2) abnormalities in immune mechanisms, possibly leading to an autoimmune disease; 3) and genetic factors which could be directly or indirectly responsible for the disease.

The hypothesis that dilated cardiomyopathy results, at least in some cases, from a viral infection, with or without an ongoing chronic autoimmune process, is based on a series of clinical, serological and molecular data. However, recent studies based on nucleic acid hybridization and polymerase chain reaction on hearts of patients with dilated cardiomyopathy, produced conflicting results. In some studies, enteroviral nucleic acids were present in nearly 70% [9] of cases, while in others [10], they were virtually absent, and in few reports, a nearly equivalent number of positives for the presence of enterovirus was found in patients and in controls [11]. In spite of these limitations, the overall data support the hypothesis that enteroviral infections are, at least in a subgroup of patients, etiologically linked to dilated cardiomyopathy. Moreover, other viruses could be implicated in the pathogenesis of the disease. However, the real prevalence of virus persistence, the role of different diagnostic techniques, and the possible mechanisms of myocardial damage are still open problems, which need further studies and clarification.

The role of genetic factors in dilated cardiomyopathy was often underestimated in the past, but more recent surveys [12-14] have clearly shown the importance of genetic transmission, with a frequency of familiarity of more than 30%.

The clinical and morphological features of familial dilated cardiomyopathy and the patterns of inheritance in the affected families are very variable, suggesting a vast heterogeneity at genetic level: this means that different mutations or different genes could cause the same disease. In most of the families, the disease is transmitted with a monogenic autosomal dominant pattern and with the typical features of left ventricular dysfunction and dilation. The penetrance (i.e. the proportion of affected individuals who manifest the disease) is "incomplete" and correlates with the patient's age (so called age-related penetrance or delayed age of onset). In our series, the penetrance was estimated to be 10% from 0 to 20 years, 34% from 20 to 30, 60% from 30 to 40 and 90% in those over 40. In other families, however, the pattern of transmission could be classified as X-linked, matrilineal, or recessive. Polygenic inheritance resulting from mutations in different genes has also been proposed.

Finally, the demonstration of autoantibodies against myosin heavy chain, beta-1 receptor and adenine nucleotide translocator suggests that autoimmunity is involved in causing myocardial damage in a substantial percentage of patients with dilated cardiomyopathy [15].

Considering the clinical features of dilated cardiomyopathy, the dilatation of the ventricles has been always considered the most important characteristics. Furthermore, prognosis appeared to correlate with ventricular size. An exception is represented by mildly dilated cardiomyopathy firstly described by Keren at al [16]: this form is characterized by severe left ventricular dysfunction, severe heart failure, and poor outcome irrespective of the small heart size and myofibrillar preservation.

Hypertrophic Cardiomyopathy

Hypertrophic cardiomyopathy (HCM) is characterized by unexplained left and/or right ventricular hypertrophy, which may assume a variety of distributions, but is usually asymmetric and involves the left ventricular septum. The left ventricular volume is normal or reduced, and systolic gradients are common. Histological features include a typical focal myocyte and myofibrillar disarray. The disease can be asymptomatic, or lead to heart failure, but the most important clinical features are arrhythmia and sudden death, particularly in the young patient population.

The incidence of HCM has been estimated to be 2.5/100,000 person-year, and the prevalence 20/100,000 population, respectively [8].

A large series of studies demonstrated that hypertrophic cardiomyopathy is

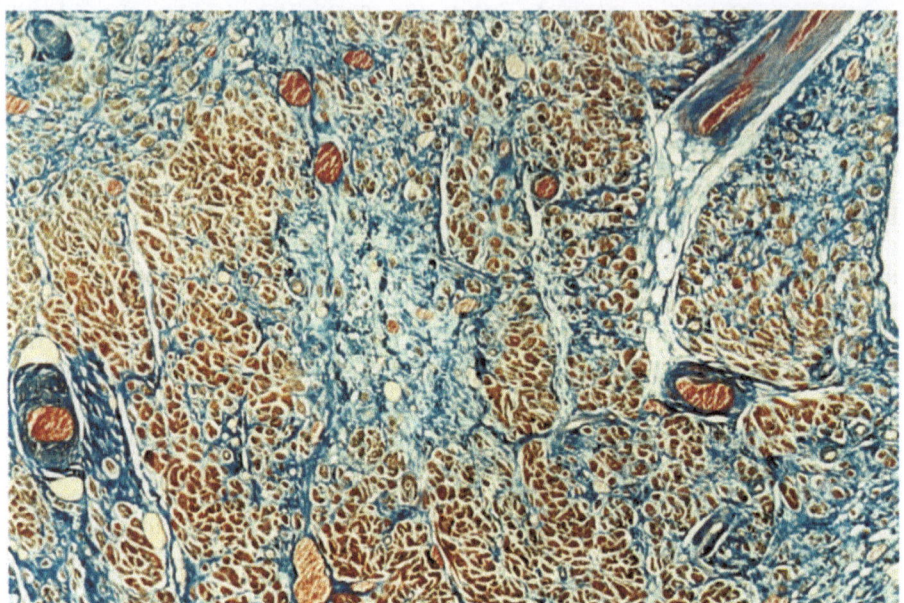

Fig. 1. Endomyocardial biopsy sample from a patient with idiopathic restrictive cardiomyopathy shows marked interstitial and perivascular fibrosis (Azan-Mallory stain; magnification 40 x; fibrosis in blue)

frequently (more than in 50% of cases) a hereditary disease with autosomal dominance and variable expression and prevalence [17]. The recent application of molecular genetic techniques to well documented large families revealed a heterogeneous disorder caused by different mutations of different genes located on chromosome 1, 3, 7, 11, 12, 14, 15. Mutations of these genes result in apparently similar clinical disease entities.

It is clear now, that these genes encode different components of the cardiac sarcomers as beta cardiac myosin heavy chain, alpha tropomyosin, cardiac troponin T, cardiac myosin binding protein C, essential and regulatory myosin light chain. It can be hypothesized that mutations of other genes encoding components of the contractile apparatus could lead to the same phenotype. Moreover, the involvement of different genes and/or specific mutations within them may determine a phenotypic heterogeneity and influence the natural history of the disease [18].

Restrictive Cardiomyopathy

Restrictive cardiomyopathy is a rare form. The first WHO/ISFC [3] report considered only two forms of restrictive cardiomyopathy, i.e. endomyocardial fibrosis (without hypereosinophilia) and the Loffler's cardiomyopathy (endocarditis parietalis fibroplastica), a condition which should be referred as to eosinophilic endomyocardial disease. However, recently some authors [19, 20] described some patients in whom neither endomyocardial fibrosis nor hypereosinophilia were present; in these cases the cause of the restrictive pathophysiology was localized in the myocardium. The histological changes observed were not uniform. They frequently included slight to severe interstitial fibrosis (Fig.1), a moderate hypertrophy and/or a certain degree of disarray. In a minority of cases the myocardium, obtained by endomyocardial biopsy, was apparently normal.

Arrhythmogenic Right Ventricular Cardiomyopathy/Dysplasia

Arrhythmogenic right ventricular cardiomyopathy/dysplasia is a new nosological entity that was not considered in the 1980 classification. This is a heart muscle disease characterized by a progressive atrophy of the myocardium with adipose or fibro-adipose substitution which involves exclusively (or predominantly) the right ventricular wall (Fig. 2). Inflammatory changes may be present. From a clinical point of view, disease onset is usually characterized by ventricular arrhythmia of right ventricular origin (of left bundle branch block morphology), and, sometimes, by symptoms of right heart failure.

Depolarization and repolarization changes, such as inverted T waves in right precordial leads, epsilon waves, and late potentials at signal averaged

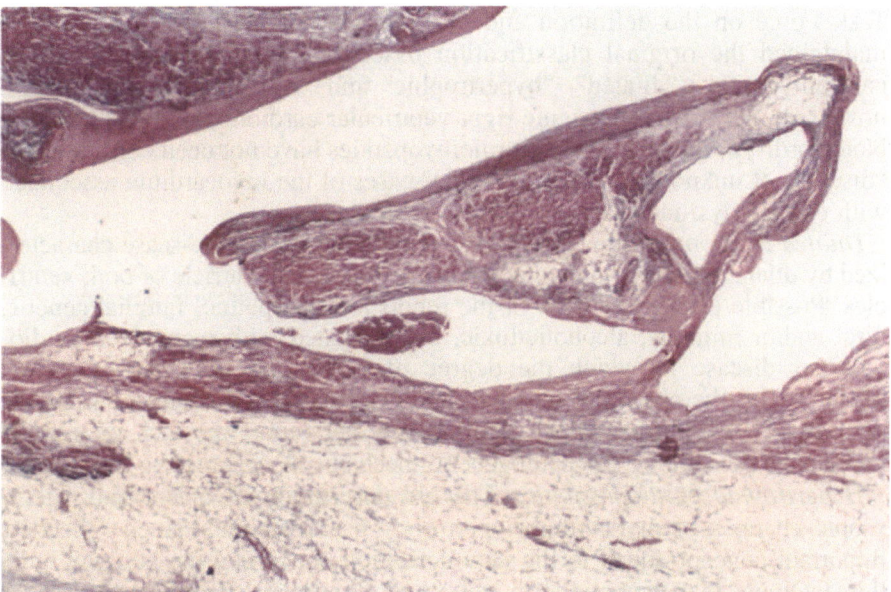

Fig. 2. Histological section of the right ventricle free wall in a patient with arrhythmogenic right ventricular dysplasia. The muscle component is replaced by fatty tissue and subendocardial connective tissue (Hematoxylin Eosine stain; magnification 2.5 x)

electrocardiogram are frequently found. Structural and functional alterations of the right ventricle can be detected by echocardiography, angiography, magnetic resonance imaging or radionuclide scintigraphy. These alterations can be localized (dyskinetic bulges, segmental dilatation or hypokinesia) or diffuse. However, the gold standard for diagnosis is the histological demonstration of a fatty or fibro-fatty substitution of right ventricular myocardium [21].

At present, the true incidence of the disease is unknown and is probably underestimated. Interestingly, also in this form a genetic trait is common, and can be detected in at least 30% of cases. The variability of penetrance and of clinical expression indicates genetic heterogeneity, suggesting that different genes are likely to be responsible for the disease phenotype.

The 1995 Classification - Progress and Doubts

In the 15 years between 1980 and 1995, relevant advances in the field of cardiomyopathies have been made. In fact, new forms of cardiomyopathies have been identified and the etiology and pathogenesis of some cardiomyopathies have been clarified, indicating a more complex situation than previously suspected. Moreover, the concept of "cardiomyopathy" as a heart muscle disease of unknown cause has became inadequate due to the progress in the knowledge of the etiology and, on the other hand, to the widespread use and the extensive meaning of the term cardiomyopathy.

According with these considerations, the "Report of the 1995 WHO/ISFC Task Force on the definition and classification of cardiomyopathies" [4] maintained the original classification based on the three main forms of cardiomyopathy ("dilated", "hypertrophic" and "restrictive"), but added a novel one, the "arrhythmogenic right ventricular cardiomyopathy" (Table 1). Noteworthy, in the new report, cardiomyopathies have not been considered as "diseases of unknown cause", but "as diseases of the myocardium associated with cardiac dysfunction".

Dilated cardiomyopathy: the disease is now defined as a disease characterized by dilatation and impaired contraction of the left ventricle or both ventricles. Possible etiologies listed in the report are: idiopathic, familial/genetic, viral and/or immune, alcoholic/toxic, or associated with recognized cardiovascular disease in which the degree of myocardial dysfunction is not explained by the abnormal loading conditions or by the extent of ischemic damage [4]. It is still evident from the present report the lack of definite knowledge concerning the pathogenetic mechanisms causing the disease.

Hypertrophic cardiomyopathy: The old description of macro and microscopic changes of myocardial hypertrophy has been maintained. The new important concept added to the new definition concerned the etiology, with the statement that "mutations in sarcomeric contractile protein genes cause disease".

Restrictive cardiomyopathy: According to the recent advances in the etiology, pathogenesis and pathophysiology of the disease, restrictive filling and

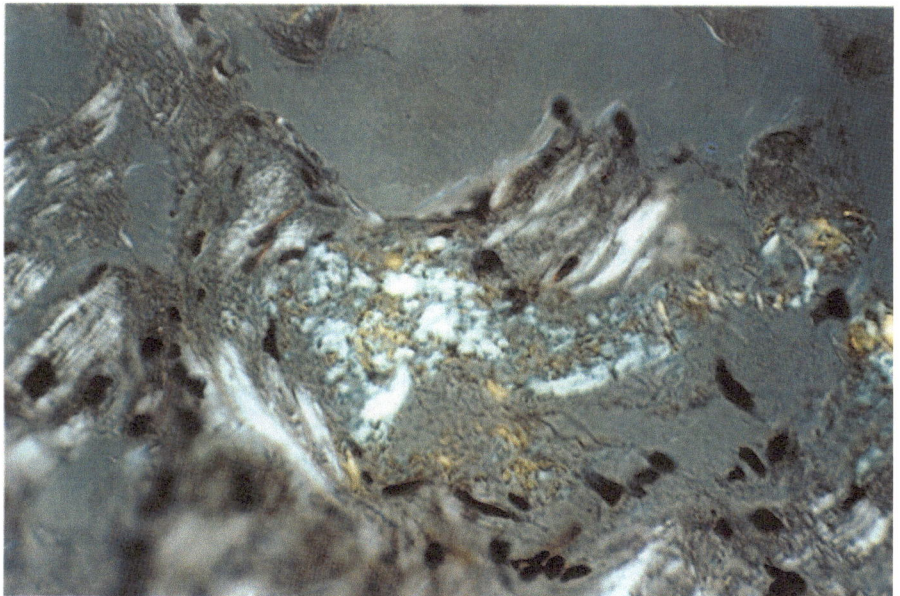

Fig. 3. Fluorescent microscopy shows brightly fluorescent (yellow-green) amyloid adjacent to and surrounding individual myocytes (Congo Red Stain, magnification 150 x)

reduced diastolic volume, in the presence of normal or nearly normal systolic function and wall thickness, were considered essential for the diagnosis, while the presence of increased interstitial fibrosis was included as optional criterion.

It may be idiopathic or associated with other diseases (e.g. amyloidosis, hemocromatosis, endomyocardial disease with or without hypereosinophilia) (see Tables 1 and 2; Figs. 3 and 4).

Arrhythmogenic right ventricular cardiomyopathy: The anatomical and clinical characteristics and the familial occurrence as described by the Task Force of the ESC/ISFC [21] were fully accepted.

Unclassified Cardiomyopathies: A subset of cases, even if rare, present with a heart muscle disease, which cannot fit into any of the previous groups (e.g.

Table 2. Diseases associated with restrictive cardiomyopathy

– Amyloidosis
– Hemochromatosis
– Glycogenosis
– Neoplastic Infiltrations
– Pseudoxantoma Elasticum
– Collagen Diseases
– Sarcoidosis
– Radiation Therapy
– Anthracycline Therapy

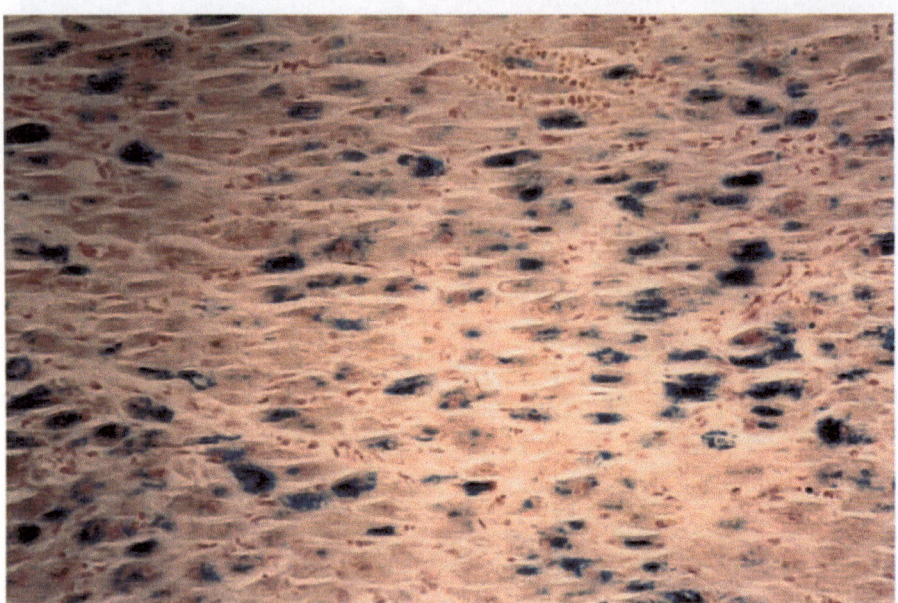

Fig. 4. Intramyocellular iron deposits in a case of familial hemocromatosis with cardiac involvement (Bleu Prussia stain; magnification 100 x)

fibroelastosis, noncompacted myocardium, systolic dysfunction with minimal dilatation, mitochondrial involvement). These patients should be grouped in the *unclassified cardiomyopathies*. Moreover, the Task Force [4] recognized that arrhythmias and conduction disease may be "primary myocardial disorders", but since we still lack definite diagnostic criteria, these entities were not strictly included in the group of cardiomyopathies.

Specific Cardiomyopathies: Under this definition are grouped the heart muscle diseases associated with specific cardiac or systemic disorders, previously called *specific heart muscle diseases*. Different types of specific cardiomyopathies are listed in Table 1, but a few need a more detailed presentation.

– Ischemic cardiomyopathy: This refers specifically to a form of dilated cardiomyopathy with impaired contractile performance which is *not explained by the extent of coronary artery disease or ischemic damage*.

– Valvular cardiomyopathy: This group includes valvular heart diseases where the ventricular dysfunction is *out of proportion to the abnormal loading conditions*.

– Hypertensive cardiomyopathy: This is characterized by left ventricular hypertrophy in association with features of dilated or restrictive cardiomyopathy with cardiac failure.

– Inflammatory cardiomyopathy: This term defines *myocarditis in association with myocardial dysfunction*. Myocarditis is diagnosed according to histological, immunological and immunohistochemical criteria.

Over time, the 1980 WHO/ISFC classification of cardiomyopathies became inadequate and it was a diffuse opinion [20, 22] that a revision was necessary.

In fact, novel forms of heart muscle diseases were identified and relevant advances in the knowledge of the etiology have been made (Table 3) [23, 24].

The 1995 WHO/ISFC Task Force [4] identified and recognized this evolution, changing the concept of *cardiomyopathy* from a disease of *unknown cause* to a disease of the myocardium which could be *idiopathic or secondary to different etiologies, associated with cardiac dysfunction*, an evolution which has been accepted previously by a large part of the cardiological community. In our opinion, a modern classification (Table 4) should integrate basic and clinical sciences, maintaining the term cardiomyopathy followed by an anathomical or a physiopathological definition.

Certainly, some questions still remain unsolved and some clinical settings are still unclear. Considering ischemic cardiomyopathy, this has been defined [4] as *a dilated cardiomyopathy with impaired contractile performance not explained by the extent of coronary artery disease and ischemic damage*. However, in certain cases it may be very difficult to identify the primary pathogenetic mechanism causing dilatation, in other words to distinguish the effects of ischemic damage from an underlying myocardial disorder. An example are patients with a previous myocardial infarction and progressive dilatation, or patients with severe global dilatation, hypokinesia and only subcritical coronary stenosis at angiography.

Similarly, in some patients with valvular cardiomyopathy, it may be difficult to establish, in cases with an apparent moderate regurgitation and relevant dilatation and hypokinesia, the pathogenetic role of volume overload.

Table 3. Molecular genetics of cardiomyopathies (modified from [23] and [24])

	Chromosomal Location	Cardiac Protein
Hypertrophic Cardiomyopathy	1q3	Troponin T
	3q3	Essential myosin light chain
	7q3	HCMP + WPW
	11p11.2	Myosin binding protein C
	12q	Regulatory myosin light chain
	14q11	Beta myosin heavy chain
	15q2	Alfa tropomyosin
Dilated Cardiomyopathy	1q1-p1	Unknown
	1q31-q32	Unknown
	3p22-p25	Unknown
	9q13-q22	Unknown
	Xp21	Dystrophin
ARVD	1q42-q43	Unknown
	2q31-q35	Unknown
	14q12-q22	Unknown
	14q23-q24	Unknown
	17	Unknown

HCMP, Hypertrophic Cardiomyopathy; ARVD, Arrhythmogenic Right Ventricular Cardiomyopathy/Dysplasia; WPW, Wolff-Parkinson-White.

Table 4. Proposed modern terminology of cardiomyopathies

Fix term	Anatomical or physiopathological definition	Etiology
Cardiomyopathy	Dilated Hypertrophic Restrictive Arrhythmogenic right ventricular CMP/dysplasia Unclassified	Viral Genetically det. Immunologically det. Specific Idiopathic

Moreover, new clinical entities have not been considered yet, but should be included among cardiomyopathies. An example is the *tachycardia-induced cardiomyopathy*, in which a long lasting high rate supraventricular or ventricular tachycardia may cause dilatation and dysfunction of the heart.

Even with these limitations, the new classification of the cardiomyopathies represents an important progress and a useful tool, both in the clinical context and for research purposes. However, further modifications can be expected in the future with the continuous advances in understanding of etiology and pathogenesis of these diseases.

This concept is fully expressed in the words that J.F. Goodwin wrote in 1982: "Since any classification is necessarily incomplete and acts as a bridge between complete ignorance and total understanding in any biological system, further modification and changes are likely to occur as knowledge advances " [25].

Acknowledgment. Long-standing, friendly and fruitful cooperation with Prof. F. Silvestri and Dr. R. Bussani of Pathology Dept., University of Trieste, Italy is acknowledged.

References

1. Bridgen W (1957) Uncommon myocardial diseases: the non-coronary cardiomy-opathies. Lancet 2:1179-1184, 1243-1249
2. Goodwin JK, Gordon H, Hollman A, Bishop MB (1961) Clinical aspects of cardiomy-opathy. Br Heart J 1:69-79
3. Report of the International Society and Federation of Cardiology/World Health Organization. Task Force on the definition of cardiomyopathies (1980) Br Heart J 44:672-673
4. Report of the 1995 World Health Organization/International Society and Federation of Cardiology. Task Force on the Definition and Classification of Cardiomyopathies. Circulation (1996) 93:841-842
5. Bagger JP, Baandrup U, Rasmussen K, Moller M, Vesterlund Y (1984) Cardiomyopa-thy in western Denmark. Br Heart J 52:327-331
6. Rakar S, Sinagra G, Di Lenarda A, Poletti A, Bussani R, Silvestri F, Camerini F (1997) Epidemiology of dilated cardiomyopathy. A prospective post-mortem study of 5252 necropsies. Eur Heart J 18:117-123
7. Williams DG, Olsen EGJ (1985) Prevalence of overt dilated cardiomyopathy in two regions of England. Br Heart J 54:153-155
8. Codd MB, Sugrue DD, Gerts BJ, Melton III LJ (1989) Epidemiology of idiopatic dilat-ed and hypertrophic cardiomyopathy. Circulation 80:564-572
9. Petitjean J, Kopecka H, Freymuth F, Langlard JM, Scanu P, Galateau F, Bouhour JB,

Ferriere M, Charbonneau P, Komajda M (1992) Detection of enteroviruses in endomyocardial biopsy by molecular approach. J Med Virol 37:76-82

10. Grasso M, Arbustini E, Silini E, Diegoli M, Percivalle E, Ratti G, Bramerio M, Gavazzi A, Vigano M, Milanessi G (1992) Search for coxsackievirus B3 RNA in idiopathic dilated cardiomyopathy using gene amplification by polimerase chain reaction. Am J Cardiol 69:658-664

11. Fujioka S, Koide H, Kitaura Y, Deguchi H, Kawamura K (1995) Analysis of enterovirus genotypes using single-strand conformation polymorphisms of polymerase chain reaction products. J Virol Methods 51:253-258

12. Michels VV, Moll PP, Miller FA, Tajik AJ, Chu JS, Driscoll DJ, Burnett JC, Rodeneffer RJ, Cheesbro JN, Tazelaar H (1992) The frequency of familial dilated cardiomyopathy in a series of patients with idiopatic dilated cardiomyopathy. N Engl J Med 326:77-82

13. Mestroni L, Miani D, Di Lenarda A, Silvestri F, Buşsani R, Filippi G, Camerini F (1990) Clinical and pathologic study of familial dilated cardiomyopathy. Am J Cardiol 65:1449-1453

14. Rocco C, Gregori D, Miocic S, Di Lenarda A, Sinagra G, Caforio AL, Vatta M, Matulic M, Zerjal T, Giacca M, Mestroni L (1997) New insights into the genetics of dilated cardiomyopathy. Circulation [Suppl.] 96:I-696

15. Caforio ALP, Keeling PJ, Zachara E, Mestroni L, Camerini F, Mann JM, Boltazzo GF, McKenna WJ (1994) Autoimmunity in dilated cardiomyopathy:evidence from family studies. Lancet 344:773-777

16. Keren A, Gottlieb S, Tzivoni D, Stern S, Yarom R, Billingham ME, Popp RL (1990) Mildly Dilated Congestive Cardiomyopathy. Use of prospective diagnostic criteria and description of the clinical course without heart transplantation. Circulation 81:506-517

17. Schwartz K, Mercadier JJ (1996) Molecular and cellular biology of heart failure. Curr Opin Cardiol 11:227-236

18. Watkins H, Rosenzweig A, Hwang D-SH,Levi T, McKenna W, Seidman CE, Seidman JG (1992) Characteristics and prognostic implication of myosin missense mutations in familial hypertrophic cardiomyopathy. N Engl J Med 326:1108-1114

19. Siegel RJ, Shah PK, Fishbein MC (1984) Idiopatic restrictive cardiomyopathy. Circulation 70:165-169

20. Boffa GM, Thiene G, Nava A, Dalla Volta S (1991) Cardiomyopathy:a necessary revision of the WHO classification. Int J Cardiol 30:1-7

21. McKenna WJ, Thiene G, Nava A, Fontaliran F, Blomstrom-Lundqvist C, Fontaine G, Camerini F (1994) Diagnosis of arrhythmogenic right ventricular dysplasia/cardiomyopathy. Br Heart J 71:215-218

22. Camerini F, Mestroni L, Perkan A, Pinamonti B, Sinagra G (1993) La classificazione delle cardiomiopatie: È opportuna una revisione? G Ital Cardiol 23:729-733

23. Malik MSA, Watkins H (1997) The molecular genetics of hypertrophic cardiomyopathy. Curr.Opinion Cardiol 12:295-302

24. Mestroni L, Giacca M (1997) Molecular genetics of dilated cardiomyopathy. Curr Opinion Cardiol 12:303-309

25. Goodwin JF (1982) The frontiers of cardiomyopathy.Br Heart J 48:1-18.

HYPERTROPHIC CARDIOMYOPATHY

The Clinical Significance of Genetic Testing in Familial Hypertrophic Cardiomyopathy

C. Seidman

Introduction

Over the past decade there has been substantial progress in understanding the molecular basis of several inherited cardiovascular disorders. Definition of the chromosome location of disease genes, identification of these genes, and characterization of different mutations within these disease genes has been the focus of many,molecular laboratories around the world. Translation of this new, fundamental genetic knowledge about human disorders, into improved clinical diagnosis and care of individuals affected by these disorders has become a new frontier in medicine. This translation is often hampered by a limited understanding by physicians of the difficulties of molecular genetic technologies and a failure by researchers to comprehend the complexities of clinical manifestations of disease. Despite these intrinsic problems, the effort of integrating basic science and medicine in hypertrophic cardiomyopathy has particular merit because the complex molecular genetics of this disease may account for the diverse clinical manifestations of this pathology. The paper will review our current understanding of the genetic basis for hypertrophic cardiomyopathy and discuss the impact this research has on clinical diagnosis and management.

Molecular Genetics

Familial hypertrophic cardiomyopathy (FHC) is usually inherited as an autosomal dominant trait (Fig. 1). Affected individuals have a 50% chance of transmitting the disorder to their offspring, whereas the offspring of unaffected individuals are at no risk of developing this disorder. This mode of inheritance has enabled molecular genetic studies to identify the chromosome location of genes that are mutated in individuals with hypertrophic cardiomyopathy. Seven chromosomes have been demonstrated to contain an FHC gene. Estimates of the contribution of each disease gene to the overall incidence of FHC, while somewhat imprecise, suggest that mutations in β cardiac myosin heavy chain (chromosome 14ql), cardiac troponin T (chromosome lq31) and cardiac myosin binding protein-C (chromosome 11p13-q13) account for approximately two thirds of all cases [1-3]. Mutations in α tropomyosin

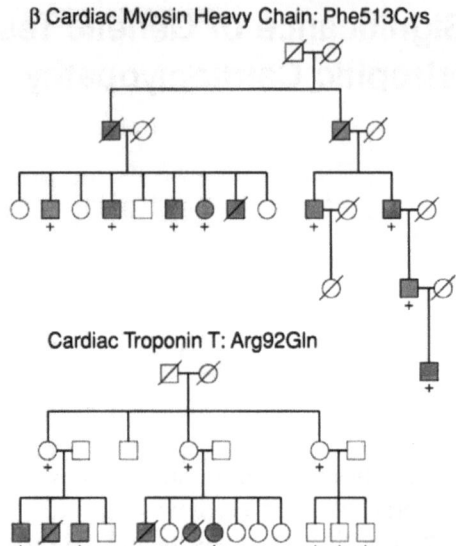

Fig. 1. Cardiac hypertrophy in FHC caused by a β cardiac myosin heavy chain or cardiac troponin T missense mutation. Pedigree symbols denote sex (squares, male; circles, female) and clinical affection status (solid, affected, open, unaffected, stippled, unknown) based on echocardiographic finding of cardiac hypertrophy. The presence of β cardiac myosin heavy chain gene mutations Phe513Cys or cardiac troponin T mutation Arg92Gln, is indicated (+). Note that some individuals with the cardiac troponin T mutation had no clinically significant cardiac hypertrophy (left ventricular wall thickness ≤13 mm)

(chromosome 15q2), myosin essential light chain (chromosome 3p) and the ventricular regulatory light chain (chromosome 12q2) contribute to less than 10% of all cases [2,4]. Another FHC gene has been localized to chromosome 7 [5], however its identity remains unknown. Because each of these disease genes encodes a component of the cardiac contractile apparatus, FHC can be viewed as a disease of the sarcomere.

Several different types of mutations have been identified in these FHC genes (Table 1). Missense mutations, which substitute a novel amino acid for that normally encoded, are the only gene defects identified to cause FHC in the β cardiac myosin heavy chain and α tropomyosin genes. In contrast missense mutations, splice site mutations, and small deletions and insertions have been identified in cardiac troponin T and cardiac myosin binding protein-C. To date, only three FHC mutations have been identified in the ventricular regulatory and essential light chains.

Clinical Correlates of Genetic Studies

The diversity of gene defects that cause FHC has prompted investigation of whether genotype predicts disease expression in FHC. The clinical manifestations of FHC are quite heterogeneous. Disease onset, severity of cardiac hypertrophy, and survival vary considerably between families. Further, few clinical findings have been identified that aid in risk stratification of affected individuals at risk for the most serious complications of the disorder, particularly sudden death. Although an incomplete compendium, correlation of genotype and clinical manifestations of disease (Table 1) has provided several insights into the variable natural history of FHC.

Although the demonstration of cardiac hypertrophy by two-dimensional echocardiography is generally considered to be the *sine quo non* for diagnosing FHC, this is not a universal manifestation of all FHC gene defects. Figure 1 contrasts genetic data and echocardiographic findings of cardiac hypertrophy in two families with FHC. Mutations in the β cardiac myosin heavy chain gene typically cause significant increases in myocardial mass, which are readily demonstrable by two-dimensional echocardiography. A mean maximal left ventricular wall thickness equal to 23.7 ± 7.7 mm was found in affected individuals from families with different myosin mutations [6]. In contrast, mutations in cardiac troponin T can result in only modest increase in myocardial mass, thus confounding clinical diagnosis. One study demonstrated the mean maximal left ventricular wall thickness resulting from six different cardiac troponin T mutations was 16.7 ± 5.5 mm, but noted that some adults with these mutations had normal cardiac wall thickness [2]. Cardiac myosin binding protein-C mutations are associated with late onset myocardial hypertrophy, which may not be demonstrable until after the fifth decade of life [3].

Identification of individuals with FHC who are at risk for sudden and unex-

Table 1. Genotype and phenotype in hypertrophic cardiomyopathy

Gene	Chromosome	Mutation Type	Hypertrophic Response	Survival	Reference
Cardiac troponin T	1q31	missense; splice site; insertion; deletion	modest; can be subclinical	generally poor	
Myosin essential light chain	3 p	missense	mid ventricular thickening	unknown	[4]
Unknown	7	unknown	unknown	unknown	
Myosin binding protein-C	11p13-q13	missense; splice site; insertion; deletion	late onset; can be subclinical until mid life	generally good	[3]
Regulatory light chain	12q2	missense	mid ventricular thickening	unknown	[4]
β cardiac myosin heavy chain	14ql	missense	moderate to severe	variable; mutation specific	[1,6,8,9]
α tropomyosin	15q2	missense	variable	good	[2,10]

pected death can be extremely difficult. Often the best clinical predictor of premature death is a malignant family history [7]. This clinical observation, perhaps provided the first recognition that genotype is an important predictor of outcome in FHC. Life expectancy in different FHC mutations has combined data from single large families and from multiple small unrelated families who bear the same mutation. This compilation has minimized the influence that different genetic backgrounds, different environments, and different life styles have on survival. Data indicate that survival in FHC due to a β cardiac myosin heavy chain gene defect is mutation specific [8,9]; some markedly shorten survival while others are associated with near normal life expectancy. Cardiac troponin T mutations are often associated with a high incidence of premature death [2]. In contrast prognosis in FHC caused by either α tropomyosin [10] or cardiac myosin binding protein-C [3] is good.

Conclusions

Molecular genetic studies have demonstrated distinct mutations in sarcomere genes that cause hypertrophic cardiomyopathy. The diverse genetic etiologies of FHC account in part for the variable clinical manifestations of disease. Gene based diagnosis is the most accurate mechanism for defining affection status, and is particularly important for diagnosis in FHC associated with only modest cardiac hypertrophy. The complexity of providing rapid genotype information remains problematic, and in part is due to the number and complexity of distinct gene mutations that can cause hypertrophic cardiomy- opathy. Development and commercialization of technologies should enable accurate and preclinical diagnosis in families and may help in risk stratifica- tion and management of patients.

Acknowledgment. This work was supported by grants from the Howard Hughes Medical Institutes and the National Institutes of Health.

References

1. Watkins H, Rosenzweig A, Hwang DS, Levi T, McKenna W, Seidman CE, Seidman JG (1992) Characteristics and prognostic implications of myosin missense mutations in familial hypertrophic cardiomyopathy. N Engl J Med 326: 1108-1114
2. Watkins H, McKenna WJ, Thierfelder L, Suk J, Anan R, O'Donoghue A, Spirito P, Matsumori A, Moravec CS, Seidman JG, Seidman CE (1995) The role of cardiac troponin T and α-tropomyosin mutations in hypertrophic cardiomyopathy. N Engl J Med 332:1058-1064
3. Niimura H, Bachinski LL, Watkins H, Thierfelder L, Chudley AE, Anastasakis A, Toutouzas P, Elstein E, Liew, C-C, Liew J, Rakowski H, Wigle ED, Zhao M, McKen- na W, Sole M, Roberts R, Seidman JG, Seidman CE (1997) Human cardiac myosin binding protein C mutations cause late-onset familial hypertrophic cardiomyopathy; submitted.
4. Poetter K, Jiang H, Hassanzadeh S, Master SR, Chang A, Dalakas MC, Rayment I, Sellers JR, Fananapazir L, Epstein ND (1996) Mutations in either the essential or regu- latory light chains of myosin are associated with a rare myopathy in human heart and skeletal muscle. Nature Genet 13:63-69

5. MacRae CA, Ghaisas N, Kass S, Donnelly S, Basson CT, Watkins H, Anan R, Their-
felder LH, McGarry K, Rowland E, McKenna W, Seidman, JG, Seidman CE (1995)
Familial hypertrophic cardiomyopathy with Wolff-Parkinson-White syndrome maps to
a locus on chromosome 7q3. J Clin Invest 96:1216-1220
6. Solomon SD, Wolff S, Watkins H, Ridker PM, Come P, Seidman CE, McKenna WJ,
Lee RT (1993) Left ventricular hypertrophy and morphology in familial hypertrophic
cardiomyopathy associated with mutations in the β myosin heavy chain gene. J Am
Coll Cardiol 22:498-505
7. Maron BJ, Lipson LC, Roberts WC, Savage DD, Epstein SE (1978) "Malignant" hypertrophic cardiomyopathy: Identification of a subgroup of families with unusually
frequent premature death. Am J Cardiol 41:1133-1139
8. Fananapazir L, Epstein ND (1994) Genotype-phenotype correlations in hypertrophic
cardiomyopathy. Circulation 89:22-32
9. Anan R, Greve G, Thierfelder L, Watkins H, McKenna WJ, Solomon S, Vecchio C,
Shono H, Nakao S, Tanaka H, Mares A, Towbin JA, Spirito P, Roberts R, Seidman JG,
Seidman CE (1994) Prognostic implications of novel beta cardiac myosin heavy chain
gene mutations that cause familial hypertrophic cardiomyopathy. J Clin Invest 93:280.
10. Coviello DA, Maron BJ, Spirito P (1996) Clinical features of hypertrophic cardiomyopathy caused by mutation of a "hot spot" in the α tropomyosin gene. J Am Coll Cardiol 29:635-640

The Italian Multicentric Study on Hypertrophic Cardiomyopathy: I. Natural History and Clinical Course of Unselected Patients

F. Cecchi, I. Olivotto, A. Montereggi, E. Lazzeroni, G. P. Chiriatti, L. Beretta, E. Giagnoni, G. Renosto, M. Ciaccheri, G. Castelli and A. Dolara, on behalf of the Italian Study Group on Cardiomyopathies (SPIC), Subproject on Hypertrophic Cardiomyopathy

In the past 8 years since the last Florence meeting, four major issues have emerged in the field of hypertrophic cardiomyopathy (HCM), namely genetic testing, pacemaker therapy, epidemiological data and outcome studies from unselected populations [1]. Among these, epidemiologic studies have shown that HCM is more common than previously thought, with a prevalence of about 0.2% [3]. Also, in contrast with what was once thought based on selected tertiary referral center populations [4], the majority of HCM patients in the general population has been shown to be asymptomatic and non-obstructive [1, 4]. Further natural history studies are therefore crucial in order to evaluate the clinical outcome and prognosis in unselected HCM populations, and to assess the appropriate strategies for clinical management of the disease. After we reported in 1989 the good clinical outcome of 157 patients with HCM followed at the Careggi Hospital in Florence [5], a multicentric study was set up including a large study group of patients from 5 non-referral institutions in Central and Northern Italy. The aim of our study was to determine the annual mortality rate for cardiovascular causes, the clinical deterioration rate and the occurrence of cardiovascular events in a large unselected population with HCM.

Methods

Patient Selection and Study Protocol

The study included all patients with a diagnosis of HCM followed at our institutions between 1963 and 1992, who were evaluated clinically on at least 2 occasions and were followed for at least 1 year. Diagnosis of HCM was based on echocardiographic identification of a hypertrophied, nondilated left ventricle in the absence of another cardiac or systemic disease capable of producing the magnitude of left ventricular hypertrophy present in that patient [3]. In those study patients who had been evaluated before echocardiography was introduced into our clinical practice in 1977, the diagnosis of HCM was made by virtue of the typical clinical, ECG, phonocardiographic, hemodynamic and angiographic findings, but was subsequently confirmed by echocardiography. Patients with the following were excluded: 1) associated valvular or congenital heart disease; 2) documented coronary artery disease; and 3) systemic hypertension (documentation of blood pressure $\geq$ 170/100 mmHg on 3 consecutive measurements) [4]. The final study group consisted of 330 consecutive patients with HCM, distributed as follows: Florence, 202; Parma, 49; Pescia; 40 Milan, 29; Treviso, 10. The initial evaluation for the purpose of this study was considered as the date of the first diagnosis of HCM in each patient. Data were collected in a computerized database which was periodically updated. End-points for the study were cardiovascular death and main cardiovascular events which included atrial fibrillation, peripheral embolization, abrupt worsening of congestive symptoms often with acute pulmonary edema, syncope, conduction abnormalities requiring a permanent pacemaker, or bacterial endocarditis with cardiovascular complications. For the purpose of this study, we have considered sudden death to be unexpected, non-traumatic and occurring within one hour from the onset of symptoms. Death occurring unexpectedly and suddenly in the clinical context of congestive heart failure was not regarded as a sudden death in this analysis [4].

Ages at initial evaluation ranged from 1 to 80 years (mean 42 ± 16); 33 patients (10%) were < 20 years and 39 (12%) were > 60 years. Ages at the most recent evaluation ranged from 13 to 90 years (mean 51 ± 16). Follow-up period from the time of diagnosis was 1 to 30 years (mean 9.5 ± 5.6); 226 patients (68%) were men. After initial identification, patients were followed in a standard fashion at about one-year intervals with clinical examination, two-dimensional echocardiogram, 12-lead ECG, 24-48 hour ambulatory Holter ECG and exercise test. Cardiac catheterization and electrophysiologic studies were performed only in a selected subgroup of patients.

Medical Treatment Strategies

Treatment strategies for the study patients were directed toward control of symptoms, arrhythmias, left ventricular outflow obstruction and the prevention of peripheral embolization. Patients with angina and/or congestive symptoms were treated with beta-adrenergic blocking agents (usually nadolol 80/160 mg/day) if evidence of resting outflow obstruction was present, or calcium channel blockers (usually verapamil 240-360 mg/day or nifedipine 30-60 mg/day) if obstruction was absent. In selected patients with repeated runs of nonsustained ventricular tachycardia or atrial fibrillation, in association with outflow obstruction, beta-blocking agents were administered in low doses (nadolol 40 mg/day) and in combination with amiodarone (average 200 mg/day). In patients with atrial fibrillation, sinus rhythm was usually restored by amiodarone alone or in association with DC cardioversion, after optimal anticoagulation was achieved with warfarin. In the presence of severe congestive symptoms or heart failure, diuretic agents (e.g. furosemide, thiazides) or ACE-inhibitors were often also administered. Asymptomatic patients did not receive drug treatment except in the presence of additional clinical variables regarded as risk factors, such as resting outflow obstruction, (beta-adrenergic blocking agents) or repetitive nonsustained runs of ventricular tachycardia (amiodarone).

Statistical Analysis

Statistical analysis was performed by using a Student's t test for comparison of normally distributed data. Fisher's exact test and χ^2 tests were used to analyze categorical data. Univariate analysis for survival and event free curves were performed by using Kaplan-Meier estimates . The association of some variables with survival time was also evaluated individually, by univariate test, and jointly following a forward stepwise entry approach, thus revealing the entry order of covariates which are added on the basis of the largest increase in the joint test statistic (Cox regression). Statistical analysis was performed using procedures in Statistical Package for the Social Sciences (SPSS, SPSS inc., Chicago). The required level of significance was $p < 0.05$.

Results

Mortality Data

The general features of our study population are reported in Table 1. Of the 330 study patients, 18 (5%) died from cardiovascular causes related to HCM; therefore, the annual mortality rate for the total follow-up period was 0.57%. Of the 18 cardiovascular deaths, 4 were sudden and unexpected, while the remaining 14 occurred in the context of congestive heart failure (Fig. 1). The Kaplan-Meier survival curve for our population showed a 5 and 10-year survival of 98% and 95%, respectively. At multivariate analysis, the only independent predictors associated with cardiovascular mortality were a severe functional limitation at diagnosis (New York Heart Association (NYHA) functional class III-IV; $p = 0.001$), and left atrial dimensions ($p < 0.01$). On the other hand, the presence of factors such as basal left ventricular outflow obstruction, syncope on nonsustained ventricular tachycardia were not associated with increased mortality [1,6].

Table 1. Clinical and demographic features of an unselected population of 330 patients with hypertrophic cardiomyopathy

	n	%
Male	226	68
Age at diagnosis (years)	42±16	
Family history of HCM/SD	146	44
Resting LVOT gradient ≥ 30 mmHg	74	22
Maximum left ventricular thickness (mm)	22±5	
NYHA III-IV at diagnosis	31	9
Atrial fibrillation during follow-up	81	25
Nonsustained ventricular tachycardia	94	28

HCM, hypertrophic cardiomyopathy; LVOT, left ventricular outflow tract; NYHA, New York Heart Association; SD, sudden death.

Symptomatic Status and Cardiovascular Events

Of the 330 study patients, the majority (195 patients; 59%) showed a stable/benign clinical course, defined as absence of 1) cardiovascular death, 2) worsening of functional status (from NYHA I-II to NYHA III-IV), and 3) cardiovascular events; among these 159 patients, 135 remained asymptomatic in NYHA class I (Fig. 1). The remaining 135 patients (41%) showed a severe/progressive course, including the 18 patients who died and 117 (36%) with worsening of functional status and cardiovascular events (Fig. 1). The annual rate of patients with cardiovascular events was 10%, with 3.7% new patients experiencing a first cardiovascular event each year. The Kaplan-Meier event-free curve for our population showed a 5 and 10-year event-free rate of 82% and 67%, respectively.

Natural History of Untreated Patients

A subgroup of 92 patients (28%) never received treatment, either because they were asymptomatic (84; 91%), or because they refused (8; 9%). All patients were in NYHA class I-II at the time of diagnosis, their maximum LV thickness was 21 ± 5 mm, and 11 (12%) had significant left ventricular outflow tract obstruction (gradient ≥ 30 mmHg). Of these 92 patients, only 2 died during the follow-up period (2%), both suddenly and unexpectedly. Annual mortality rate in this particular subgroup was therefore 0.2%. One additional patient from this subgroup deteriorated to NYHA class III, and 7 patients (8%) had major cardiovascular events during follow-up.

Discussion

In the last five years several studies have shown that HCM is a disease whose

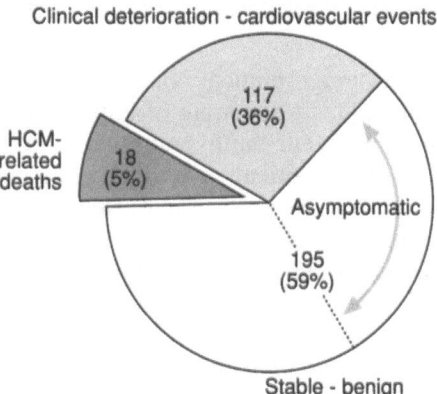

Fig. 1. Clinical course of an unselected population of 330 patients with hypertrophic cardiomyopathy during a 9.5-year average follow-up

prevalence is higher and whose prognosis is more benign than previously thought [1-3,6-8]. As the degree of selection of the patient population studied diminished, both these concepts became progressively clearer. In this perspective, the real profile of HCM in the general population can only be derived from studies performed on unselected patient populations with the disease, which was the aim of the Italian Multicentric Study on HCM.

The data presented show that, in our population, HCM is associated with a relatively favourable long-term prognosis, with an annual mortality rate for HCM-related causes below 1%. This is substantially different from the majority of published reports appearing before 1990, that generally described mortality rates, due primarily to sudden death, in the range of 2% to 6%, with an average of about 4% [3,6]. However, these data are in agreement with the annual mortality rate observed by the Florence group in 1989, and in fact the disease appears to be even more benign than reported at that time [5]. In particular, sudden and unexpected death was a rare event, occurring in only 1.2% of patients during a 9.5 year follow-up; the most common cause of death was related to congestive heart failure and its complications [4]. In the subgroup of asymptomatic patients who never received any treatment during follow-up (nearly 30% of the total population), the true natural history was assessed, revealing a particularly benign prognosis with only 2 deaths and 7 cardiovascular events in the overall period. Patients with symptoms at the time of diagnosis had a more severe prognosis, which is the subject of the paper by Lazzeroni et al. in this book.

Besides a favourable long-term survival, the majority of our patients (59%) also showed a remarkably stable clinical course, without clinical deterioration (progression to NYHA III-IV) or major cardiovascular events. However, one tenth of the patients each year did suffer a cardiovascular event, with considerable impact on their health and quality of life. Therefore, while patients with no symptoms and absence of risk factors, such as a malignant family history, should be reassured and encouraged to lead a normal life, HCM patients will often require careful follow-up and non-invasive testing in order to identify early markers of disease progression, and will need timely intervention in the not unlikely occurrence of an acute event, such as syncope or atrial fibrillation [4].

Reasons to explain the benign clinical course described in our population include a possible benign genetic substrate of Italian patients with HCM and the effect of treatment. We favour the hypothesis that a largely conservative but careful management of our patients may have influenced significantly the natural history of the disease: in particular by the routine use of low-dose amiodarone treatment, in HCM patients with multiple-repetitive nonsustained ventricular tachycardia and/or atrial fibrillation [4,9].

In conclusion, HCM is a more frequent disease than previously thought, and is associated with a relatively benign prognosis in unselected patient populations. The vast majority of patients are asymptomatic or with mild symptoms, and constitute a subgroup with particularly benign outcome. Overall cardiovascular mortality is low, and mostly related to congestive heart failure; sudden and unexpected death is rare. However, life quality may be affected by functional status deterioration and by the frequent occurrence of cardiovascular events requiring hospitalization.

References

1. Spirito P, Seidman CE, McKenna WJ, Maron BJ (1997) The management of hypertrophic cardiomyopathy. N Engl J Med 336:775-785
2. Maron BJ, Gardin JM, Flack JM, Gidding SS, Kurosaki TT, Bild DE (1995) Prevalence of hypertrophic cardiomyopathy in a general population of young adults: echocardiographic analysis of 4111 subjects in the CARDIA study. Circulation 92:530-533
3. Maron BJ, Bonow RO, Cannon RO, Leon MB, Epstein SE (1987) Hypertrophic cardiomyopathy: Interrelation of clinical manifestations, pathophysiology, and therapy. N Engl J Med 316:780-789 and 844-852
4. Cecchi F, Olivotto I, Montereggi A, Santoro G, Dolara A, Maron BJ (1995) Hypertrophic cardiomyopathy in Tuscany: clinical course and outcome in an unselected population. J Am Coll Cardiol 26:1529-1536
5. Cecchi F, Montereggi A, Squillantini G, Zuppiroli A, Dolara A (1990) The natural history and clinical course of hypertrophic cardiomyopathy. In: G Baroldi, F Camerini, JF Goodwin (eds) Advances in Cardiomyopathies. Springer-Verlag, Berlin Heidelberg New York, pp 25-31
6. Maron BJ, Cecchi F, McKenna WJ (1994) Risk factors and current status of risk stratification profiles for sudden cardiac death in patients with hypertrophic cardiomyopathy. Br Heart J, 72 [Suppl]:S13-18
7. Kofflard MJ, Waldstein DJ, Vos J, ten Cate FJ (1993) Prognosis in hypertrophic cardiomyopathy: Long-term follow-up in a large, unselected outpatient population. Am J Cardiol 72:939-943
8. Spirito P, Chiarella F, Carratino L, Berisso MZ, Bellotti P, Vecchio C (1989) Clinical course and prognosis of hypertrophic cardiomyopathy in an outpatient population. N Engl J Med 320:749-755
9. McKenna WJ, Oakley CM, Krikler DM, Goodwin JF (1985) Improved survival with amiodarone in patients with hypertrophic cardiomyopathy and ventricular tachycardia. Br Heart J 53:412-416

The Italian Multicentric Study on Hypertrophic Cardiomyopathy: II. Prognostic Assessment in Symptomatic Patients

E. Lazzeroni, I. Olivotto, F. Cecchi, G.P. Chiriatti, A. Sachero and G. Renosto, on behalf of the Italian Study Group on Cardiomyopathies (SPIC), Subproject on Hypertrophic Cardiomyopathy

Introduction

The morphological, functional, and genetic abnormalities are heterogeneous in different patient populations with hypertrophic cardiomyopathy (HCM) [1-8]; as a consequence, the natural history and the clinical course are extremely variable and prognostic evaluation is a challenging task in the individual patient.

Most data about the natural history of HCM come from tertiary centre series introducing a selection bias that had a substantial impact on the perception of disease severity [1, 9-20]. Conversely, reports on outpatient or general population series show a more benign course of HCM [6, 20-27]. However, long-term prognostic studies of unselected symptomatic patients are still scarce. The purpose of the present study was to assess the prognostic factors associated with adverse cardiovascular events and mortality among a large group of symptomatic patients, representing a subset of an unselected patient population with HCM.

Methods

Study protocol: the aim of the Italian Multicentric Cardiomyopathy Study (SPIC), the criteria for the diagnosis of HCM and the study protocol used during the follow-up of our study population have been fully described previously in this book (Cecchi et al.).

Patient selection: for the particular purpose of this study, out of the 330 consecutive patients enrolled in the SPIC, only those patients with symptoms at diagnosis were selected. Therefore, the study group consisted of 237 patients who had symptoms at initial evaluation (150 males and 87 females; age 44 ± 15 years, ranging from 1 to 74). Mean follow-up duration for this group was 9.7 ± 5 years.

Statistical analysis: statistical analysis was performed by using a Student's t test for comparison of normally distributed data. Fisher's exact test and χ^2 tests were used to analyze categorical data. Univariate analysis for survival and event-free curves were performed by using Kaplan-Meier estimates. The association of some variables with survival time was also evaluated individually, by univariate test, and jointly following a forward stepwise entry approach, thus revealing the entry order of covariates which are added on the basis of the largest increase in the joint test statistic (Cox regression). Statistical analysis was performed using the procedure in Statistical Package for the Social Sciences (SPSS, SPSS inc., Chicago). The required level of significance was $p < 0.05$.

Results

Baseline Characteristics

The clinical, echocardiographic and Holter findings of the study group are reported in Table 1. At first evaluation, the most common symptoms were palpitations and dyspnea (occurring in 57 % and 50% of patients respectively); angina was reported by about one third (32%), and syncope by 11% of these patients. The great majority (87%) had only mild functional limitation (NYHA class I-II) (Table 1).

As compared with patients who were asymptomatic at diagnosis, sympto-

Table 1. Clinical, echocardiographic and ambulatory Holter findings in the 330 patients with hypertrophic cardiomyopathy

Features at diagnosis	Asymptomatic patients (n = 93)	Symptomatic patients (n = 237)	p value
Clinical Data			
Age (yrs.)	34±17	44 ±15	< 0.001
Sex (Male/Female)	76/17	150/87	< 0.002
FH of HCM and/or SD	47 (50%)	99(42%)	n.s.
NYHA Class I - II	93(100%)	206(87%)	-
NYHA Class III - IV	0	31(13%)	-
Syncope	0	26 (11%)	-
Angina	0	77 (32%)	-
Dyspnea	0	118 (50%)	-
Palpitations	0	136 (57%)	-
Echocardiographic data			
Max. LV Thickness (mm.)	21±5	23±5	< 0.02
LVEDD (mm.)	45±6	43±23	< 0.05
Fractional shortening (%)	41±8	37±9	< 0.05
LAD (mm.)	37±6	43±9	< 0.001
Resting LVOT gradient ≥ 30 mmHg	8 (9%)	66 (31%)	< 0.0001
24 to 48 hours Holter data			
Ventricular Tachycardia	16 (18%)	78 (34%)	< 0.01
Chronic Atrial Fibrillation	1 (1%)	21 (9%)	< 0.05
Duration of Follow-up (years)	8.9 ±5.9	9.7±5.4	n.s.

FH, family history; LAD, left atrium dimension; LV, left ventricle; LVEDD, left ventricular end-diastolic dimension; LVOT, left ventricular outflow tract; SD, sudden death; n.s. not significant.

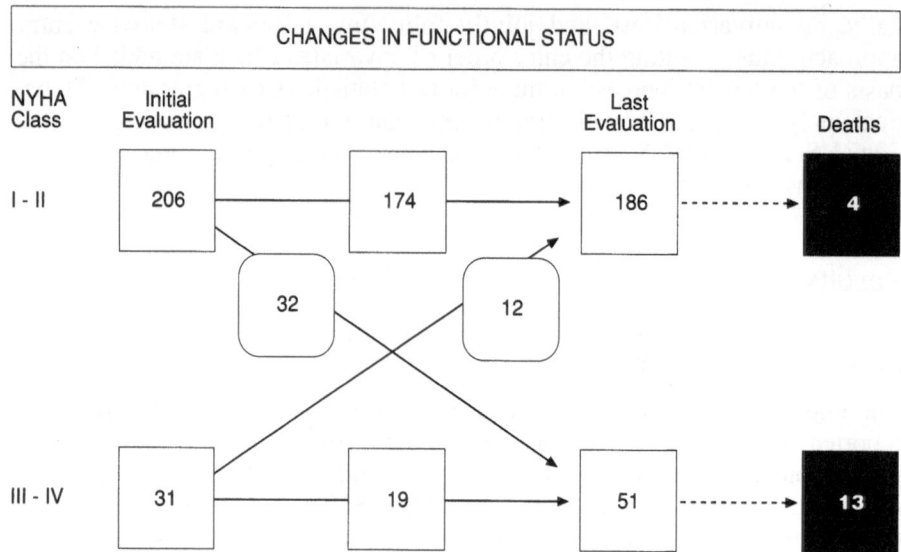

Fig. 1. Changes in functional status during follow-up in 237 patients with hypertrophic cardiomyopathy symptomatic at diagnosis

matic patients were characterized by older age and prevalence of female gender (Table 1). Moreover, symptomatic patients showed a greater left ventricular wall thickness, smaller end-diastolic left ventricular diameter, larger left atrial diameter, higher prevalence of left ventricular outflow tract obstruction, greater prevalence of chronic atrial fibrillation and of nonsustained ventricular tachycardia at Holter ECG (Table 1).

Follow-up Data: Cardiovascular Events, Functional State and Mortality

During a mean follow-up period of 9.7 years, 114 of the 237 symptomatic patients (48%) had one or more adverse cardiovascular events: 66 patients (23%) had atrial fibrillation, 27 (11%) syncope, 25 (10%) congestive heart failure, 25 (10%) peripheral embolization, 13 (5%) bradyarrhythmias or conduction abnormalities requiring permanent pacemaker insertion, 10 (4%) underwent myotomy-myectomy, 9 (4%) had acute myocardial ischemia or infarction, and 10 patients (4%) had other less frequent events.

Changes in functional status between the initial and most recent clinical evaluation are reported in Figure 1. Of the 237 patients symptomatic at diagnosis, 43% had a stable clinical course, 22% showed a worsening of NYHA class and the remaining 35% showed an improvement.

Out of 237 symptomatic patients 17 (7.2%) died of cardiovascular causes as compared to 1 among the 93 asymptomatic patients: 4 deaths were sudden and unexpected (mean age 40 ± 9 years) while 13 were related to congestive heart failure (mean age 62 ± 16 years). Annual mortality rate was therefore 0.7% in this group, as compared to 0.12% among asymptomatic patients.

Prognostic Determinants in Symptomatic Patients

At univariate analysis the following clinical and instrumental variables, evaluated at diagnosis, were significantly associated with subsequent cardiovascular events: age, severe functional limitation (NYHA class III-IV) symptoms, symptomatic reduced fractional shortening, left atrial dilatation, runs of non-sustained ventricular tachycardia at Holter, and chronic atrial fibrillation. At multivariate analysis only older age at diagnosis, NYHA functional class III-IV, and syncope were independent predictors of cardiovascular events (Table 2).

Among the same variables, 5 were associated with cardiovascular mortality at univariate analysis: NYHA functional class III-IV, maximal left ventricular thickness, reduced fractional shortening, atrial dilatation, chronic atrial fibrillation, and nonsustained, but repetitive, runs of ventricular tachycardia. Advanced functional limitation (III-IV NYHA class), degree of left ventricular hypertrophy and left atrial dilatation were the only independent predictors of cardiovascular mortality by multivariate analysis (Table 3).

Comparison between Symptomatic and Asymptomatic Patients

When compared to asymptomatic patients, patients who were symptomatic at diagnosis showed a greater tendency towards clinical worsening of the functional status: 22% progressed to NYHA classes III-IV as compared to 12% in the asymptomatic group. The proportion of patients with at least one cardio-

Table 2. Relation of clinical, echocardiographic and Holter findings in the 237 symptomatic patients with hypertrophic cardiomyopathy to subsequent cardiovascular events

Variable at diagnosis	Univariate analysis	Multivariate analysis
Clinical Data	p	p
Age (yrs.)	< 0.0001	< 0.0001
Sex	n.s.	n.s.
F H of HCM and/or SD	n.s.	n.s.
III-IV NYHA Class	< 0.0001	< 0.0002
Syncope	< 0.0001	< 0.0005
Angina	< 0.01	n.s.
Dyspnea	< 0.001	n.s.
Palpitations	< 0.005	n.s.
Echocardiographic Data		
Max. LV Thickness (mm.)	n.s.	n.s.
LVEDD (mm.)	n.s.	n.s.
Fractional shortening (%)	< 0.05	n.s.
Resting LVOT gradient (mmHg)	n.s.	n.s.
LAD (mm.)	< 0.0001	n.s.
24 to 48 Hours Holter Data		
Ventricular Tachycardia	< 0.05	n.s.
Chronic Atrial Fibrillation	< 0.0005	n.s.

For abbreviations, see Table 1.

Table 3. Relation of clinical, echocardiographic and Holter findings in 237 symptomatic patients with hypertrophic cardiomyopathy to mortality

Variable at diagnosis	Univariate analysis	Multivariate analysis
Clinical Data	*p*	*p*
Age (yrs.)	n.s.	n.s.
Sex	n.s.	n.s.
F H of HCM and/or SD	n.s.	n.s.
III-IV NYHA Class	< 0.0001	< 0.001
Echocardiographic Data		
Max. LV Thickness (mm.)	< 0.02	< 0.05
LVEDD (mm.)	n.s.	n.s.
Fractional shortening (%)	< 0.05	n.s.
Resting LVOT gradient (mmHg)	n.s.	n.s.
LAD (mm.)	< 0.002	< 0.02
24 to 48 Hours Holter Data		
Ventricular Tachycardia	< 0.05	n.s.
Chronic Atrial Fibrillation	< 0.05	n.s.

For abbreviations, see Table 1.

vascular event was higher in the symptomatic group (48% vs. 6%; $p < 0.0001$), and so was cardiovascular mortality (7.2% vs 1.1%; $p < 0.05$). Kaplan-Meier analysis showed that the presence of symptoms at diagnosis was associated with reduced event-free survival ($p < 0.0001$, Fig. 2), and increased cardiovascular mortality ($p < 0.05$, Fig. 3).

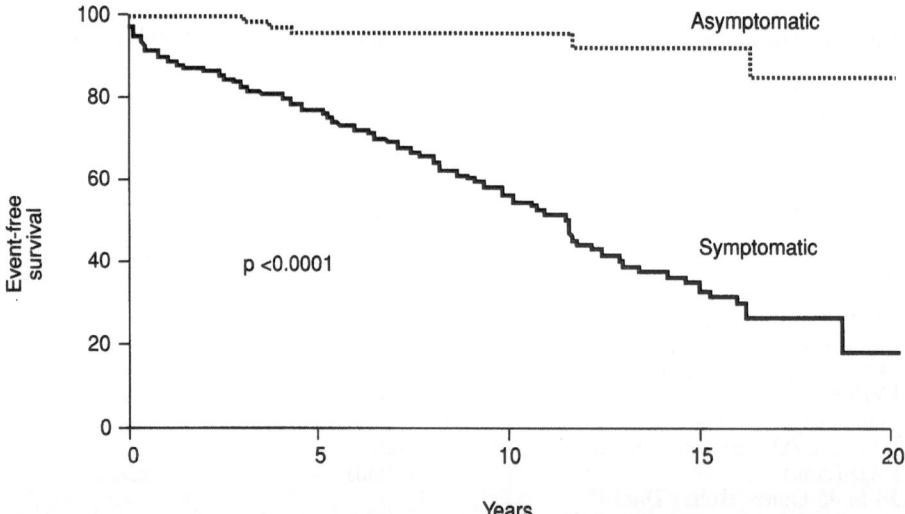

Fig. 2. Event-free survival in 330 unselected patients with hypertrophic cardiomyopathy. Kaplan-Meier curve shows increased event rate in 237 symptomatic as compared to 93 asymptomatic patients

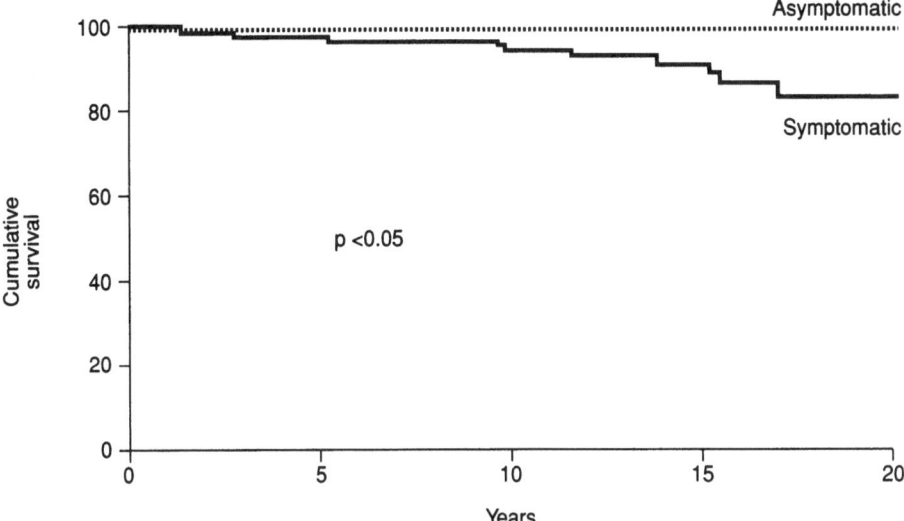

Fig. 3. Cumulative survival in 330 unselected patients with hypertrophic cardiomyopathy. Kaplan-Meier curve shows increased cardiovascular mortality in 237 symptomatic as compared to 93 asymptomatic patients

Discussion

A great diversity of morphologic, functional, genetic and clinical expression characterizes patients with HCM [1-8]. Hypertrophy can be localized to one segment of the left ventricle or involve all segments of both ventricles, and the clinical spectrum may vary, in patients with the same morphologic appearance, from the absence of symptoms to severe functional limitation [1-3,5,6].

The majority of the studies on prognosis published in the major cardiology journals have come from only two tertiary referral centers [23,27] and their reported annual mortality varies from 2% to 6%. Patients in these studies were characterized by young age at diagnosis, malignant family history, severe symptoms, high prevalence of obstructive forms, and sudden death [1,9-20]. Accordingly, these patients reflect the more severe face of the disease. On the other hand, more recent studies based on patients from non-referral centers [6, 21-26] reported a substantially lower annual mortality ranging from 0% to 1%. Indeed, these patients reflect the population of HCM patients which is usually seen in general and local hospitals. All these studies concluded that the natural history of HCM may be less severe than previously reported.

The present study was conducted in a large group of symptomatic patients out of an unselected HCM population, who where followed for an average of almost 10 years and represented all age groups. Our data show that the presence of symptoms at diagnosis is associated with increased cardiovascular mortality and occurrence of adverse events related to the disease, as compared to asymptomatic patients, although the long-term prognosis remains relatively benign in these patients (Fig. 3). Moreover, patients with symptoms are more prone to develop worsening of functional status in the long-term, although almost 50% remain clinically stable and a sizeable subset may improve with appropriate management.

The only independent predictors of mortality in our study group were the presence of moderate to severe functional limitation (NYHA class III-IV), left atrial enlargement, and degree of left ventricular hypertrophy. These findings reflect the fact that severe and progressive heart failure was the most frequent cause of death in our population, with an annual mortality of 0.5%, while sudden death was infrequent (0.2% annual mortality) and significantly lower than previously reported by others [1,9-20]. Such a low incidence of sudden and unexpected death is only in part explained by the strict definition criteria for sudden death used in this study [25], while it more probably reflects the real prevalence of sudden death in unselected populations and, possibly, the beneficial effect of amiodarone treatment in high-risk patients.

In conclusion, our results show that, in an unselected HCM population, the presence of symptoms at diagnosis is associated with a moderately increased mortality as compared with asymptomatic patients, but the long-term prognosis remains in these patients more favorable than previously described. However, symptomatic patients represent a subset at high risk for adverse cardiac events who, in approximately one fourth of cases, will develop severe functional limitation (NYHA class III-IV). Routine monitoring of symptomatic status and left atrial dimension may be useful for an early identification of patients prone to clinical deterioration.

References

1. Frank S, Braunwald E (1968) Idiopathic hypertrophic subaortic stenosis: clinical analysis of 126 patients with emphasis on the natural history. Circulation 37:759-787
2. Goodwin JF. (1970) Congestive and hypertrophic cardiomyopathies: a decade of study. Lancet 1:732-739
3. Wigle ED, Sasson Z, Henderson MA, et al. (1985) Hypertrophic cardiomyopathy: the importance of the site and the extent of hypertrophy: a review. Prog Cardiovasc Dis 28:1-83
4. Maron BJ, Spirito P, Wesley Y, Arce J (1986) Development and progression of left ventricular hypertrophy in children with hypertrophic cardiomyopathy. N Engl J Med 315:610-614
5. Maron BJ, Bonow RO, Cannon RO III, Leon MB, Epstein SE (1987) Hypertrophic cardiomyopathy: interrelations of clinical manifestations, pathophysiology, and therapy. N Engl J Med 316:780-844
6. Spirito P, Chiarella F, Carratino L, Berisso MZ, Bellotti P, Vecchio C, (1989) Clinical course and prognosis of hypertrophic cardiomyopathy in an outpatient population. N Engl J Med 320:749-761
7. Louie EK, Edwards LC III (1994) Hypertrophic cardiomyopathy. Prog Cardiovasc Dis 36:275-308
8. Wigle ED, Rakowski Hypertrophy, Kimball BP, Williams WG (1995) Hypertrophic cardiomyopathy: clinical spectrum and treatment. Circulation 92:1680-1682
9. Shah PM, Adelman AG, Wigle ED, et al (1973) The natural (and unnatural) history of hypertrophic obstructive cardiomyopathy. Circ Res 34,35 [Suppl II]: II-179-185
10. Maron BJ, Roberts WC, Epstein SE (1982) Sudden death in hypertrophic cardiomy-

opathy: profile of 78 patients. Circulation 65:1388-1394

11. Swan DA, Bell B, Oakley C, Goodwin J (1971) Analysis of symptomatic course and prognosis and treatment of hypertrophic obstructive cardiomyopathy. Br Heart J 33:671-675

12. Hardarson T, De La Calzada CS, Curiel JF (1973) Prognosis and mortality of hypertrophic obstructive cardiomyopathy. Lancet 2:1462-1464

13. Loogen F, Kuhn H, Gietzen F, Losse B, Schulte HD, Bircks W (1983) Clinical course and prognosis of patients with atypical hypertrophic obstructive and hypertrophic nonobstructive cardiomyopathy. Eur Heart J 4 [Suppl. F]:145-151

14. Hect GM, Panza JA, Maron BJ (1992) Clinical course of middle-aged asymptomatic patients with hypertrophic cardiomyopathy. Am J Cardiol 69:935-940

15. McKenna WJ, Deanfield JE (1984) Hypertrophic cardiomyopathy: an important cause of sudden death. Arch Dis Child 59:971-976

16. Maron BJ, Lipson LC, Roberts WC, Savage DD, Epstein SE. (1978) "Malignant" hypertrophic cardiomyopathy: identification of a subgroup of families with unusually frequent premature deaths. Am J Cardiol 41:1133-1140

17. Fiddler GI, Tajik AJ, Weidman WH, McGoon DC, Ritter DG, Giuliani ER (1978) Idiopathic hypertrophic subaortic stenosis in the young. Am J Cardiol 42:793-799

18. Cecchi F, Maron BJ, Epstein SE (1989) Long-term outcome of patients with hypertrophic cardiomyopathy successfully resuscitated after arrest. J Am Coll Cardiol 13:1283-1288

19. McKenna WJ, Camm AJ (1989) Sudden death in hypertrophic cardiomyopathy: assessment of patients at high risk. Circulation 80:1489-1494

20. Maron BJ, Henry WL, Clark CE, Redwood DR, Roberts WC, Epstein SE (1976) Asymmetric septal hypertrophy in childhood. Circulation 53:9-14

21. Shapiro LM, Zezulka A (1983) Hypertrophic cardiomyopathy: a common disease with a good prognosis: five year experience of a district general hospital. Br Heart J 50:530-533

22. Kofflard MJ, Waldstein DJ, Vos J, ten Cate FJ (1993) Prognosis in hypertrophic cardiomyopathy observed in a large clinic population. Am J Cardiol 72:939-943

23 Maron BJ, Spirito P (1993) Impact of patient selection biases on the perception of hypertrophic cardiomyopathy and its natural history. Am J Cardiol 72:970-972

24. Spirito P, Rapezzi C, Autore C, et al. (1994) Prognosis of asymptomatic patients with hypertrophic cardiomyopathy and nonsustained ventricular tachicardia. Circulation 90:2743-2747

25. Cecchi F, Olivotto I, Montereggi A, Santoro G, Dolara A, Maron BJ (1995) Hypertrophic cardiomyopathy in Tuscany: clinical course and outcome in an unselected regional population. J Am Coll Cardiol 26:1529-1534

26. Cannan CR, Reeder GS, Bailey KR, Melton LJ III, Gersh BJ (1995) Natural history of hypertrophic cardiomyopathy: a population based study, 1976 through 1990. Circulation 92:2488-2495

27. Spirito P, Seidman CE, McKenna WJ, Maron BJ (1997) The management of hypertrophic cardiomyopathy. N Engl J Med 11:775-785

Detection and Clinical Consequences of Myocardial Ischemia and Reduced Coronary Reserve

P.G. Camici

Myocardial Ischemia in Patients with Hypertrophic Cardiomyopathy

Chest pain suggestive of reversible myocardial ischemia is a common symptom in patients with hypertrophic cardiomyopathy (HCM) [1]. The ischemic nature of the chest pain, which most often occurs in patients with angiographically normal coronary arteries, could be demonstrated by the presence of reversible perfusion defects on thallium-201 scanning [2]. In addition, net lactate release and a reduced coronary vasodilator reserve during atrial pacing have been reported [3]. The mechanisms of myocardial ischemia in any individual patient with HCM is difficult to determine *in vivo*, but a number of pathophysiological features, including increased myocardial mass [4], reduced capillary density [5] and "small vessel disease" [6] may compromise myocardial blood flow sufficiently to cause a mismatch between oxygen supply and demand. HCM is also characterized by abnormalities of left ventricular diastolic function that have the potential to cause myocardial ischemia [7,8].

Since the interventricular septum is the region of the left ventricle which is most severely affected by macroscopic hypertrophy in patients with HCM, the abnormalities of the coronary vasodilator reserve in the territory of the great cardiac vein, which predominantly drains blood from the anteroseptal region of the left ventricle, were interpreted as a mere consequence of myocyte hypertrophy. A number of observations, however, indicate that the anatomic and functional abnormalities of the myocardium and the coronary circulation do not necessarily follow the geography of macroscopic tissue hypertrophy. For instance, morphological abnormalities of cardiac muscle and intramural coronary arteries have been reported in myocardial regions with normal wall thickness [6] and diastolic wall motion abnormalities have been demonstrated in these regions [9].

The Coronary Circulation Is Dysfunctional in Both Hypertrophied and Nonhypertrophied Myocardium

Positron emission tomography (PET) allows the noninvasive measurement of regional myocardial blood flow. Using PET we have measured myocardial blood flow and the coronary vasodilator reserve (the ratio of myocardial blood flow measured during pharmacologically-induced coronary vasodilatation and resting blood flow) which is an indirect index of coronary microvascular function, in patients with HCM and asymmetrical hypertrophy. Myocardial blood flow could be measured simultaneously in the hypertrophied septum and the nonhypertrophied free wall [10]. The results of this study demonstrated that, despite angiographically normal coronary arteries, the coronary vasodilator reserve was severely blunted in HCM patients not only in regions of macroscopic hypertrophy, but also in the nonhypertrophied myocardium.

Microvascular Dysfunction Is More Severe in HCM Patients Who Develop Systolic Dysfunction

The above results were later confirmed in a larger patient population [11] (Fig. 1). Since a minority of patients (5% to 10%) with HCM develop progressive dilatation of the left ventricle with systolic dysfunction, and eventually die of congestive heart failure later in the course of the disease, in the latter study [11] we aimed to ascertain whether any relation existed between left ventricular dysfunction and the abnormal coronary microvascular function.

We found that HCM patients in advanced NYHA classes had lower dipyridamole flows (NYHA class I = 1.57 ± 0.64 vs NYHA class II = 1.52 ± 0.58

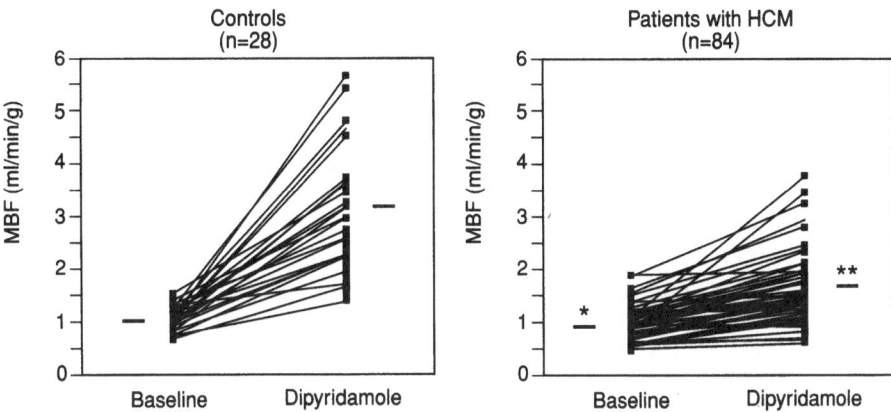

Fig. 1. Individual values of mean left ventricular myocardial blood flow (MBF) measured at baseline and following I.V. dipyridamole (0.56 mg/kg) infusion in 28 sex and age matched control subjects *(left panel)* and 84 patients with hypertrophic cardiomyopathy (HCM) *(right panel)*. Following dipyridamole, MBF in patients with hypertrophic cardiomyopathy increased significantly less than in controls. Regional analysis in HCM showed that the increase in MBF following dipyridamole was similarly blunted in the hypertrophied septum and the nonhypertrophied left ventricular free wall. * = $p < 0.05$; and ** = $p < 0.01$ vs relative values in controls

vs NYHA class III = 0.96 ± 0.32 ml/min/g; ANOVA, $p < 0.05$) and coronary vasodilator reserve (NYHA class I = 1.93 ± 0.64 vs NYHA class II = 1.69 ± 0.54 vs NYHA class III = 1.40 ± 0.43; ANOVA, $p < 0.05$). A significant negative correlation between left ventricular end-systolic diameter and dipyridamole flow was present. In addition, a significant positive correlation between fractional shortening and dipyridamole flow was demonstrated and patients with abnormal left ventricular function (fractional shortening < 29%) had lower dipyridamole flows (1.07 ± 0.43 vs 1.58 ± 0.62 ml/min/g, $p < 0.01$).

Evidence of Subendocardial Hypoperfusion

The limited spatial resolution of currently available PET cameras precludes the determination of transmural myocardial blood flow distribution in myocardium of normal thickness. In some patients with HCM, however, the presence of particularly severe myocardial hypertrophy offers the possibility of selectively assessing myocardial blood flow in the subendocardial and subepicardial layers.

We have demonstrated that in patients with HCM there is evidence of transmural maldistribution of myocardial blood flow with a reduced subendocardial to subepicardial flow ratio following dipyridamole infusion [12]. In a subsequent study, evidence of subendocardial underperfusion was found in 3 of 7 patients with interventricular septal thickness > 25 mm while off treatment [13]. More recently, myocardial blood flow at baseline and following dipyridamole was measured in 15 HCM patients using oxygen-15 labelled water and PET [14]. Subendocardial (endo) and subepicardial (epi) flows were assessed in the septum (thickness 25.4 ± 5.8 mm). Studies in animals using radioactive microspheres [15] have demonstrated that the ratio endo-flow/epi-flow (the endo/epi ratio), which is an index of the heterogeneity of transmural myocardial blood flow distribution, is approximately 1, both during autoregulation and during maximal coronary vasodilation (range 0.8 to 1.2) suggesting a rather even blood flow distribution across the left ventricular wall. Arbitrarily, ratios of < 0.8 in our patients were taken as an index of subendocardial underperfusion. At baseline the endo/epi ratio in the septum was uniform (1.13 ± 0.18), but following dipyridamole it decreased to 0.93 ± 0.24 ($p < 0.01$ vs baseline) and 5/15 (33%) patients had a ratio < 0.8 (Fig. 2). Thus, dipyridamole-induced subendocardial underperfusion could be demonstrated in one third of the patients in this series.

Possible Mechanisms of Coronary Microvascular Dysfunction

The small coronary arterioles below 450 μm in diameter are the principal determinants of coronary vascular resistance and a 50% drop in perfusion pressure, relative to aortic, may be observed in vessels between 70 and 440 μm in diameter. The latter observation is consistent with 40%-50% of total

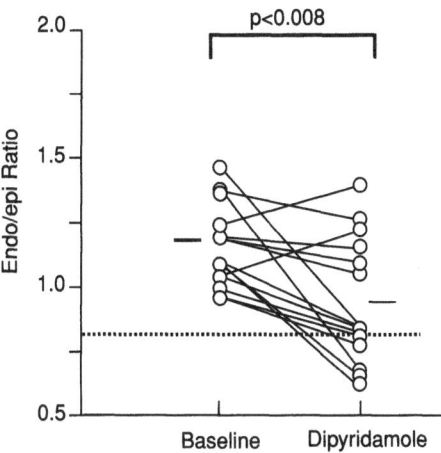

Fig. 2. The individual subendocardial/subepicardial (endo/epi) flow ratios measured in the interventricular septum of 15 patients with hypertropic cardiomyopathy at baseline and following dipyridamole stress are reported. The broken line indicates an endo/epi ratio of 0.8 on the vertical axis. See text for more details

coronary vascular resistance being located in pre-arterioles greater than 100 μm. Nearly all of the remaining resistance lies in vessels less than 100 μm in diameter, which are also those responsible for autoregulation of myocardial blood flow [16]. In theory a reduction in the caliber of the small coronary arterioles could be due to a series of different mechanisms including: 1) active vasoconstriction or loss of vasodilator capacity, 2) remodelling of the vessel wall (e.g. medial hypertrophy with lumen/wall ratio reduction), 3) abnormal intramyocardial pressure (i.e., increased extravascular resistance).

1- Active Vasoconstriction or Loss of Vasodilator Capacity
It has been proposed that constriction of the small vessels can be induced by: a) the drop in perfusion pressure distal to the epicardial stenosis, b) endothelial dysfunction, and c) neurohumoral factors (e.g. endothelin, neuropeptide Y, serotonin). In addition, the small coronary arterioles receive autonomic innervation and their diameter may be altered by stimulation of these nerves [16].

2- Remodelling of the Vessel Wall
The structural remodelling of the coronary microcirculation, as that observed in hypertensive heart disease [17-19] and HCM [6], includes changes in the arteriolar wall and a relative reduction in the total number of vessels, probably as a consequence of the disproportionate growth of myocytes, without a corresponding increase in the available blood supply. Medial thickening of intramural coronary arteries in myocardial biopsy specimens from humans with hypertension has recently been confirmed: an increase in the wall/lumen ratio correlates with the increase in the resistance to coronary blood flow, and the reduction in coronary flow reserve. These clinical data confirm previous

reports in post-mortem specimens where marked thickening of arterioles of 50-200 μm had been reported in patients with chest pain and hypertensive heart disease [17-19].

3- Abnormal Intramyocardial Pressure (i.e., increased extravascular resistance) Both in the presence of coronary autoregulation and during maximal coronary vasodilatation the subendocardial to subepicardial flow ratio is close to unity [20-23]. This occurs despite the higher extravascular intramyocardial pressure which is present in the subendocardial myocardium, and is probably due to a greater vascularity in this layer [24]. During maximal vasodilatation, however, if coronary perfusion pressure falls below the "subendocardial opening pressure" (i.e. the perfusion pressure required to open the subendocardial vessels, which is higher than the pressure required to open the subepicardial vessels) selective subendocardial hypoperfusion occurs [24]. This will produce a drop in the subendocardial to subepicardial ratio to levels below 0.8 (transmural steal). A greater fall of perfusion pressure below the "subepicardial opening pressure" will cause transmural hypoperfusion [24].

In the case of HCM, remodeling of the vessel wall and increased extravascular pressures seem to be the principal mechanisms responsible for microvascular dysfunction and subendocardial underperfusion. This may explain, at least in part, the mechanisms of action of some of the drugs currently used in the treatment of HCM [25].

References

1. Pasternac A, Noble J, Steulens Y, Elie R, Henschke C, Bourassa MG (1982) Pathophysiology of chest pain in patients with cardiomyopathy and normal coronary arteries. Circulation 65:778-789
2. O'Gara PT, Bonow RO, Maron BJ, Damske BA, Van Lingen A, Bacharach SL, Larson SM, Epstein SE (1987) Myocardial perfusion abnormalities in patients with hypertrophic cardiomyopathy: assessment with Thallium-201 emission computed tomography. Circulation 76:1214-1223
3. Cannon RO, Rosing DR, Maron BJ, Leon MB, Bonow RO, Watson RM, Epstein SE (1985) Myocardial ischemia in patients with hypertrophic cardiomyopathy: contribution of inadequate vasodilator reserve and elevated left ventricular filling pressures. Circulation 71: 234-243
4. Scheler S, Motz W, Strauer BE (1992) Transient myocardial ischaemia in hypertensives: the missing link with left ventricular hypertrophy. Eur Heart J 13 [Suppl D]:62-65
5. O'Gorman DJ, Sheridan DJ (1991) Abnormalities of the coronary circulation associated with left ventricular hypertrophy. Clin Sci 81:703-713
6. Maron BJ, Wolfson JK, Epstein SE, Roberts WC (1986) Intramural ("small vessel") coronary artery disease in hypertrophic cardiomyopathy. J Am Coll Cardiol 8:545-557
7. Bonow RO, Vitale DF, Maron BJ, Bacharach SL, Frederick TM, Green MV (1987) Regional left ventricular asynchrony and impaired global left ventricular filling in hypertrophic cardiomyopathy: effect of verapamil. J Am Coll Cardiol 9:1108-1116
8. Bonow RO, Dilsizian V, Rosing DR, Maron BJ, Bacharach SL, Green MV (1985) Verapamil-induced improvement in left ventricular diastolic filling and increased exercise tolerance in patients with hypertrophic cardiomyopathy: short- and long-term effects. Circulation 72:853-864
9. Spirito P, Maron BJ, Chiarella F, Bellotti P, Tramarin R, Pozzoli M (1985) Diastolic abnormalities in patients with hypertrophic cardiomyopathy: relation to magnitude of

left ventricular hypertrophy. Circulation 72:310-316

10. Camici PG, Chiriatti G, Lorenzoni R, Bellina CR, Gistri R, Italiani G, Parodi O, Salvadori PA, Nista N, Papi L, L'Abbate A (1991) Coronary vasodilation is impaired in both hypertrophied and nonhypertrophied myocardium of patients with hypertrophic cardiomyopathy: a study with nitrogen-13 ammonia and positron emission tomography. J Am Coll Cardiol 17:879-886

11. Lorenzoni R, Gistri R, Cecchi F, Chiriatti G, Elliott P, McKenna WJ, Camici PG (1997) The coronary vasodilator reserve is more severely impaired in patients with hypertrophic cardiomyopathy and left ventricular dysfunction. J Am Coll Cardiol 29:462 (abstr)

12. Camici PG, Cecchi F, Gistri R, Montereggi A, Salvadori P, Dolara A, L'Abbate A (1991) Dipyridamole-induced subendocardial underperfusion in hypertrophic cardio-myopathy assessed by positron-emission tomography. Coronary Artery Disease 2:837-841

13. Gistri R, Cecchi F, Choudhury L, Montereggi A, Sorace O, Salvadori PA, Camici PG (1994) Effect of verapamil treatment on absolute myocardial blood flow in hypertrophic cardiomyopathy. Am J Cardiol 74:363-368

14. Choudhury L, Ryan MP, Page CA, Boyd H, Elliott P, McKenna WJ, Camici PG (1994) Does verapamil favourably alter transmural myocardial blood flow distribution in hypertrophic cardiomyopathy? Eur Heart J 15:507 (abstr)

15. Hoffman JI (1987) Transmural myocardial perfusion. Progress in Cardiovascular Diseases XXIX:429-464

16. De Silva R, Camici PG (1994) Role of positron emission tomography in the investigation of human coronary circulatory function. Cardiovasc Res 28:1595-1612

17. Strauer BE, Schwartzkopff B, Motz W, Vogt M (1991) Coronary vascular changes in the progression and regression of hypertensive heart disease. J Cardiovasc Pharmacol 18 [Suppl 3]: S20-7

18. Schwartzopff B, Motz W, Frenzel H, Vogt M, Knauer S, Strauer E (1993) Structural and functional alterations of the intramyocardial coronary arterioles in patients with arterial hypertension. Circulation 88:993-1003

19. Folkow B (1990) "Structural factor" in primary and secondary hypertension. Hypertension 16:89-101

20. Domenech RJ, Hoffman JIE, Noble MIM, Saunders KB, Henson JR, Subijanto S (1969) Total and regional coronary blood flow measured by radioactive microspheres in conscious and anesthetized dogs. Circ Res 25:581-596

21. Bache RJ, Cobb FR, Greenfield JC (1974) Myocardial blood flow distribution during ischemiainduced vasodilatation in the unanesthetized dog. J Clin Invest 54:1462-1472

22. Cobb FR, Bache RJ, Greenfield JC (1974) Regional myocardial blood flow in awake dogs. J Clin Invest 53:1618-1625

23. Buckberg GD, Fixler DE, Archie JP, Hoffman JIE (1972) Experimental subendocardial ischemia in dogs with normal coronary arteries. Circ Res 30:67-81

24. L'Abbate A, Marzilli M, Ballestra AM, Camici PG, Trivella MG, Pelosi G, Klassen GA (1980) Opposite transmural gradients of coronary resistance and extravascular pressure in the working dog's heart. Cardiovasc Res 14:21-29

25. Camici PG (1997) Microcirculation: what is the role of calcium antagonists? Eur Heart J 18 [Suppl A]:A51-A55

Identification and Management of High Risk Patients with Hypertrophic Cardiomyopathy

P.M. Elliott and W.J. McKenna

Introduction

Hypertrophic cardiomyopathy (HCM) is a primary heart muscle disorder caused by mutations in genes encoding cardiac sarcomeric proteins. The pathological hallmarks of the disease, namely myocardial hypertrophy, myocyte disarray and fibrosis, result in a diverse pathophysiology that includes myocardial ischaemia, diastolic dysfunction, ventricular and atrial arrhythmia, and congestive cardiac failure [1]. While it has been long recognised that sudden death is a complication of the disease, the identification and treatment of patients at risk of dying suddenly remains a contentious issue.

This chapter briefly reviews current data on clinical risk stratification and gives a personal perspective on the management of high risk patients.

Epidemiology and Natural History

Most studies suggest that the prevalence of HCM in the general population is approximately 1:500 [2-6]. While symptoms may occur at any age, myocardial hypertrophy usually develops during periods of rapid somatic growth, sometimes during the first year of life, but more typically during adolescence [7].

De novo myocardial hypertrophy in early middle age is not reported, but idiopathic or "inappropriate" left ventricular hypertrophy in patients over 60 years old is well described [8-10].

While the natural history of HCM is characterised by an age-related progression of symptoms in parallel with gradual deterioration in left ventricular function, less than 10% of patients develop overt congestive cardiac failure [11]. However, this slow decline may be complicated throughout life by sudden death, with an annual incidence ranging from 2%-4% in tertiary referral centres to approximately 1% in regionally based populations [12-14]. The most vulnerable period for sudden death is adolescence, with estimates of 4%-6% annual mortality in some series [15-16]. Sudden death in the first decade of life is thought to be relatively uncommon, but data in this age group are limited [17].

Rationale for Risk Stratification

Although the annual incidence of sudden death in HCM is relatively low, the fact that most deaths occur in young, asymptomatic individuals gives this particular complication a disproportionate significance to affected families and the wider community. The rationale for clinical risk stratification in patients with HCM is based on the fact that the incidence of other causes of cardiovascular mortality in HCM is low, and thus, if sudden death can be prevented, the natural history of the disease for most patients is relatively benign. The absence of risk factors also facilitates reassurance of low risk individuals.

Markers of Sudden Death Risk

A number of clinical observations are associated with an increased risk of sudden death in patients with HCM.

Genetic Risk Markers

Six HCM related loci have been identified in genes encoding cardiac sarcomeric proteins; β-myosin (chromosome 14), Troponin-T (chromosome 1), octropomyosin (chromosome 15), myosin binding protein C (chromosome 11), and the essential and regulatory myosin light chains [18-21]. A further locus on chromosome 7 has been identified in a family with Wolff-Parkinson-White syndrome [22].

While preliminary studies indicate that individual mutations may be associated with different prognoses [23] (Fig.1), it is clear that the expression of disease in individuals with the same mutation is highly variable, implying that other genetic and/or environmental factors must have a role in determining the phenotype.

Clinical History

While many sudden deaths occur in patients that have no or only minor symptoms, there are important aspects of the clinical history that indicate an increased risk. In children and adolescents recurrent unexplained syncope (particularly during exertion) and a family history of premature sudden death are highly specific markers of risk [1,15,16]. Young patients with severe symptoms are also more vulnerable to sudden death.

Morphological Predictors of Risk

Although the magnitude of left ventricular hypertrophy does not directly relate to prognosis [24], symptomatic patients with particularly severe (more than 3-3.5 cm) and diffuse hypertrophy may be at greater risk of sudden death. Similarly, while there is no conclusive evidence that the presence of left ventricular

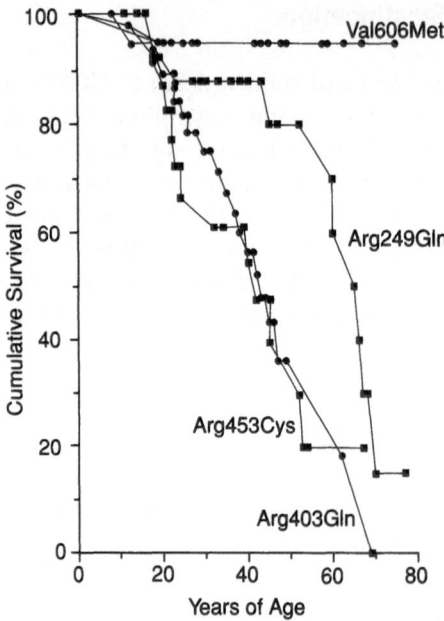

Fig. 1. Kaplan-Meier survival curves for the members of four families with different point mutations in the β-myosin gene (from [23])

outflow gradients *per se* influence prognosis, severe outflow tract obstruction (>100 mmHg) may have a role in triggering fatal ventricular arrhythmia.

Exercise Blood Pressure

Abnormal blood pressure responses occur in approximately 25% of patients with HCM during exercise [25] and are associated with a family history of sudden death and small left ventricular cavity dimensions. In patients less that 40 years of age, the presence of an abnormal blood pressure response is associated with a higher mortality (Fig. 2) [26]. The underlying mechanism for the abnormal response is uncertain, but inappropriate vasodilatation in non-exercising muscles may be responsible [27].

Arrhythmias and Prognosis

Pooled data from two studies [28-29] indicate that, in patients with HCM, non-sustained ventricular tachycardia (NSVT) is associated with an increased risk of sudden death. However, its value as a single risk marker is limited by a modest positive predictive accuracy of 22% and a low incidence in children. More recently some workers have suggested that NSVT is prognostically significant only when repetitive, or when it occurs in symptomatic patients [30].

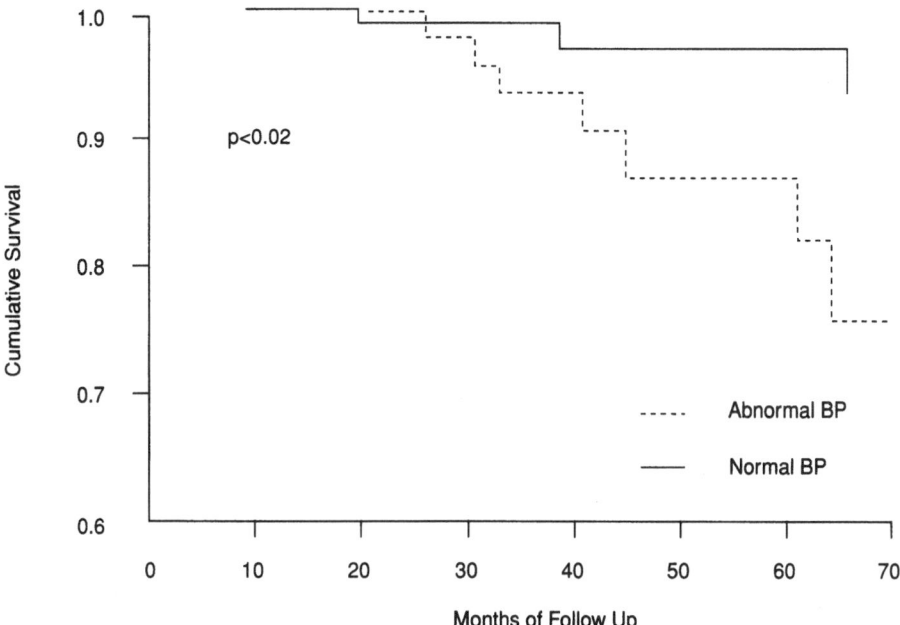

Fig. 2. Relation of exercise blood pressure response to cumulative survival in patients aged less than 40 years of age (adapted from [26]). BP, blood pressure

In the past, the onset of atrial fibrillation was thought to signal a poor prognosis. However, one retrospective study has shown that the 5 year survival in patients with atrial fibrillation is similar to age and sex matched patients that remain in sinus rhythm [31] .

Non-invasive Electrophysiological Techniques

A number of studies have shown that QT and QTc intervals are increased in patients with HCM, but QT prolongation appears to relate to maximal left ventricular wall thickness (possibly due to variable volumes of repolarising tissue) [32-35] and is not by itself of particular value in risk stratification. The sensitivity of QT measurement may be increased by assessing its dynamic behaviour and relationship to preceding RR intervals, and one study has shown that the QT/RR regression relationship is steeper when compared to normal controls. However, the QT/RR slope did not discriminate between high and low risk patients [34]. There are conflicting data on the significance of QT dispersion in HCM with regard to sudden death, but ongoing work should clarify its value as a risk marker.

Abnormal signal averaged electrocardiograms are more common in patients with HCM and NSVT, but are not associated with other clinical risk factors or an increased incidence of sudden death [36]. Similarly, while both global and specific vagal components of heart rate variability are reduced in patients with NSVT [37], abnormal heart rate variability does not identify those patients who go on to have a catastrophic cardiac event.

Programmed Ventricular Stimulation

Approximately a third of patients have inducible sustained ventricular tachycardia during programmed electrical stimulation [38]. While some studies have suggested that inducible ventricular tachycardia is associated with a higher risk of cardiac events, the response to ventricular stimulation in any patient depends on the protocol that is employed. Thus, while aggressive protocols using three or more premature stimuli induce sustained polymorphic ventricular tachycardia in 30%-40% of patients, their predictive accuracy for sudden death is low [38,39]. As ventricular arrhythmias are not infrequently associated with haemodynamic collapse in patients with HCM, and most patients at risk can be identified using safer non-invasive testing, it is our view that conventional programmed stimulation has no role in routine evaluation of patients with HCM.

Electrocardiogram Fractionation

The precise nature of the arrhythmogenic substrate in HCM is unknown, but it is likely that myocyte disarray and myocardial fibrosis cause dispersion of conduction velocities and refractory periods within the myocardium and thereby predispose to reentrant tachycardia. In comparison with controls and HCM patients with no clinical risk factors for sudden death, patients with HCM and a history of ventricular fibrillation have marked prolongation ("fractionation") of paced electrocardiograms recorded in the right ventricle at relatively long extrastimulus coupling intervals [40]. The value of this observation in prospectively identifying high risk patients is currently being studied.

Triggers for Sudden Death

As most deaths in patients with HCM are sudden and unexpected the sequence of events leading up to cardiac arrest are rarely documented. Nevertheless, data from case reports and anecdotal experience in referral centres suggest that there are a number of potential initiating mechanisms for sudden death including paroxysmal atrial fibrillation, sustained monomorphic ventricular tachycardia, conduction system disease, accessory pathways and myocardial ischaemia. When present, therapy designed to attenuate or abolish "triggers" for sudden death should be started.

Management of the High Risk Patient

Data on the survival of patients following successful resuscitation from

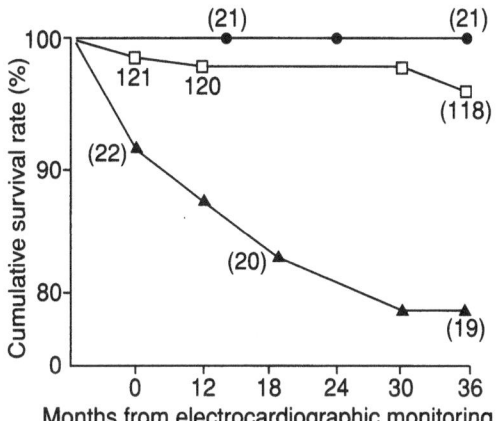

Fig. 3. Survival curves for patients with non-sustained ventricular tachycardia during ambulatory electrocardiography treated with conventional antiarrhythmic drugs (▲) or amiodarone (●), and for patients without non-sustained ventricular tachycardia (□) (from [42])

ventricular fibrillation are limited, but it is generally accepted that the incidence of further catastrophic cardiac events is relatively low, even when patients are treated in a nonsystematic fashion [41]. Unfortunately, most patients with HCM do not survive their first episode of ventricular fibrillation and there is, therefore, a strong case for initiating prophylactic therapy in those individuals who are at risk. Although conclusive data on the relative value of different markers of sudden death risk are not available, patients with several risk markers should always be considered for prophylactic therapy. Low dose amiodarone is the only drug that has been shown to reduce the incidence of sudden death in patients with NSVT (Fig. 3) [42], and it has been our practice to consider its use in all patients with two or more conventional risk factors (Table 1). The drug's potential side effects are minimised by using low doses (100-300 mg/day) and by regular determination of blood levels of the parent compound and its metabolites. An increasing number of high risk patients, receive implantable cardioverter/defibrillators but these devices are costly, and have socioeconomic implications for individual patients with respect to insurance and employment. While implantable cardioverter/defibrillators are probably the most appropriate therapy in patients that have survived ventricular fibrillation, further work is necessary to clarify their role in patients without such a history.

Table 1. Risk factors for sudden death in hypertrophic cardiomyopathy

1. Family history of premature sudden death
2. Recurrent unexplained syncope (particularly when associated with exertion)
3. Abnormal exercise blood pressure response (in patients aged less than 40 years)
4. Non-sustained ventricular tachycardia during 48 hour ambulatory ECG monitoring

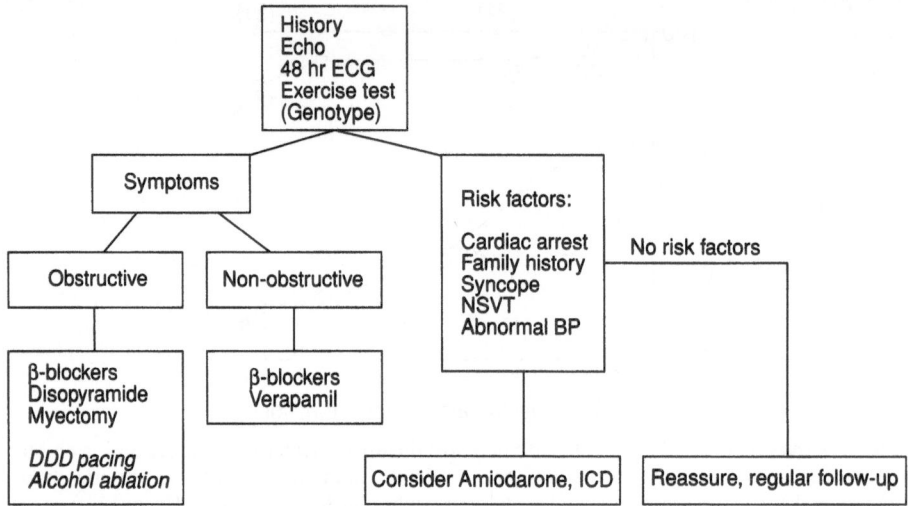

Fig. 4. Schematic summary of the management of hypertrophic cardiomyopathy, with respect to symptomatic treatment and risk stratification.
ICD, implantable cardioverter-defibrillator; NSVT, nonsustained ventricular tachycardia; BP, blood pressure; DDD, dual chamber pacing

Summary

The two principle aims of therapy in patients with HCM are the relief of symptoms and the prevention of disease related complications, the most important of which is sudden death (Fig. 4). While there are some legitimate areas of uncertainty concerning the identification and treatment of high risk patients, clinical risk stratification is feasible and effective therapies are available. As ongoing research refines current management algorithms, then "unexpected" deaths in patients known to have the disease should be preventable.

References

1. Spirito P, Seidman CE, McKenna WJ, Maron BJ (1997) The management of hypertrophic cardiomyopathy. N Engl J Med 336:775-785
2. Hada Y, Sakamoto T, Amano K, Yamaguchi T, Takenaka K, Takahashi H, Takikawa R, Hasegawa I, Takahashi T, Suzuki J-I, Sugimoto T, Saito K-I (1987). Prevalence of hypertrophic cardiomyopathy in a population of adult Japanese workers as detected by echocardiographic screening. Am J Cardiol 59:183-184
3. Savage DD, Castelli WP, Abbott RD, Garrison RJ, Anderson SJ, Kanell WB, Feinleib M (1983) Hypertrophic cardiomyopathy and its markers in the general population: the great masquerader revisited: the Framingham Study. J Cardiovasc Ultrason 2:41-47
4. Maron BJ, Gardin JM, Flack JM, Gidding SS, Kurosaki TT, Bild DE (1995) Prevalence of hypertrophic cardiomyopathy in a population of young adults. Echocardiographic analysis of 4111 subjects in the CARDIA study. Coronary Artery Risk Development in (Young) Adults. Circulation 92:785-789
5. Codd MB, Sugrue DD, Gersh BJ, Melton LJ (1989) Epidemiology of idiopathic dilated and hypertrophic cardiomyopathy: a population based study in Olmsted County, Minnesota, 1975-1984. Circulation 80:564-572

6. Maron BJ, Peterson EE, Maron MS, Peterson JE (1994) Prevalence of hypertrophic cardiomyopathy in an outpatient population referred for echocardiographic study. Am J Cardiol 73:577-580

7. Maron BJ, Spirito P, Wesley Y, Arce J (1986) Development or progression of left ventricular hypertrophy in children with hypertrophic cardiomyopathy: identification by two-dimensional echocardiography. N Engl J Med 315:610-614

8. Topol EJ, Traill TA, Fortuin NJ (1985) Hypertensive hypertrophic cardiomyopathy of the elderly. N Engl J Med 312:277-283

9. Fay WP, Taliercio CP, Ilstrup DM, Tajik AJ, Gersh BJ (1990) Natural history of hypertrophic cardiomyopathy in the elderly. J Am Coll Cardiol 16:821-826

10. Lewis JF, Maron BJ (1994) Clinical and morphology expression of hypertrophic cardiomyopathy in patients ≥ 65 years of age. Am J Cardiol 73:1105-1111

11. Spirito P, Maron BJ, Bonow RO, Epstein SE (1987) Occurrence and significance of progressive left ventricular wall thinning and relative cavity dilatation in hypertrophic cardiomyopathy. Am J Cardiol 60:123-129

12. McKenna WJ, Deanfield J, Faruqui A, England D, Oakley C and Goodwin J (1981) Prognosis in hypertrophic cardiomyopathy. Role of age and clinical, electrocardiographic and haemodynamic features. Am J Cardiol 47:532-538

13. Spirito P, Chiarella F, Carratino L, Zoni-Berisso M, Bellotti P, Vecchio C (1989) Clinical course and prognosis of hypertrophic cardiomyopathy in an outpatient population. N Engl J Med 320:749-755

14. Cecchi F, Olivotto I, Montereggi A, Santoro G, Dolara A, Maron BJ (1995) Hypertrophic cardiomyopathy in Tuscany: Clinical course and outcome in an unselected regional population. J Am Coll Cardiol 26:1529-1536

15. McKenna WJ, Franklin RCG, Nihoyannopoulos P, Robinson KC, Deanfield JE (1988) Arrhythmia and prognosis in infants, children and adolescents with hypertrophic cardiomyopathy. J Am Coll Cardiol 11:147-153

16. McKenna WJ, Deanfield JE (1984) Hypertrophic cardiomyopathy: an important cause of sudden death. Arch Dis Childhood 59:971-975

17. Maron BJ, Tajik AJ, Ruttenberg HD, Graham TP, Atwood GF, Victorica BE, Lie JT, Roberts WC (1982) Hypertrophic cardiomyopathy in infants: clinical features and natural history. Circulation 65:7-17

18. Jarcho JA, McKenna WJ, Pare JA, Solomon SD, Holcombe RF, Dickie S, Levi T, Donis Keller H, Seidman JG, Seidman CE (1989) Mapping a gene for familial hypertrophic cardiomyopathy to chromosome 14q 1. N Engl J Med 321:1372-1378

19. Thierfelder L, Watkins H, MacRae C, Lamas R, McKenna WJ, Vosberg HP, Seidman JG, Seidman CE (1994) Alpha-tropomyosin and cardiac troponin T mutations cause familial hypertrophic cardiomyopathy: a disease of the sarcomere. Cell 77:701-712

20. Bonne G, Carrier L, Bercovici J, Cruaud C, Richard P, Hainque B, Gautel M, Labeit S, James M, Beckmann J et al (1995) Cardiac myosin binding protein C gene splice acceptor site mutation is associated with familial hypertrophic cardiomyopathy. Nature Genetics 11:438-440

21. Poetter K, Jiang H, Hassanzadeh S, Master SR, Chang A, Dalakas MC, Rayment I, Sellers JR, Fananapazir L, Epstein ND (1996) Mutations in either the essential or regulatory light chains of myosin are associated with a rare myopathy in human heart and skeletal muscle. Nature Genetics 13:63-69

22. MacRae CA, Ghaisas N, Kass S, Donnelly S, Basson CT, Watkins HC, Anan R, Thierfelder LH, McGarry K, Rowland E et al (1995) Familial hypertrophic cardiomyopathy with Wolff-Parkinson-White syndrome maps to a locus on chromosome 7q3. J Clin Invest 96:1216-1220

23. Watkins H, Rosenzweig A, Hwang D, Levi T, McKenna W, Seidman CE, Seidman JG (1992) Characteristics and prognostic implications of myosin missense mutations in familial hypertrophic cardiomyopathy. N Engl J Med 326:1108-1114

24. Spirito P, Maron BJ (1990) Relation between extent of left ventricular hypertrophy and occurrence of sudden cardiac death in hypertrophic cardiomyopathy. J Am Coll Cardiol 15:1521-1526

25. Frenneaux MP, Counihan PJ., Caforio A, Chikamori T, McKenna WJ (1990) Abnormal

blood pressure response during exercise in hypertrophic cardiomyopathy. Circulation 82:1995-2002

26. Sadoul N, Prasad K, Slade AKB, Elliott PM, McKenna WJ (1997) Abnormal blood pressure response during exercise is an independent marker of sudden death in young patients with hypertrophic cardiomyopathy. Circulation (in press).

27. Counihan PJ, Frenneaux MP, Webb DJ, McKenna WJ (1991) Abnormal vascular responses to supine exercise in hypertrophic cardiomyopathy. Circulation 84:686-696

28. McKenna WJ, England D, Doi Y, Deanfield JE, Oakley CM, Goodwin JF (1981) Arrhythmia in hypertrophic cardiomyopathy. 1. Influence on prognosis. Br Heart J 46:168-172

29. Maron BJ, Savage DD, Wolfson JK, Epstein SE (1981) Prognostic significance of 24 hour ambulatory electrocardiographic monitoring in patients with hypertrophic cardiomyopathy: A prospective study. Am J Cardiol 48:252-257

30. Spirito P, Rapezzi C, Autore C, Bruzzi P, Bellone P, Ortolani P, Fragola PV, Chiarella F, Zoni-Berisso M, Branzi A et al (1994) Prognosis of asymptomatic patients with hypertrophic cardiomyopathy and nonsustained ventricular tachycardia. Circulation 90:2743-2747

31. Robinson K, Frenneaux MP, Stockins B, Karatasakis G, Poloniecki J, McKenna WJ (1990) Atrial fibrillation in hypertrophic cardiomyopathy: A longitudinal study. J Am Coll Cardiol 15:1279-1285

32. Dritsas A, Sabarouni E, Gilligan D, Nihoyannopoulos P, Oakley CM (1992) QT Interval abnormalities in hypertrophic cardiomyopathy. Clin Cardiol 15:739-742

33. Yanagisawa-Miwa A, Inoue I, Sugimoto T (1991) Diurnal change in QT intervals in dilated and hypertrophic cardiomyopathy. Am J Cardiol 67:1428-1430

34. Fei L, Slade AK, Grace AA, Malik M, Camm AJ, McKenna WJ (1994) Ambulatory assessment of the QT interval in patients with hypertrophic cardiomyopathy: risk stratification and effect of low dose amiodarone. Pacing and Clin Electrophys 17:2222-2227

35. Buja G, Miorelli M, Turrini P, Melacini P, Nava A (1993) Comparison of QT dispersion in hypertrophic cardiomyopathy between patients with and without ventricular arrhythmias and sudden death. Am J Cardiol 72:973-976

36. Kulakowski P, Counihan PJ, Camm AJ, McKenna WJ (1993) The value of time and frequency domain, and spectral temporal mapping analysis of the signal averaged electrocardiogram in identification of patients with hypertrophic cardiomyopathy at increased risk of sudden death. Eur Heart J 14:941-950

37. Counihan PJ, Fei L, Bashir Y, Farrell TG, Haywood GA, McKenna WJ (1993) Assessment of heart rate variability in hypertrophic cardiomyopathy. Association with clinical and prognostic features. Circulation 88:1682-1690

38. Fananapazir L, Chang AC, Epstein SE, McAreavey D (1992) Prognostic determinants in hypertrophic cardiomyopathy: Prognostic evaluation of a therapeutic strategy based on clinical, holter, hemodynamic and electrophysiological findings. Circulation 86:730-740

39. Kuck KH, Kunze KP, Schluter M, Nienaber CA, Costard A (1988) Programmed electrical stimulation in hypertrophic cardiomyopathy. Results in patients with and without cardiac arrest or syncope. Eur Heart J 92:177-185

40. Saumarez RC, Slade AKB, Grace AA, Sadoul N, Camm AJ, McKenna WJ (1995) The significance of paced electrocardiogram fractionation in hypertrophic cardiomyopathy. A prospective study. Circulation 91:2762-2768

41. Cecchi F, Maron BJ, Epstein SE (1989) Long-term outcome of patients with hypertrophic cardiomyopathy successfully resuscitated after cardiac arrest. J Am Coll Cardiol 13:1283-1288

42. McKenna WJ, Oakley CM, Krikler DM et al (1985) Improved survival with amiodarone in patients with hypertrophic cardiomyopathy and ventricular tachycardia. Br Heart J 53:412-416

Hypertrophic Cardiomyopathy and Sudden Death in the Young: a Pathologist's View

C. Basso, D. Corrado, A. Angelini and G. Thiene

Introduction

Hypertrophic cardiomyopathy (HCM) is a highly arrhythmogenic primary heart muscle disease. Clinical manifestations are variable ranging from a benign asymptomatic course to severe heart failure and cardiac arrest. Ventricular arrhythmias, palpitations and syncope are frequent signs and symptoms. Sudden, unexpected cardiac arrest is a pending catastrophe in the natural history of HCM.

In this chapter, after a brief review of pathology, pathophysiology and natural history, we will deal with prevalence and peculiar substrates of sudden death in the young with HCM. The occurrence of sudden death in the athlete affected by HCM will also be considered.

Pathology

Left ventricular concentric hypertrophy, whether asymmetric or symmetric, with increased heart weight not explained by any cause of overload, is the usual finding [1]. Asymmetric septal hypertrophy (Fig.1), located either in the basal portion or in the mid septum, and bulging into the left ventricular outflow tract, is by far the most frequent variety [2,3]. Other localised forms of asymmetric hypertrophy at the apex and free wall have been reported [4]. The whole echocardiographic spectrum of asymmetric HCM has been recently described [5].

The asymmetric septal variety almost regularly shows an endocardial plaque, mirror image to the septal leaflet of the mitral valve, which is pushed against the bulging hypertrophic septum during the systolic anterior motion (Fig.2).

The symmetric form of HCM is less frequent (nearly 10%-20%) and usually does not exhibit a subaortic endocardial plaque [5,6]. It seems less severe than the asymmetric one, since it has been observed mostly in old patients with HCM.

Congenital coronary artery anomalies, either in the origin or along with the epicardial course (intramural course) have been reported in association with HCM [6,7]. They may contribute to precipitate cardiac arrest through an ischemic event.

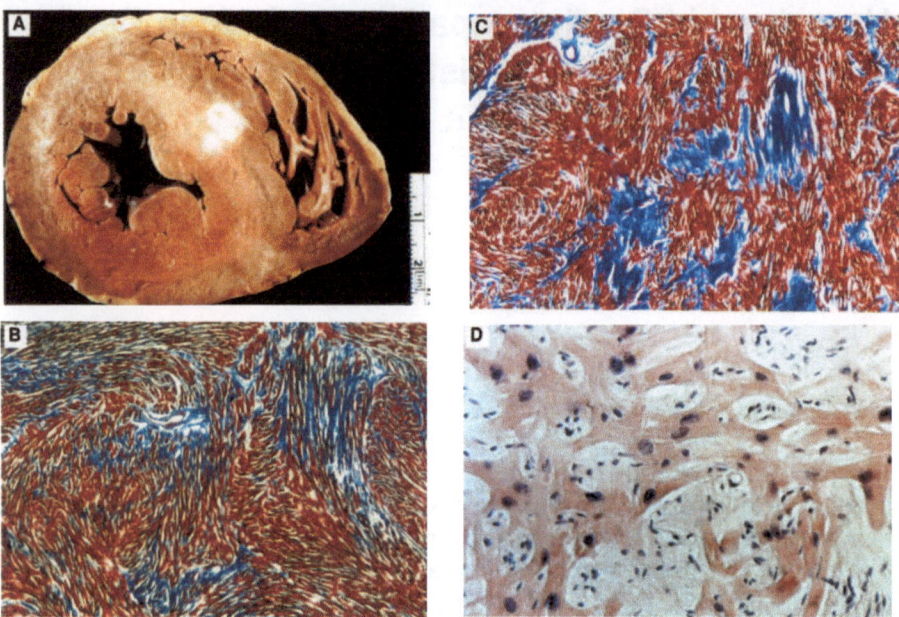

Fig. 1. Asymmetric HCM in a 20-year-old man who died suddenly. **A** Short axis view showing asymmetric septal hypertrophy and a large scar within. **B** Histology of the septum showing remarkable myocardial disarray (Azan stain x15). **C** Spots of replacement type fibrosis within the disarray (Azan stain x15). **D** High magnification of the disarray showing myocyte hypertrophy, bizzarre nuclei and interstitial fibrosis (Haematoxylin-Eosin stain x240)

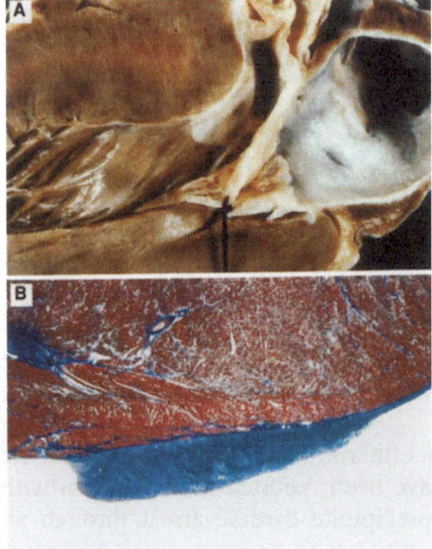

Fig. 2. Asymmetric HCM in a 15-year-old boy who died suddenly. **A** Long axis view showing septal hypertrophy with subaortic stenosis: note the fibrous plaque and the anterior mitral leaflet thickening. **B** Histology of the plaque (Azan stain x10)

Structural disorganisation of myocardial fascicles and myocytes in the forms of myocardial disarray (Fig.1B) is considered to be the pathognomonic histologic feature of HCM [1,8,9]. It is particularly evident within the hypertrophy, whether asymmetric or symmetric. Although not specific (it is a regular finding at the confluence of the ventricular septum with the free wall at the crux cordis), evidence of widespread disarray of myocardial fibers in the ventricular septum, involving at least 5% of tissue section, is considered diagnostic [8,9].

At ultrastructural level, the disarray may involve also the myofibrils and myofilaments, further providing structural evidence of the genetic sarcomeric disease [10].

Myocyte hypertrophy, bizzare nuclei and various degree of interstitial and replacement-type fibrosis are accompanying microscopic features [11-13]. Small vessel disease, in the form of intimal hyperplasia, medial hypertrophy and fragmentation of internal elastic membrane of intramural arteries, is a frequent observation [15,16], but rarely accounts for significant lumen size reduction.

Pathophysiology

The classic three dimensional structure of the myocytes, featured by myocardial disarray, is clearly a potential substrate of impaired intraventricular impulse conduction at risk of reentry and most probably accounts for the electrical instability of the ventricular myocardium in these patients [8,9]. Fibrosis exacerbates this risk by delaying the conduction.

The septal bulge accounts for significant subaortic gradient and stenosis [4]. The superimposed endocardial fibrous plaque, as well as the increasing asymmetric hypertrophy with time, progressively aggravates left ventricular outflow tract narrowing, as to require in some cases surgical relief by myectomy [17]. In recent years, non-surgical techniques for relief of outflow tract obstruction have been used, such as dual-chamber pacing and the injection of alcohol into the first major septal coronary artery [18].

Asymmetric septal hypertrophy accounts for a disarrangement of the mitral valve apparatus with displacement of the posterior papillary muscle. The functional consequence is the so called systolic anterior motion of the anterior mitral leaflet, which accounts for mitral regurgitation. During systole the anterior leaflet moves anteriorly instead of posteriorly, thus creating an incompetent orifice and friction with the septal bulge, which in turn produces the septal endocardial plaque and thickened mitral leaflet [4].

Concentric hypertrophy leads to significant left ventricular cavity size reduction, as to impair the diastolic filling [19-21]. The myocardial disarray may also interfere with ventricular compliance. Systolic performance in these patients, when subaortic stenosis is trivial, is quite preserved or even supernormal, whereas ventricular performance may be deteriorated at the time of diastole, as to account for impaired diastolic filling and cardiac failure which may even require cardiac transplantation [22].

There are HCM patients in whom the clinical pattern is merely characterised by severe ventricular restriction and congestive heart failure. The pathology experience from cardiac transplantation allowed to disclose small recipient hearts with normal ventricles and dilated atria in the setting of end-stage congestive heart failure, characterised haemodynamically by severe impairment of ventricular compliance (primary restrictive cardiomyopathy), in which the histologic background was that of typical myocardial disarray (Fig.3) [23-25]. Cardiomyopathies with restrictive physiology may be observed either with or without ventricular hypertrophy [26]. Restrictive cardiomyopathies with or without hypertrophy share the same histologic features in terms of disarray and fibrosis [23-25, 27-29]. Familial forms were also observed [30,31]. Since patients with restrictive cardiomyopathy presented familiarity for HCM, the two forms may represent two different phenotypes of the same genetic disease.

Natural history

HCM has been observed throughout the human life, from the fetus to the elderly [1]. It may be early symptomatic, as to account for sudden death or congestive heart failure even in newborns or infants [32-35]. On the contrary,

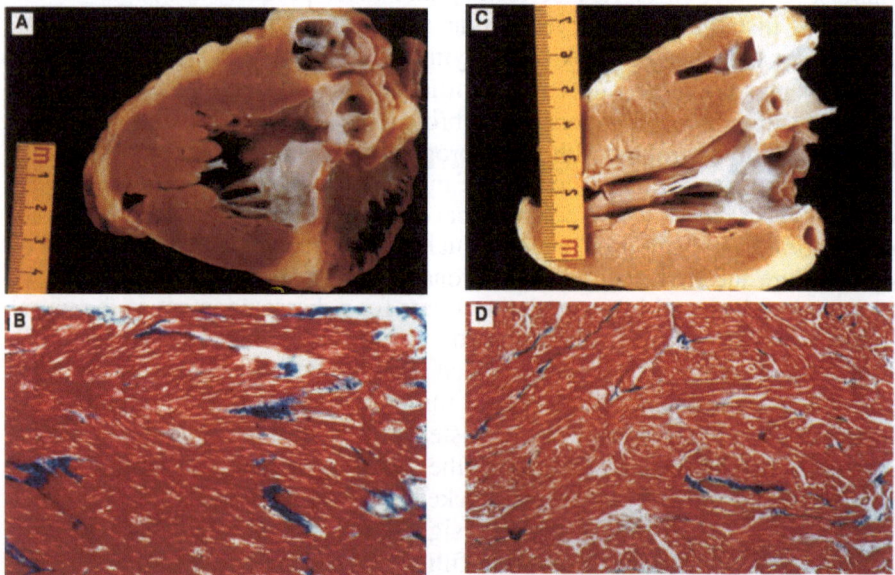

Fig. 3. Heart specimens from cardiac transplantation of patients with hypertrophic-restrictive cardiomyopathies. **A** Left ventricle normal in size and thickness in a 19-year-old boy. **B** Histology of the same, showing ventricular myocardial disarray (Azan stain, x75). **C** Asymmetric septal hypertrophy in a 28-year-old woman. **D** Histology of the same showing ventricular myocardial disarray (Azan stain, x90)

it may remain concealed or paucisymptomatic until old age with the patients dying for other cardiac or extracardiac reasons [36, 37].

Sudden death is the sword of Damocles in the natural history and especially affects the young (see below), even in the absence of previous symptoms [32-35, 39].

Congestive heart failure may be an early clinical picture, in the setting of restrictive behaviour, and may occur later both with severe concentric hypertrophy and with normal or nearly normal left ventricle (primary restrictive cardiomyopathy).

Otherwise, congestive heart failure may be explained by a dilatation of the left ventricle and impairment of ventricular contractility, as a shift from concentric to eccentric hypertrophy. Besides a decompensation of the individual myocytes, this evolution may be ascribed to extensive fibrosis by progressive loss of myocardium [22,40]. Whether this is due to ischemic damage or to apoptotic cell death remains to be ascertained.

Sudden Death in the Young and in the Athlete

In various pathological reports from the USA, HCM has been described as one of the most important, if not the leading cause, of sudden death in the young [41,42]. In the prospective clinico-pathologic study project of the Veneto Region on juvenile sudden death (≤ 35 years), in the time interval 1979-1996 we collected 269 consecutive fatal events, 243 of which were sudden cardiac deaths (Fig.4).

Seventeen patients (7%) were found at autopsy to be affected by HCM,

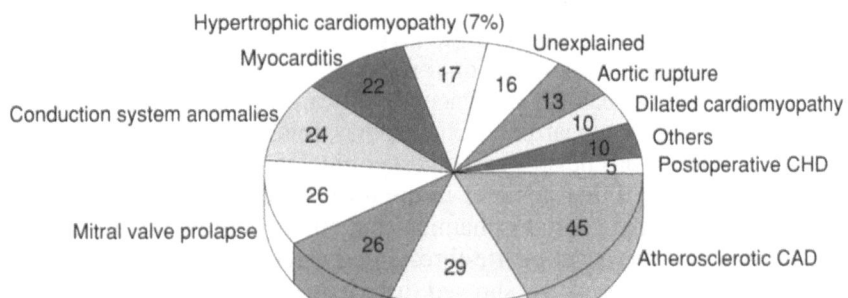

Fig. 4. Prevalence of cardiac disease causing sudden death in the young in the Veneto Region experience (1979-1996). *CAD*, coronary artery disease; *CHD*, congenital heart disease; *RVC*, right ventricular cardiomyopathy

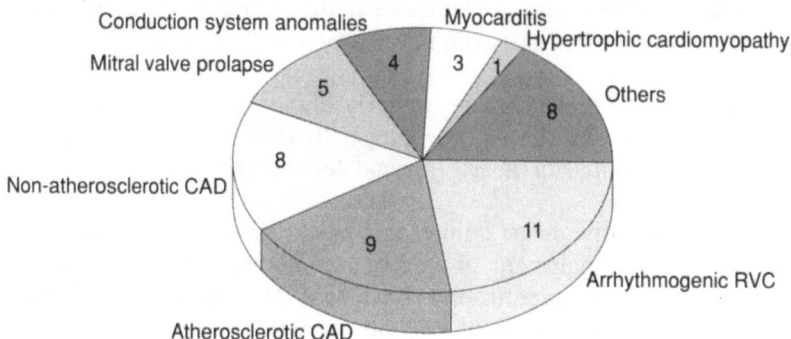

Fig. 5. Prevalence of disease causing sudden death in the athlete in the Veneto Region experience (1979-1996). *CAD*, coronary artery disease; *RVC*, right ventricular cardiomyopathy

18.5% by atherosclerotic coronary artery disease, 12.5% by arrhythmogenic right ventricular cardiomyopathy, 10.5% by non-atherosclerotic coronary artery disease and 10.5% by mitral valve prolapse.

HCM patients were 13 males and 4 females, with ages ranging from 1 to 32 years [43]. Sudden death occurred at rest in 12 and on effort in 5 patients, and was the first manifestation of disease in 12; 5 patients had previous symptoms of syncope (3 cases) and palpitations (2 cases). At post-mortem, heart weight ranged from 70 to 1000 g; hypertrophy was septal asymmetric in 10 cases and symmetric in 7. Gross examination disclosed large scars within the septal hypertrophy in 8 (Fig.1). None had obstructive atherosclerotic coronary artery disease, and 3 exhibited a deep intramyocardial course of the left anterior descending coronary artery. At histology, myocardial disarray (Fig.1 B,C,D) always exceeded 20% of the septal myocardium; myocardial fibrosis was extensive, replacement-type, in the absence of obstructive small vessel disease; signs of acute-subacute myocardial necrosis were present in 6 cases, one of them with acute regional myocardial infarction.

The underlying mechanism of syncope and cardiac arrest in patients with HCM is intriguing. Myocardial ischemia has long been incriminated, but pathologic evidence has never been reported [44,45]. Our pathologic findings of ischemic damage, either acute or in the form of myocardial scars, support the hypothesis that myocardial ischemia occurs in the natural history of HCM and contributes to the onset of life-threatening electrical instability.

Previous studies in the USA showed that HCM is the commonest cause of sudden death in young competitive athletes followed by congenital coronary arteries anomalies and Marfan syndrome [46]. In our experience, among the above mentioned 269 consecutive cases of sudden death in young people occurring in the Veneto Region from 1979 to 1996, 49 (18%) were young competitive athletes (44 males and 5 females, mean age 23.1 years) (Fig.5).

Although HCM accounted for 7.5% of sport-unrelated sudden death in the general young population (see above), it caused sport-related death in only one instance [47]. More prevalent causes of sudden death in competitive athletes included arrhythmogenic right ventricular cardiomyopathy (11 athletes, 22.4%), coronary atherosclerosis (9 athletes, 18.5%), congenital anomalies of coronary arteries (8 athletes, 16.3%)

Thus, causes of sudden death in young competitive athletes differ from those previously reported in the USA [48,49]. HCM was an uncommon cause of fatal events in athletes, most likely because exposure of the athletic population to preparticipation screening over many years resulted in identification and disqualification of the affected subjects. Arrhythmogenic right ventricular cardiomyopathy, a poorly recognised clinico-pathologic condition at risk of sport-related cardiac arrest, was the most frequently encountered cardiovascular substrate.

Acknowledgment. Supported by the Juvenile Sudden Death Target Project of the Veneto Region, Venice and by the National Council for Research, Target Project FAT.MA, Rome (Italy).

References

1. Maron BJ, Bonow RO, Cannon RO, Leon MB, Epstein SE (1987) Hypertrophic cardiomyopathy. Interrelations of clinical manifestations, pathophysiology and therapy (1). N Engl J Med 316:780-789 and 844-852
2. Teare RD (1958) Asymmetrical septal hypertrophy of the heart in young adults. Br Heart J 20:1-8
3. Braunwald E, Morrow AG, Cornell WP, Aygen MM, Hilbish TF (1960) Idiopathic hypertrophic subaortic stenosis. Am J Med 29:924-945
4. Wigle ED, Rakowski H, Kimball BP, Williams WG (1995) Hypertrophic cardiomyopathy. Clinical spectrum and treatment. Circulation 92:1680-1692
5. Klues HG, Schiffers A, Maron BJ (1995) Phenotypic spectrum and patterns of left ventricular hypertrophy in hypertrophic cardiomyopathy: morphologic observations and significance as assessed by two-dimensional echocardiography in 600 patients. J Am Coll Cardiol 26:1699-1708
6. Wigle ED, Sasson Z, Henderson MA, Ruddy TD, Fulop J, Rakowski H, Williams WG (1985) Hypertrophic cardiomyopathy: the importance of the site and the extent of hypertrophy: a review. Prog Cadiovasc Dis 28:1-83
7. Brugada P, Bar FWHM, De Zwann C, Roy D, Green M, Wellens HJJ (1982) "Sawfish" systolic narrowing of the left anterior descending coronary artery: an angiographic sign of hypertrophic cardiomyopathy. Circulation 66:800-803
8. Maron BJ, Roberts WC (1979) Quantitative analysis of cardiac muscle cell disorganization in the ventricular septum of patients with hypertrophic cardiomyopathy. Circulation 59:689-706
9. Maron BJ, Anan TJ, Roberts WC (1981) Quantitative analysis of the distribution of cardiac muscle cell disorganization in the left ventricular wall of patients with hypertrophic cardiomyopathy. Circulation 63:882-894
10. Ferrans VJ, Rodriguez ER (1983) Specificity of light and electron microscopic features of hypertrophic obstructive and nonobstructive cardiomyopathy. Qualitative, quantitative and etiologic aspects. Eur Heart J 4 [Suppl F]:9-22
11. StJohn Sutton MG, Lie JT, Anderson KR, O'Brien PC, Frye RL (1980) Histologic specificity of hypertrophic obstructive cardiomyopathy: myocardial fiber disarray and myocardial fibrosis. Br Heart J 44:433-443
12. Factor SM, Butany J, Sole MJ, Wigle ED, Williams WC, Pojkind M (1991) Patholog-

ic fibrosis and matrix connective tissue in the subaortic myocardium of patients with hypertrophic cardiomyopathy. J Am Coll Cardiol 17:1343-1351

13. Davies MJ, McKenna WJ (1995) Hypertrophic cardiomyopathy -pathology and pathogenesis. Histopathology 26:493-500
14. Maron BJ, Epstein SE, Roberts WC (1979) Hypertrophic cardiomyopathy and transmural myocardial infarction without significant atherosclerosis of the extramural coronary arteries. Am J Cardiol 43:1086-1102
15. Maron BJ, Wolfson JK, Epstein SE, Roberts WC (1986) Intramural ("small vessel") coronary artery disease in hypertrophic cardiomyopathy. J Am Coll Cardiol 8:545-557
16. Slade AKB, Saumarez RC, McKenna WJ (1993) The arrhythmogenic substrate- diagnostic and therapeutic implications: hypertrophic cardiomyopathy. Eur Heart J 14 [Suppl E]:84-90
17. Morrow AG, Brockenbrough EC (1961) Surgical treatment of idiopathic hypertrophic subaortic stenosis: technique and hemodynamic results of subaortic ventriculomyotomy. Ann Surg 154:181-189
18. Spirito P, Seidman CE, McKenna WJ, Maron BJ (1997) The management of hypertrophic cardiomyopathy. N Engl J Med 336:775-785
19. Wigle ED, Wilansky S (1987) Diastolic dysfunction in hypertrophic cardiomyopathy. Heart Failure 3:82-93
20. Maron BJ, Spirito P, Greene KJ, Wesley YE, Bonow RO, Arce J (1987) Non invasive assessment of left ventricular diastolic function by pulsed Doppler echocardiography in patients with hypertrophic cardiomyopathy. J Am Coll Cardiol 10:733-742
21. Inoue T, Morooka S, Hayashi T, Takayanagi K, Sakai Y, Fujito T, Fujinuma S, Takabatake Y (1991) Global and regional abnormalities of left ventricular diastolic filling in hypertrophic cardiomyopathy. Clin Cardiol 14:573-577
22. Shirani J, Maron BJ, Cannon III RO, Shahin S, Roberts WC (1993) Clinico-pathologic features of hypertrophic cardiomyopathy managed by cardiac transplantation. Am J Cardiol 72:434-440
23. Boffa GM, Thiene G, Nava A, Dalla Volta S (1991) Cardiomyopathy: a necessary revision of the WHO classification. Int J Cardiol 30:1-7
24. Boffa GM, Chioin R, Pellegrino PA, Scognamiglio R, Fasoli G, Razzolini R, Milanesi O, Thiene G (1983) Cardiomiopatia restrittiva primaria. Rev Lat Cardiol 4:263-275
25. Angelini A, Calzolari V, Boffa GM, Calabrese F, Valente M, Thiene G (1995) Primary restrictive cardiomyoapthy.Eur Heart J 16 [Suppl]:395 (abstr)
26. Maron BJ, Lang L, Moller JH, Edwards JE (1980) Cardiomyopathies characterized by evidence of resistence to left ventricular inflow. Cathet Cardiovasc Diag 6:29-39
27. Arbustini E, Buonanno C, Trevi P, Pennelli N, Ferrans VJ, Thiene G (1983) Cardiac ultrastructure in primary restrictive cardiomyopathy. Chest 84:236-238
28. Edwards WD (1987) Cardiomyopathies. Hum Pathol 18:625-635
29. Katritsis D, Wilmshurst PT, Wendon JA, Davies MJ, Webb-People MM (1991) Primary restrictive cardiomyopathy:clinical and pathologic characteristics. J Am Coll Cardiol 18:1230-1235
30. Aroney C, Bett N, Redford D (1988) Familial restrictive cardiomyopathy. Aust Nz J Med 18:877-878
31. Mc Kenna WJ, Stewart JT, Nihoyannopoulos P, McGinfy F, Davies MJ (1990) Hypertrophic cardiomyopathy without hypertrophy: two families with myocardial disarray in the absence of increased myocardial mass. Br Heart J 63:287-290
32. McKenna WJ, Camm AJ (1989) Sudden death in hypertrophic cardiomyopathy: assessment of patients at high risk. Circulation 80:1489-1492
33. Maron BJ, Fananapazir L (1992) Sudden death in hypertrophic cardiomyopathy. Circulation 85 [Suppl I]:57-63
34. Maron BJ, Roberts WJ, Epstein SE (1982) Sudden death in hypertrophic cardiomyopathy: a profile of 78 patients. Circulation 67:1388-1394
35. McKenna WJ, Deanfield J, Faruqui A, England D, Oakley C, Goodwin J (1981) Prognosis in hypertrophic cardiomyopathy: role of age and clinical, electrocardiographic and hemodinamic features. Am J Cardiol 47:532-538
36. Spirito P, Chiarella F, Carratino L, Berisso MZ, Bellotti P, Vecchio C (1989) Clinical course and prognosis of hypertrophic cardiomyopathy in an outpatient population. N

Engl J Med 320:749-755
37. Cecchi F, Olivotto I, Montereggi A, Santoro G, Dolara A, Maron BJ (1995) Hypertrophic cardiomyopathy in Tuscany: clinical course and outcome in an unselected regional population. J Am Coll Cardiol 26:1529-1536
38. McKenna WJ, Deanfield JE (1984) Hypertrophic cardiomyopathy. An important cause of sudden death. Arch Dis Chil 59: 971-975
39. McKenna WJ, Franklin RCG, Nihoyannopoulos P, Robinson KR, Deanfield JE (1988) Arrhythmia and prognosis in infants, children and adolescents with hypertrophic cardiomyopathy. J Am Coll Cardiol 11:147-153
40. Spirito P, Maron BJ, Bonow RO, Epstein SE (1987) Occurrence and significance of progressive left ventricular wall thinning and relative cavity dilatation in hypertrophic cardiomyopathy. Am J Cardiol 60:123-129
41. Topaz O, Edwards JE (1985) Pathologic features of sudden death in children, adolescents and young adults. Chest 87:476-482
42. Burke AP, Farb A, Virmani R, Goodin J, Smialek JE (1991) Sports-related and non sports-related sudden cardiac death in young adults. Am Heart J 121:568-575
43. Basso C, Corrado D, Nava A, Dalla Volta S (1996) Hypertrophic cardiomyopathy: pathologic evidence of myocardial ischemic injury in young sudden death victims. Circulation 94 [Suppl]:I-427 (abstr)
44. Cannon RO, Rosing DR, Maron BJ, Leon MB, Bonow RO, Watson RM, Epstein SE (1985) Myocardial ischemia in patients with hypertrophic cardiomyopathy: contribution of inadequate vasodilator reserve and elevated left ventricular filling pressures. Circulation 71:234-243
45. Dilsizian V, Bonow RO, Epstein SE, Fananapazir L (1993) Myocardial ischemia detected by thallium scintigraphy is frequently related to cardiac arrest and syncope in young patients with hypertrophic cardiomyopathy. J Am Coll Cardiol 22:796-804
46. Maron BJ, Roberts WC, McAllister HA, Rosing DR, Epstein SE (1980) Sudden death in young athletes. Circulation 62:218-229
47. Corrado D, Basso C, Thiene G (1996) Pathologic findings in victims of sport-related sudden cardiac death. Sports Exercise and Injury 2:78-86
48. Corrado D, Thiene G, Nava A, Rossi L, Pennelli N (1990) Sudden death in young competitive athletes: clinico-pathologic correlations in 22 cases. Am J Med 89:588-596
49. Thiene G, Nava A, Corrado D, Rossi L, Pennelli N (1988) Right ventricular cardiomyopathy and sudden death in young people. N Engl J Med 318:129-133

The Clinicopathologic Spectrum of Hypertrophic Cardiomyopathy. The Experience of the Italian Heart Transplant Program

G. Baroldi, C. Rapezzi, R. De Maria, E. Angelini, E. Arbustini, E. Bonacina,
C. Bosman, G. Catani, L. De Biase, E. Donegani, A. Fiocchi, G. Gagliardi, P.
Gallo, A. Gavazzi, E. Gronda, O. Leone, U. Livi, A. Parma, M. Porcu, A. Pucci,
G. Thiene and M.Viganò

Hypertrophic cardiomyopathy (HCM) is an idiopathic cardiac disease which is predominantly genetic in origin and transmitted as an autosomally dominant trait [1, 2]. The mutated genes code for altered contractile myofibrillar proteins, leading to deformed myocytes and histological evidence of extensive myocell disorganization, namely the disarray typical of hypertrophic cardiomyopathy (HCM). In the natural history of HCM end-stage heart failure is relatively infrequent and associated with a pattern of left ventricular systolic impairment with cavity dilatation, which occurrs in about 10% of patients [3, 4], with a yearly incidence of 1.5% [5]. End-stage disease may coexist with premature sudden death in family members carrying the same genetic abnormality [6]. This pattern is characterized by a particularly poor prognosis, so that heart transplantation has been advocated in this subgroup of patients.

The structural correlates of this end-stage phase of HCM have been rarely examined in the literature [7]. In ten HCM hearts excised at transplantation, an extensive myocardial scarring in the absence of coronary lesions was documented. This retrospective review aims to relate the clinical aspects in HCM patients who underwent heart transplantation in the Italian Heart Transplant Program with the pathologic findings in hearts excised at surgery and to discuss the functional significance of disarray and its role in the definition of cardiomyopathies.

Study Population

From 1985 to December 31, 1996 in eight Italian Heart Transplant Centers (Milano, Pavia, Torino, Padova, Bologna, Bergamo, Roma, Cagliari) 1950 heart transplantation procedures were performed in patients older than 15 years. Thirty-nine cases (2%) had clinically documented HCM. The indication to heart transplantation were prevailing refractory symptoms (arrhythmias, angina, etc.) in 8 cases and evolution towards left ventricular (LV) dilatation with untractable congestive heart failure in the remaining 31 cases, who are the subject of the present report. There were 24 men and 7 women with an age ranging from 15 to 63 years (mean 37 ± 14).

Clinical Findings

Detailed information on the clinical and echocardiographic history of the patients before heart transplantation was available in 20 cases with evolution towards the end-stage phase of congestive heart failure. End-stage disease was defined by the presence of a hypokinetic dilated left ventricle, with an end diastolic diameter exceeding the upper normal range for body square area, and reduced ejection fraction (<50%). Thirteen patients were men (65%). A family history of HCM was evident in 9 cases (45%). In three patients myectomy had been previously performed; in two of these cases and in two additional patients a pacemaker had been implanted. Atrial fibrillation was present in seven patients at the time of heart transplantation.

Age was 25 ± 1 years at diagnosis, 36 ± 10 years at the first documentation of LV dilatation and 38 ± 12 at transplantation. The first signs of LV dilatation and hypokinesis became evident within 14 ± 7 years after the diagnosis of HCM. The mean interval since the echo appearance of LV dilatation to heart transplantation was 3 ± 3 years (range 2 months to 9 years) (Table 1). Echocardiographic findings (Table 2) demonstrated progressive wall thinning and ventricular dilatation, associated with a decline in pump function. At transplantation, moderate impairment in left ventricular systolic function was evident; for comparison the mean ejection fraction in a series of 136 heart transplant candidates with cardiomyopathy of different nature was $24 \pm 9\%$.

In the 6 cases who had both a baseline echo at first diagnosis and a pre-transplant evaluation, LV chamber size increased by 18 ± 4 mm in diastole ($p < 0.04$ vs baseline) and 26 ± 10 mm in systole ($p < 0.04$ vs baseline), fractional shortening decreased by $25 \pm 19\%$ ($p < 0.04$ vs baseline), the septal and lateral walls thinned by 5 ± 8 and 4 ± 9 mm and left ventricular ejection fraction declined by $39 \pm 29\%$ (n = 4, $p < 0.07$ vs baseline).

Table 1. Clinical findings in 20 transplant candidates with end-stage HCM

Male gender	65%
Family history of HCM	45%
Age (years)	
at diagnosis	25 ± 1
at LV dilatation	36 ± 10
at transplantation	38 ± 12
Time interval from diagnosis to LV dilatation (years)	14 ± 7
Time interval from LV dilatation to transplantation (years)	3 ± 3

Table 2. Echocardiographic findings in HCM transplant candidates

Echocardiographic indices	first available	before surgery
Left ventricular end diastolic diameter (mm)	48±7	61±11
Left ventricular end systolic diameter (mm)	30±9	50±10
Interventricular septum thickness (mm)	21±7	15±5
Posterior wall thickness (mm)	16±8	11±3
Left ventricular ejection fraction (%)	66±22	30±12

Morphologic Findings

Detailed data on heart pathology were available in 31 cases. For each heart, weight, type and extent of gross hypertrophy were obtained. Symmetric hypertrophy was observed in 16 cases; asymmetric hypertrophy was confined to the interventricular septum in 10 cases, and to the left ventricular free wall in the remaining 5.

Heart weight

The hearts excised at transplantation are practically free of atria. In order to compare these hearts with autopsy hearts, the theoretical atrial weight, estimated approximately one-fourth of the total organ was added to the actual weight of the excised hearts (actual weight x 4/3) [8]. The adjusted heart weight in HCM was 659 ± 179 g; heart weight exceeded 750 g in 11 cases and was lower than 450 g in 3. No significant differences in respect of symmetric or asymmetric hypertrophy and presence or absence of severe dilation were observed (Table 3). HCM autopsy hearts showed a higher value than excised hearts. In our cases the non-adjusted heart weight was 518 ± 137 g, range 215-800 g. In ten reported hearts excised at transplantation the heart weight was 400 ± 110 g, range 290-650 g [7].

Wall Thickness

Thickness of the interventricular septum and left and right ventricular free wall was measured at the basal, mid-ventricular and apical level in 12 hearts, at the basal and apical level in 12 hearts and at the mid-ventricular level only in the remaining 7.

The wall thickness of the superior-anterior left ventricular wall of HCM

Table 3. Heart weight in adult hypertrophic cardiomyopathy and controls

Source	n	Heart weight (g)
Hypertrophic cardiomyopathy[a]	31	659 ± 174
symmetric hypertrophy	16	708 ± 163
asymmetric hypertrophy	15	608 ± 176
mild dilation	14	607 ± 163
severe dilation	17	702 ± 197
Autopsy hearts with hypertrophic cardiomyopathy[b]	26	591 ± 135
Excised hearts with hypertrophic cardiomyopathy[c]	10	400 ± 110
Ischemic heart disease	63	565 ± 108
Dilated cardiomyopathy	63	639 ± 155
Valvulopathy	18	827 ± 179
Normal heart (head trauma)	45	364 ± 47

[a] heart excised at transplantation with adjusted heart weight: actual weight x 4/3
[b] Reported in literature [1]
[c] Reported in literature [7]: actual weight only

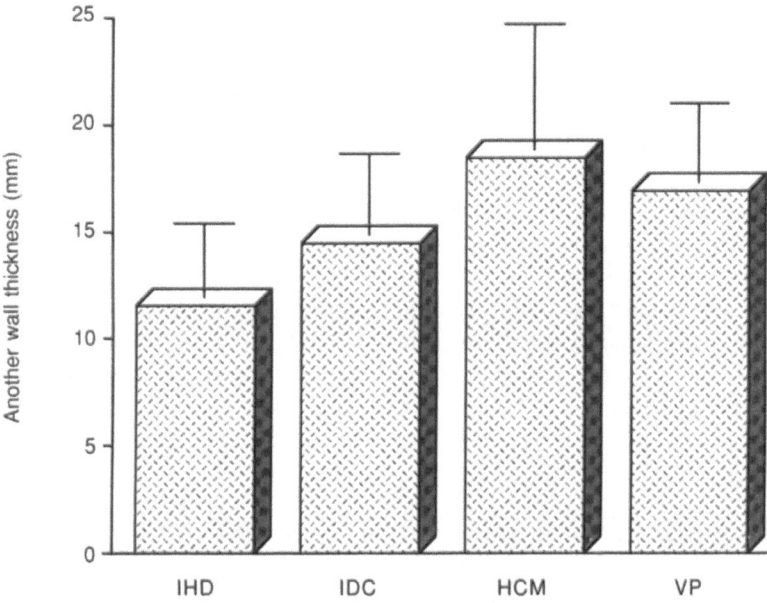

Fig. 1. Left ventricular anterior wall thickness is significantly greater in excised hearts with hypertrophic cardiomyopathy (HCM) and VP (Valvulopathy) than in ischemic heart disease (IHD) and idiopathic dilated cardiomyopathy (IDC), $p < 0.0001$

cases was similar to the excised hearts with congestive heart failure of different nature (Fig. 1). In HCM hearts with asymmetric hypertrophy confined to the interventricular septum the average septal thickness was 24 ± 6 mm, significantly higher than the one of the left ventricular free wall (16 ± 6 mm, $p < 0.001$). The reverse was observed in hearts showing asymmetric hypertrophy of the left ventricular wall (average thickness 21 ± 5 mm vs an average septal thickness of 14 ± 3 mm, $p = 0.01$). As expected, no difference was observed between these two cardiac regions in cases with symmetric hypertrophy.

Chamber Size

Moderate or severe dilatation of the left ventricle was present in 54% of patients, while it was absent or mild in 46%. In this HCM series, marked left ventricular cavity dilatation tended to be associated with a thinner anterior left ventricular wall than in hearts showing less cavity enlargement (17 ± 6 vs 19 ± 7 mm, ns). For comparison, in patients with dilated cardiomyopathy of unknown cause, absent or mild dilatation, defined as an end diastolic diameter within 15% of the upper normal value for body surface, was observed in 14% of cases [9]: in contrast to HCM, grossly dilated hearts tended to have thicker walls than mildly dilated ones (15 ± 4 vs 12 ± 2 mm, $p = 0.06$)

Histologic Findings

Myocardial Fibrosis

The majority (52%) of the total histologic sections (n=225) of the 31 cases showed mild intermyocellular and/or microfocal myocardial fibrosis (< 20% of the histological area), while relevant fibrosis involving from 20% to 50% of histologic slide area was seen in 28% of sections. Extensive scarring, defined as > 50% fibrosis was found in 16% of sections. In almost all sections myocardial fibrosis of any form and extent was associated with hypertrophy. The percent of sections with relevant (> 20%) fibrosis averaged 50 ± 37% (median 44%) and was significantly higher in cases with hypertrophic cardiomyopathy than in other excised hearts (Fig. 2). No differences in the extent of fibrosis were observed according to the type (symmetric or asymmetric) of hypertrophy.

Disarray

In all histologic sections examined the extent of disarray was less than 20% of the total histologic area in 49%, between 20%-50% in 26% and greater than 50% in 9%. Only 15% of sections did not show disarray. In the individual hearts, relevant (> 20%) disarray was present in about one third of sections (mean 37 ± 39%, median 22%). Disarray was significantly more frequent in the left than in the right ventricle ($p = 0.04$, Fig. 3), even though extensive myocardial disorganization was also found at the latter site.

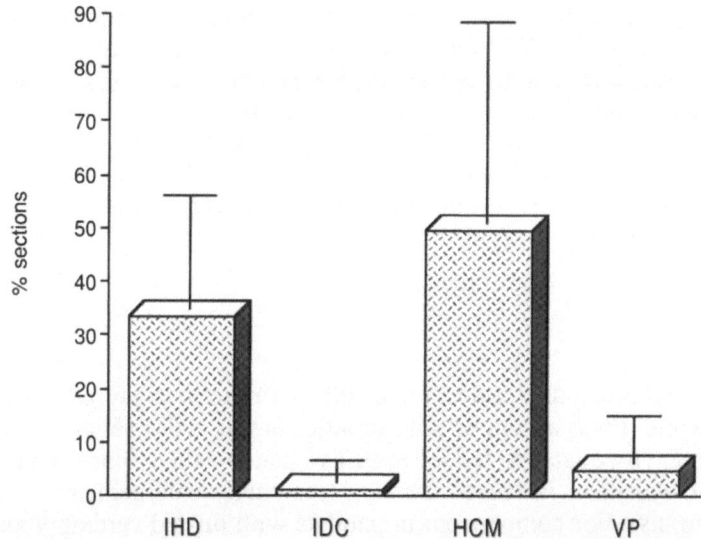

Fig. 2. The percent of histologic sections showing relevant (> 20%) fibrosis is significantly higher in excised hearts with hypertrophic cardiomyopathy (HCM) and ischemic heart disease (IHD) than in VP (Valvulopathy) and idiopathic dilated cardiomyopathy (IDC) , $p <$ 0.0001

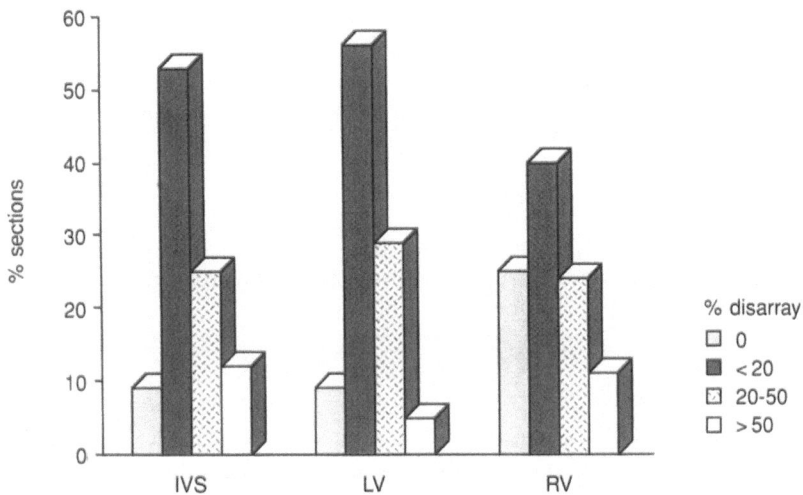

Fig. 3. Disarray is significantly more frequent in the interventricular septum (IVS) and left ventricular free wall (LV) than in the right ventricular free wall (RV), $p = 0.04$

The extent of myocyte disorganization did not correlate with severity of gross hypertrophy at any site. Wall thickness averaged 15±6 mm in regions with < 20% disarray and 14 ± 8 mm both in areas with 20% to 50% and > 50% disarray. Disarray prevailed in areas with extensive myocardial fibrosis ($p < 0.001$, Fig. 4) and was always associated with hypertrophy of normally arranged myocardial cells.

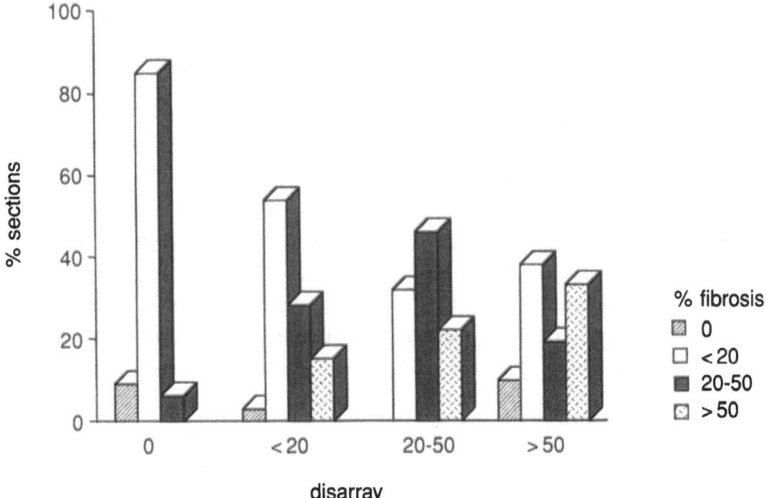

Fig. 4. Disarray is significantly more extensive in areas with higher fibrosis $p < 0.001$

Endocardial Plaque and Mitral Leaflet Thickening

An endocardial plaque was found in 74% of cases, without differences between cases showing symmetric or asymmetric hypertrophy.

Thickening of the anterior mitral valve leaflet was found in 48% of cases, and similarly distributed in symmetric or asymmetric hypertrophy.

Arteriolar Medial Hyperplasia

Arteriolar medial hyperplasia involved less than 5 vessels in 15 and ≥ 5 vessels in the remaining 7 cases presenting this abnormality; it occurred in areas with disarray and/or myocardial fibrosis.

Coronary Atherosclerosis

A functional ($\geq$ 70% lumen-diameter reduction) coronary stenosis was present as unique severe lesion of the left anterior descending branch in one heart without any associated myocardial scar. In other 16 patients minor atherosclerotic plaques were detected.

Discussion

In the Italian Heart Transplant Program, left ventricular dilatation with wall thinning and related clinical dysfunction, the so-called end-stage phase of HCM, was the most common indication for heart transplantation (79% of cases) in adults with this disease. This is in agreement with others [7], who reported progressive dilatation, pump dysfunction and refractory heart failure in nine of ten transplanted HCM patients.

The evolution towards end-stage disease occurred at a relatively young age in this series (mean 36 years), in keeping with the previous literature, where average age at dilatation ranged from to 28 to 42 years [3-7]. Although the interval from diagnosis to ventricular enlargement was long (14 years), once established, the evolution towards heart failure and hence transplantation was rapid (mean 3 years). This finding does not support the contention that progressive dilatation and wall thinning represent a late stage of HCM [10], but rather suggests that they are a complication which may occur even in young patients. Therefore careful echocardiographic follow-up is mandatory in HCM regardless of age, to screen for initial changes in chamber size.

In our series all patients presented severe symptoms (NYHA functional class IV) refractory to medical treatment for heart failure, in spite of a depression in left ventricular ejection fraction which might be considered only moderate (Table 1) when compared to transplant candidates with diseases of different nature. A possible overimposition of systolic impairment to relevant pre-existing diastolic dysfunction could explain this apparent discrepancy.

Increased left ventricular chamber size and thinning of both the septum and left ventricular free wall were observed before surgery in our cases with respect to the available baseline evaluation. Therefore, symmetrical thinning of ventricular walls could be a potential prognostic marker in the clinical follow-up of HCM patients, pointing to an unfavourable disease course.

The morphologic substrate offers little understanding of the pathophysiologic mechanisms which underly progression towards refractory heart failure in HCM. The pathways leading to heart failure in HCM are probably diverse, as is the phenotypic expression of its varying genotype mutations [1].

At gross examination, all our excised HCM hearts presented a lower wall thickness, even at the site of asymmetric hypertrophy, than 26 autopsy hearts [11], 19 of whom were from patients who had obstructive HCM. Moreover, left cavity dilation, which has been reported to occur in 9.5% of unselected HCM hearts [10], was present in 89% of our HCM cases, being moderate to severe in about half of them. This discrepancy is easily explained by the different selection of cases undergoing heart transplantation with respect to autopsy cases.

Conversely, histologic evaluation showed the pattern of myocardial disarray and fibrosis usually observed in HCM. Interstitial myocardial fibrosis is common in this disease and is likely due to a proliferation of fibrillar collagen consequent to a maximal hypertrophy of the disarranged myocells. This finding has been reported even in the absence of heart failure: myocardial fibrosis was significantly increased in autopsy hearts from HCM patients who died suddenly [12] and in subaortic myectomy specimens [13], when compared to normal non-hypertrophied or hypertrophied control hearts. Myocardial scar areas secondary to acute infarction in the absence of coronary artery disease [10] have been reported in about one-fourth of cases. Even in our excised HCM hearts relevant fibrosis was significantly more extensive than in control failing hearts with a different substrate (Fig. 2). However extensive scarring, involving >50% slide area, was much less frequent, representing only 16% of sections. Therefore, as previously noted in other diseases leading to heart failure and transplantation [14], even in HCM the amount of histologically viable myocardium far exceeds the extent of fibrosis. Probably a definite causal link between extensive myocardial replacement by fibrotic tissue and failure is limited to a minority of cases.

The secondary increase in myocardial collagen content, which leads to a stiff, non-compliant chamber certainly plays an important role in the diastolic dysfunction of HCM, but is not likely to be the main mechanism of systolic pump failure, as it is present even in non-failing HCM hearts. The assumption that loss of myocardium and fibrotic replacement will per se result in heart failure merits further investigation.

Another argument to be discussed is the meaning of ventricular dilatation in relation to global failure of the ventricle. As in dilated cardiomyopathy, refractory congestive heart failure may be associated with absent or minor dilatation [9]. In our HCM cases 46% showed the latter condition. This finding does not support the concept of stretching of myocardial cells and/or their slippage to explain thinning of wall/myocell and cavity dilatation [9].

Finally, greater importance should probably be given to an alternative pathway leading to end-stage disease: the primary role of disarray as dissynergic factor. There is a general agreement in focusing on myocell disorganization as the structural hallmark of this disease. Disarray means architectural alteration based on perpendicular or oblique hypertrophic myobridges between adjacent myocells. Found in specific areas in the normal heart, surrounding myocardial fibrosis in diseased hearts, or in a variety of conditions (Noonans, Friedreichs ataxia, Lentiginosis, Familial restrictive cardiomyopathy with disarray, etc), disarray has been interpreted as an exaggerated physiological response related to genic alterations of the myofibrillar protein apparatus [10]. In HCM disarray is generally extensive and not associated to wall thickness [15]. In particular, diffuse disarray in the absence of myocardial hypertrophy and associated with a clinical pattern of restrictive cardiomyopathy has been reported in two families [16] and observed in one case of our transplant population, namely a 28-year-old woman with a normal-sized heart who underwent heart transplantation with the clinical diagnosis of irreversible restrictive cardiomyopathy: the only lesion found in the excised heart was a typical, diffuse disarray.

If one focuses on this structural disorganization as main morphofunctional lesion of the disease, the suggestion is that disarray is the cause of an asynergic dysfunction proportional to its extent. The whole clinical spectrum of HCM may therefore range from a "restrictive" pattern to extensive symmetric or asymmetric hypertrophy, the concept being that disarrayed myocells hypertrophy, as they are forced to an endless, but useless contractility, the whole disarray region becoming an asynergic zone. In turn, segmental asynergy will trigger in other regions a compensatory hypertrophy without disarray, which may end in progressive exhaustion of myocellular contractility. When this stage occurs, the whole cardiac pump function is reduced and there are all the morphologic changes typical of congestive heart failure.

In conclusion, the outcome of hypertrophic cardiomyopathy in a small percentage of cases is due to a pattern of congestive heart failure similar to that of other diseases with a different etiologic substrate. This gives rise to the concept that congestive heart failure, when it starts, may have a common and still undetermined etiopathogenetic mechanism, independently of the primitive disease [14].

In defining the so-called hypertrophic cardiomyopathy we suggest to heighten the focus on the typical morphostructural abnormality and call this disease "disarray cardiomyopathy", a term which encompasses the whole clinical spectrum of the disease, ranging from left cavity obstruction to a restrictive pattern without cavity dilation and hypertrophy. The term hypertrophy should be restricted to the compensatory increase in size of all components of the myocardial cell and related interstitial collagen matrix changes.

References

1. Marian AJ, Roberts R (1995) Recent advances in the molecular genetics of hypertrophic cardiomyopathy. Circulation 92:1336-1347
2. Wigle ED, Rakowski H, Kimball BP, Williams WG (1995) Hypertrophic cardiomyopathy. Clinical spectrum and treatment. Circulation 92:1680-1692

3. Spirito P, Maron BJ, Bonow BO, Epstein SE (1987) Occurrence and significance of progessive left ventricular wall thinning and relative cavity dilatation in hypertrophic cardiomyopathy. Am J Cardiol 59:123-129
4. Spirito P, Maron BJ (1987) Absence of progression of left ventricular hypertrophy in adult patients with hypertrophic cardiomyopathy. J Am Coll Cardiol 9:1013-1017
5. Seiler C, Jenni R, Vassalli G, Turina M, Hess OM (1995) Left ventricular chamber dilatation in hypertrophic cardiomyopathy: related variables and prognosis in patients with medical and surgical therapy. Br Heart J 74:508-516
6. Hecht GM, Klues HG, Roberts WC, Maron BJ (1993) Coexistence of sudden cardiac death and end-stage heart failure in familial hypertrophic cardiomyopathy. J Am Coll Cardiol 22:489-497
7. Shirani J, Maron BJ, Cannon RD, Shahin S, Roberts WC (1993) Clinicopathologic features of hypertrophic cardiomyopathy managed by cardiac transplantation. Am J Cardiol 72:434-440
8. Reiner L (1968) Gross examination of the heart. In: Gould SE (ed) Pathology of the Heart and Blood Vessels, 3rd ed. Thomas CC, Springfield, Ill, p 1136
9. Baroldi G, De Maria R, Silver MD (1996) Pathology of dilated cardiomyopathy of unknown cause. Heart failure 12:98-127
10. Davies MJ, McKenna WJ (1995): Hypertrophic cardiomyopathy. Pathology and pathogenesis. Histopathology 26:493-500
11. Teare D (1958) Asymmetrical hypertropy of the heart in young adults. Br Heart J 20:1-8
12. Unverferth DV, Baker PB, Pearce LI, Lautman J, Roberts WC (1987) Regional myocyte hypertrophy and increased interstitial myocardial fibrosis in hypertrophic cardiomyopathy. Am J Cardiol 59:932-936
13. Factor SM, Butany J, Sole MJ, Wigle ED, Williams WC, Rojkind M (1991) Pathologic fibrosis and matrix connective tissue in the subaortic myocardium of patients with hypertrophic cardiomyopathy. J Am Coll Cardiol 17:1343-1351
14. Baroldi G, Silver MD, De Maria R, Pellegrini A (1998) Pathology and pathogenesis of congestive heart failure. A quantitative morphologic study of 144 hearts excised at transplantation. Pathogenesis (in press)
15. Maron BJ, Wolfson JK, Roberts WC (1992) Relation between extent of cardiac muscle cell disorganization and left ventricular wall thickness in hypertrophic cardiomyopathy. Am J Cardiol 70:785-790
16. McKenna, WJ, Stewart JT, Nihoyannopoulos P, Mc Ginty F, Davies MJ (1990) Hypertrophic cardiomyopathy without hypertrophy: 2 families with myocardial disarray in the absence of increased myocardial mass. Br Heart J 63:287-290

Medical Treatment Options in Hypertrophic Cardiomyopathy

P. Spirito and P. Bellone

Introduction

Hypertrophic cardiomyopathy (HCM) is a complex cardiac disease characterized by marked left ventricular hypertrophy and a great diversity in its functional alterations and clinical course [1-3]. In the 1960s, shortly after the initial contemporary descriptions of HCM, diagnosis was based on physical examination and cardiac catheterization. While these diagnostic approaches tended to emphasize the role of dynamic left ventricular outflow obstruction in the pathophysiology of the disease, some investigators had already focused on diastolic dysfunction and impaired left ventricular filling as the dominant functional alteration in HCM [4,5]. With the advent of echocardiography, it became clear that the great majority of patients have the nonobstructive form of the disease [6]. In the 1980s, metabolic, nuclear and necropsy studies drew attention to myocardial ischemia as another important functional alteration in HCM [7-10]. At present, pharmacologic therapy directed toward improving diastolic filling and possibly reducing myocardial ischemia represents the principal treatment for relieving symptoms in most patients [11] (Fig. 1). Invasive interventions focused on abolition of the outflow gradient are applied to a minority of patients (probably 5% or less of the overall HCM population) who have both outflow obstruction and severe symptoms unresponsive to medical therapy [11]. In the present discussion, we will address the issue of the pharmacologic treatment of symptoms of heart failure in HCM.

Medications

Medical treatment for HCM was first introduced in the 1960s in the form of the beta-adrenergic blocking agent propranolol. The beneficial effects of this drug on symptoms (principally, dyspnea and chest pain) and exercise tolerance appear to be due largely to a decrease in heart rate with consequent prolongation of diastole and increased passive ventricular filling [12,13]. By reducing the inotropic state, propranolol may also lessen myocardial oxygen demand and decrease left ventricular outflow gradient during exercise, when sympathetic tone is increased [12-13]. Standard doses of oral propranol in

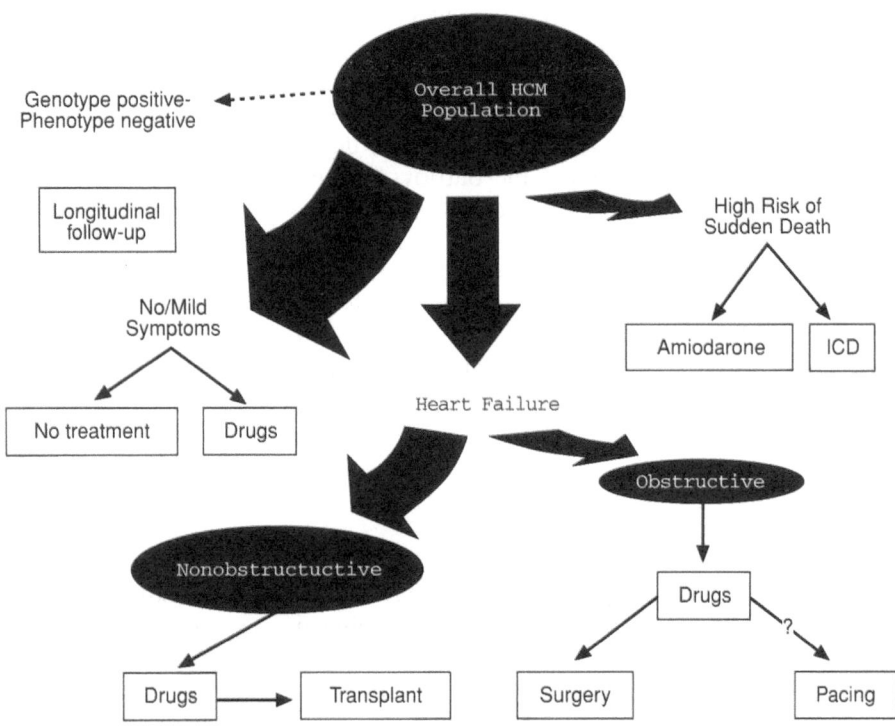

Fig. 1. Principal clinical presentations of hypertrophic cardiomyopathy and corresponding treatment strategies. The size of the arrows represents an estimate (based on the available literature) of the proportion of patients with hypertrophic cardiomyopathy in each subgroup. The dashed arrow indicates the present uncertainties regarding the size of this subgroup, and the question mark indicates the present uncertainties regarding the therapeutic efficacy of pacing (from [11])

HCM range from 160 to 360 mg per day. Long-acting and cardioselective beta-blocking agents have also been used extensively in the management of patients with HCM even in the absence of direct documentation of their efficacy in this disease.

Beta-blockers remained the sole pharmacologic option for patients with HCM until the introduction of the calcium channel blockers in the late 1970s. Verapamil has been the most extensively used calcium channel blocker in HCM (standard doses, 240 to 480 mg per day). This drug exerts favorable effects on symptoms of dyspnea and chest pain, and increases exercise capacity by improving left ventricular filling through a direct effect on the diastolic properties of the ventricle, and probably by reducing myocardial ischemia [2,11,14,15]. Other calcium antagonists such as nifedipine and diltiazem have also been utilized sporadically in the treatment of patients with HCM. Because of its potent vasodilator actions, however, nifedipine may have deleterious hemodynamic effects in this disease, particularly in patients with outflow obstruction [16]. Diltiazem appears to have beneficial effects in HCM, but experience with this drug is limited [17].

In 1982, disopyramide was introduced as a treatment for patients with obstructive HCM and severe symptoms unresponsive to standard medical therapy [18]. This drug, administered in oral doses of 600 to 800 mg per day, has the potential to decrease the outflow gradient by virtue of its negative inotropic properties [18,19]. In many patients, however, the initial hemodynamic and clinical benefits decrease with time [19]. Because disopyramide may reduce atrio-ventricular conduction time and thus increase ventricular rate during paroxysmal atrial fibrillation, it is prudent to combine this drug with beta-blockers administered in low doses. The potential pro-arrhythmic effects of disopyramide are also of concern and have probably limited the widespread use of this drug.

Patient Management

In patients with HCM, pharmacologic therapy with beta-blockers and verapamil has traditionally been administered in an empirical fashion, based on subjective perception of benefit rather than objective assessment of effect on exercise capacity. Such judgements are often challenging given the day-to-day variability in symptoms often reported by HCM patients. Also, drug treatment strategies are not standardized and reflect, in part, the experience and biases of individual investigators. Most favor beta-blocking drugs over verapamil as the initial treatment in patients with exertional dyspnea and fatigue, although it is probably not of critical importance which of these drugs is used first. Some investigators also tailor drug selection to hemodynamic state, confining administration of verapamil to patients without outflow obstruction and using beta-blockers and/or disopyramide in patients with obstruction; others administer verapamil selectively to those patients with chest pain as the predominant symptom. There is no evidence that beta-blockers and verapamil given together are advantageous over the use of either drug alone.

Patients who fail to respond to beta-blocking therapy often experience symptomatic improvement with verapamil. In some patients, the improvement with verapamil could also be due, in part, to the withdrawal of beta-blockers and their associated side-effects [20]. In the presence of a large outflow gradient and/or markedly elevated pulmonary pressures, verapamil should be used with caution since its vasodilatory effects may lead to severe hemodynamic consequences [1,2,11].

Patients with particularly severe symptoms of heart failure despite treatment with beta-blockers or verapamil may show symptomatic improvement with administration of diuretic agents [1,2,11]. However, since many of these patients have diastolic dysfunction and require relatively high filling pressures to achieve adequate left ventricular filling, it is advisable to administer diuretics with caution.

Treatment of End-stage HCM

Some patients with HCM and severe heart failure have evolved to a phase that is generally described as "end-stage". This evolution in the natural history of HCM has been reported to occur in about 15% of patients with

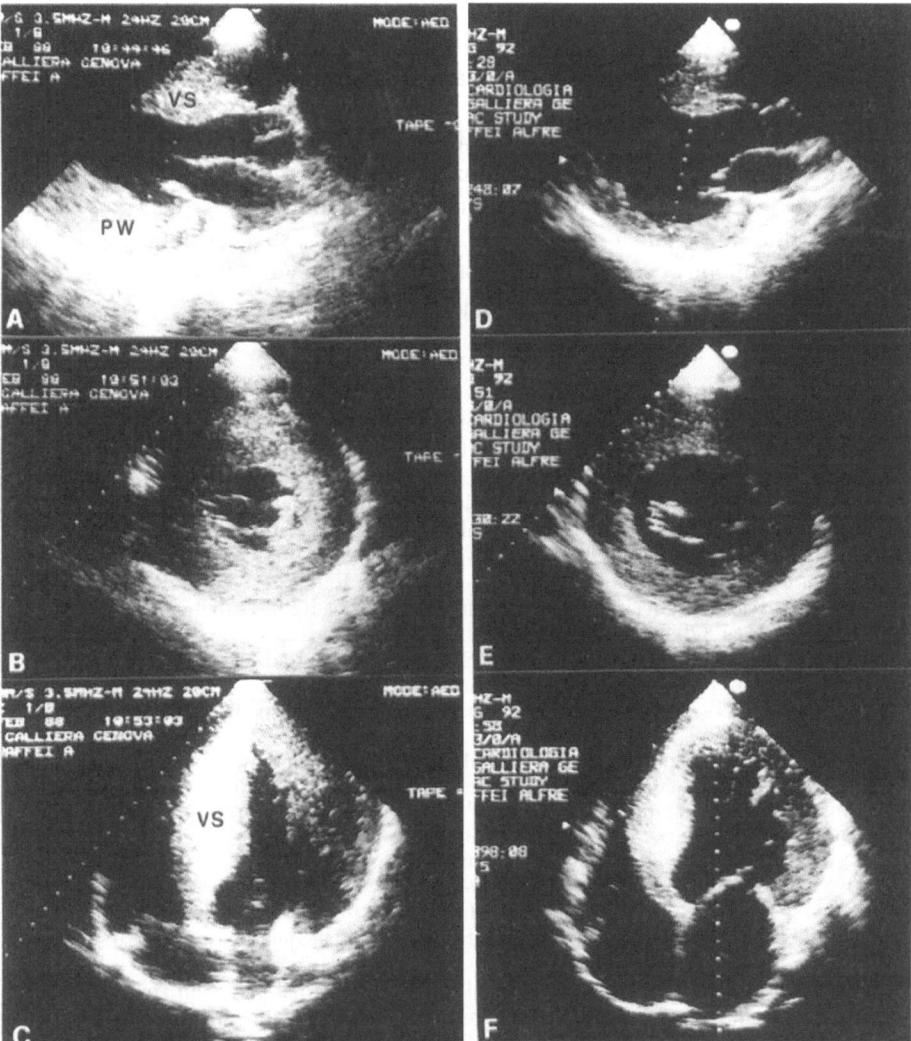

Fig. 2. Stop frames of the initial (A-C) and most recent (D-F) echocardiogram obtained during diastole in a patient with hypertrophic cardiomyopathy who developed progressive left ventricular wall thinning, cavity dilatation and systolic dysfunction. In A-C, at 19 years of age, septal and posterior wall thickness measure 32 mm, diastolic cavity dimension is 42 mm. In D-F, five years later, septal and posterior wall thickness have decreased substantially (to 22 and 18 mm, respectively) and the left ventricular cavity is dilated (70 mm) (from [23])

symptoms of heart failure [21,22], usually during mid-life, and is characterized by substantial left ventricular remodeling with progressive wall thinning, relative cavity enlargement and systolic dysfunction (Fig. 2). All the patients in the end-stage phase are without outflow obstruction, since those with the obstructive form of HCM loose the outflow gradient as the ventricle undergoes wall thinning and cavity dilatation. Histologically, the left ventricular wall is characterized by extensive scarring. The precise mechanisms responsible for the progression to end-stage are unknown; however, several metabolic, nuclear imaging and necropsy studies have demonstrated the presence of myocardial ischemia in HCM [7-10]. Therefore, it is likely that chronic myocardial ischemia leading to myocardial cell death and replacement fibrosis plays a role in this evolution.

In patients in the end-stage phase of HCM, drug treatment has to be redirected from beta-blockers or verapamil to the standard therapy for heart failure associated with systolic dysfunction, including diuretics, converting enzyme inhibitors and digitalis [1,2,11]. In many such patients, however, medical treatment becomes insufficient to control symptoms and heart transplantation emerges as the only therapeutic option.

References

1. Wigle ED, Sasson Z, Henderson MA, et al (1985) Hypertrophic cardiomyopathy: the importance of the site and the extent of hypertrophy: a review. Prog Cardiovasc Dis 28:1-83
2. Maron BJ, Bonow RO, Cannon RO III, Leon MB, Epstein SE (1987) Hypertrophic cardiomyopathy: interrelations of clinical manifestations, pathophysiology, and therapy. N Engl J Med 316:780-789, and 844-852
3. Spirito P, Chiarella F, Carratino L, Zoni-Berisso M, Bellotti P, Vecchio C (1989) Clinical course and prognosis of hypertrophic cardiomyopathy in an outpatient population. N Engl J Med 320:749-755
4. Stewart S, Mason DT, Braunwald E (1968) Impaired rate of left ventricular filling in idiopathic hypertrophic subaortic stenosis and valvular aortic stenosis. Circulation 37:8-14
5. Goodwin JF (1970) Congestive and hypertrophic cardiomyopathies: a decade of study. Lancet 1:731-739
6. Maron BJ, Gottdiener JS, Epstein SE (1981) Patterns and significance of distribution of left ventricular hypertrophy in hypertrophic cardiomyopathy. A wide-angle, two-dimensional echocardiographic study of 125 patients. Am J Cardiol 48:418-428
7. Thompson DS, Naqvi N, Juul SM et al (1980) Effects of propranolol on myocardial oxygen consumption, substrate extraction, and hemodynamics in hypertrophic obstructive cardiomyopathy. Br Heart J 44:488-498
8. Cannon RO III, Rosing DR, Maron BJ et al (1985) Myocardial ischemia in patients with hypertrophic cardiomyopathy: contribution of inadequate vasodilator reserve and elevated left ventricular filling pressures Circulation 71:234-243
9. O'Gara PT, Bonow RO, Maron BJ, et al (1987) Myocardial perfusion abnormalities in patients with hypertrophic cardiomyopathy: assessment with thallium-201 emission computed tomography. Circulation 47:1214-1223
10. Maron BJ, Wolson JK, Epstein SE, Roberts WC (1986) Intramural ("small vessel") coronary artery disease in hypertrophic cardiomyopathy. J Am Coll Cardiol 8:545-557
11. Spirito P, Seidman CE, McKenna WJ, Maron BJ (1997) The management of hypertrophic cardiomyopathy. N Eng J Med 336:775-785
12. Harrison DC, Braunwald E, Glick G, Mason DT, Chidsey CA, Ross J Jr (1964) Effects of beta adrenergic blockade on the circulation, with particular reference to observations in patients with hypertrophic subaortic stenosis. Circulation 29:84-98

13. Flamm MD, Harrison DC, Hancock EW (1968) Muscular subaortic stenosis: prevention of outflow obstruction with propranolol. Circulation 38:846-858
14. Rosing DR, Kent KM, Maron BJ, Epstein SE (1979) Verapamil therapy: a new approach to the pharmacologic treatment of hypertrophic cardiomyopathy. II. Effects on exercise capacity and symptomatic status. Circulation 60:1208-1213
15. Bonow RO, Rosing DR, Bacharach SL, et al (1981) Effects of verapamil on left ventricular systolic function and diastolic filling in patients with hypertrophic cardiomyopathy. Circulation 1981;64:787-796
16. Betocchi S, Cannon RO III, Watson RM, et al (1985) Effects of sublingual nifedipine on hemodynamics and systolic and diastolic function in patients with hypertrophic cardiomyopathy. Circulation 72:1001-1007
17. Betocchi S, Piscione F, Losi MA, et al (1996) Effects of diltiazem on left ventricular systolic and diastolic function in hypertrophic cardiomyopathy. Am J Cardiol 78:451-457
18. Pollick C (1982) Muscular subaortic stenosis: hemodynamic and clinical improvement after disopyramide. N Engl J Med 307:997-999
19. Wigle ED, Rakowski H, Kimball BP, Williams WG (1995) Hypertrophic cardiomyopathy. Clinical spectrum and treatment. Circulation 92:1680-1692
20. Gilligan DM, Chan WL, Stewart RA, Oakley CM (1991) Adrenergic hypersensitivity after beta-blocker withdrawal in hypertrophic cardiomyopathy. Am J Cardiol 68:766-772
21. Spirito P, Maron BJ (1987) Absence of progression of left ventricular hypertrophy in adult patients with hypertrophic cardiomyopathy. J Am Coll Cardiol 9:1013-1017
22. Spirito P, Maron BJ, Bonow RO, Epstein SE (1987) Occurrence and significance of progressive left ventricular wall thinning and relative cavity dilatation in hypertrophic cardiomyopathy. Am J Cardiol 60:123-129
23. Spirito P, Bellone P (1994) Natural history of hypertrophic cardiomyopathy. Br Heart J 72[Suppl]:510-512

DDD Pacing in Hypertrophic Cardiomyopathy: State of the Art

S. Betocchi, M.A. Losi, C. Briguori and M. Chiariello

Introduction

Hypertrophic cardiomyopathy (HCM) is a primary myocardial disease, whose typical pathophysiological features include normal systolic dynamics, impaired diastolic function [1-4], and, in about one fourth of patients, left ventricular (LV) outflow tract obstruction [5-8].

Treatment for LV outflow tract obstruction has for decades relied upon the surgical resection of a septal wedge (myotomy-myectomy) [9]. This approach has shown to provide symptomatic benefit and improvement in prognosis, especially if associated with appropriate medical therapy [7]. The potential role of pacing in the treatment of obstruction has been pioneered in the mid seventies [10-12]. It was not until 1992 that sequential right atrioventricular (AV) pacing with short AV delay (i.e. apical pre-excitation) gained momentum in the treatment of patients with obstructive HCM [13-14]. AV pacing diminishes the outflow gradient by inducing septal systolic asynchrony: qualitative and quantitative analysis of motion of the upper septum shows that the width of the outflow tract is increased, thereby reducing the outflow tract gradient [14-15].

Acute Hemodynamic Effects

Effects on LV Outflow Tract Obstruction

AV pacing reduces the degree of LV outflow tract gradient in most patients with obstructive HCM (up to 80%) [13]. Efficacy of AV pacing in reducing obstruction depends on the AV interval: apical preexcitation is necessary to that effect [14, 16]. Long AV intervals are ineffective, whereas too short intervals may interfere with filling and reduce cardiac output [14, 16]: AV intervals of 80 to 100 ms lower the degree of obstruction without altering the filling dynamics in most patients [16].

Effects on LV Systolic Function and Hemodynamics

AV pacing minimally affects ejection fraction [15] but decreases cardiac output [19]: these findings could be interpreted as evidence of a modest negative inotropic effect of AV pacing. In contrast, the reduction in LV outflow tract gradient achieved by AV pacing is beneficial in that it increases aortic pressure [12].

Effects on LV Diastolic Function

It has been shown in the experimental animal [17] and in patients with coronary artery disease [18] that asynchrony induced by AV pacing impairs active diastolic function (both isovolumetric relaxation and early filling). If the same was true for patients with HCM, AV pacing would worsen diastolic function in a category of patients, those with obstructive HCM, in whom it is already jeopardized [1-4]. Two studies that appeared almost simultaneously have shown that acute AV pacing impairs the time constant of isovolumetric relaxation [15, 19]; this occurs despite a decrease in LV outflow tract gradient and, therefore, of LV systolic pressure [15]. Because the time constant of isovolumetric relaxation is inversely related to afterload [20], it should have been shortened by a reduction in LV systolic pressure. In addition, the maximal rate of LV filling decreased [15], despite an increase in the filling pressure [15, 19], whereas in this setting filling should have been faster [21]. These findings indicate that AV pacing damages the active part of diastole in an acute study. The elevation in the filling pressure, in addition, is potentially detrimental as it may induce symptoms of congestive heart failure.

Chronic Effects

Long-term Hemodynamic Effects

LV outflow tract gradient decreases with permanent stimulation in atrial synchronized ventricular pacing mode [13] and it keeps decreasing over time [22-23]. The decrease in LV outflow tract gradient is associated with a progressive decrease in LV systolic pressure and an increase in aortic pulse pressure. Filling pressure and cardiac output do not change in the long-term [22]. Interestingly, such hemodynamic changes are also observed when the pace-maker is turned off [22]. The mechanism for this finding is unclear: a pacing-induced "plastic remodeling" of the left ventricle has been advocated. This hypothesis, however, has not been confirmed by analysis of LV anatomy: Fananapazir and coworkers [22] have observed a pacing-induced reduction in septal thickness in about one fourth of their patients, while Jeanrenaud and coworkers have seen no changes in LV anatomy [14].

In a small group of pediatric patients with symptomatic HCM, acute and chronic DDD pacing lowers LV outflow tract gradient and decreases pulmonary artery wedge pressure [24]. This latter result conflicts with previous studies [15, 19]

In patients with angina, a DDD pacing-induced reduction in global coronary blood flow has been observed by positron emission tomography [25]; this decrease is associated with a homogenization in regional coronary blood

flow (i.e. there are fewer differences among regions). The clinical significance of this finding is unclear.

The impairment in diastolic function, which has been found in acute studies, persists over the long term: left atrial fractional shortening, an index
closely related to LV end-diastolic pressure, is significantly impaired after
pacemaker implant as compared to the baseline and to a group of age-
matched patients with HCM; such impairment persists significantly up to 3
months, and a nonsignificant trend is evident up to two years [26]. The clinical significance of such pacing-induced diastolic dysfunction is yet to be
clarified.

Clinical Outcome

The effects of DDD pacing on functional capacity are still controversial [13-
14, 22]. According to a study of a large cohort, symptomatic status is
improved over the long term in approximately 90% of patients; angina
pectoris, dyspnea, palpitation, and pre-syncope all decrease after DDD pacing
and exhibit a further decrease in some patients at late follow-up [22]; the
improvement of symptoms, however, is totally unrelated to the hemodynamic
effects of pacing, namely decrease in obstruction [23]. A few patients (about
10%) do not benefit from chronic DDD pacing for several reasons, including
persistent obstruction and accelerated AV conduction (this latter precluding
from pacing at long-enough AV intervals) [22]. A recently published study
analyzed the effect of DDD pacing on symptoms and on objective exercise
tolerance in a double blind, randomized, cross-over way [27]. Patients were
studied before and after pacemaker implant, in DDD and AAI pacing modes
(this latter was set at a very low rate, and is equivalent to the pacemaker being
turned off). These Authors observed an improvement in symptoms over the
baseline during DDD pacing in about 60% of patients, but also in about 40%
of patients in AAI pacing mode; furthermore, exercise capacity, as assessed by
peak oxygen consumption, was unchanged in either pacing mode as compared
to the baseline. These findings suggest a placebo effect that is responsible, at
least in part, for the improvement in symptoms seen with DDD pacing.

Unanswered Questions

Mortality

The main goals of treatment for any disease are reduction in mortality and
improvement in the quality of life. The efficacy of DDD pacing in lowering
mortality (particularly sudden death, the leading cause of death in HCM) is
still unknown: few studies have been published that include relatively small
populations of patients followed up for short time intervals. Because many
patients with obstructive HCM are young and, if implanted, are likely to
experience many years of DDD pacing, studies available thus far appear inadequate in addressing this issue.

Symptoms

The controversial effects on symptoms suggest that a placebo effect of pacemaker implant cannot be ruled out. Larger controlled studies are needed to draw conclusions on this topic.

Acute AV pacing appears associated with a negative inotropic effect. If this effect persists in the long term, the possibility that DDD pacing leads to LV dilatation should be assessed in large long-term studies.

The influence of pacing-induced diastolic dysfunction on clinical status and on prognosis needs further investigation: a negative lusitropic effect could be counterbalanced in the short term by the decrease in obstruction in some patients, while it may determine symptoms of heart failure in others; it would be important to identify patients who will benefit from DDD pacing before implant.

References

1. Sanderson JE, Gibson DG, Brown DJ, Goodwin JF (1977) Left ventricular filling in hypertrophic cardiomyopathy. Br Heart J 39:661-670
2. Bonow RO, Frederick TM, Bacharach SL, Green MV, Goose PW, Maron BJ, Rosing DR (1983) Atrial systole and left ventricular filling in patients with hypertrophic cardiomyopathy. Am J Cardiol 51:1386-1391
3. Betocchi S, Bonow RO, Bacharach SL, Rosing DR, Maron BJ, Green MV (1986). Isovolumic relaxation period in hypertrophic cardiomyopathy: assessment by radionuclide angiography. J Am Coll Cardiol 7:74-81
4. Hess OM, Murakami T, Krayenbuehl HP (1986) Does verapamil improve left ventricular relaxation in patients with myocardial hypertrophy? Circulation 74:530-543
5. Maron BJ, Gottdiener JS, Arce J, Rosing DR, Wesley YE, Epstein SE (1985) Dynamic subaortic obstruction in hypertrophic cardiomyopathy: analysis by pulsed Doppler echocardiography. J Am Coll Cardiol 6:1-15
6. Maron BJ, Epstein SE (1986). Clinical significance and therapeutic implications of the left ventricular outflow tract pressure gradient in hypertrophic cardiomyopathy. Am J Cardiol 58: 1093-1096
7. Seiler C, Hess OM, Schoenbeck M, Turina J, Jenni R, Turina M, Krayenbuehl HP (1991). Long-term follow-up of medical versus surgical therapy for hypertrophic cardiomyopathy: a retrospective study. J Am Coll Cardiol 17:634-642
8. Kaltenbach M, Hopf R, Kober G, Bussman WD, Keller M, Paterson Y (1979) Treatment of hypertrophic cardiomyopathy with verapamil. Br Heart J 42:35-42
9. Morrow AG, Fogarty TJ, Hannah H III, Braunwald E (1968) Operative treatment in idiopathic hypertrophic subaortic stenosis: techniques and the results of preoperative and postoperative clinical and hemodynamic assessment. Circulation 37:589-596
10. Hassenstein P, Walther H, Dittrich J (1975) Haemodynamische Veränderungen durch einfache und gekoppelte Stimulation bei Patienten mit obstruktiver Kardiomyopathie. Verh Dtsch Ges Inn Med 81:170-173
11. Duck HJ, Hutschemeister W, Paneau H, Trenckmann H (1984) Atrio-ventricular stimulation with reduced AV-delay time as a therapeutic principle in hypertrophic obstructive cardiomyopathy. Z Gesamte Inn Med 39:437-447
12. McDonald K, McWilliam E, O'Keeffe B, Maurer B (1988) Functional assessment of patients treated with permanent dual chamber pacing as a primary treatment for hypertrophic cardiomyopathy. Eur Heart J 9:893-898
13. Fananapazir L, Cannon RO III, Tripodi D, Panza JA (1992) Impact of dual-chamber permanent pacing in patients with obstructive hypertrophic cardiomyopathy with symptoms refractory to verapamil and β-adrenergic blocker therapy. Circulation 85:2149-2161
14. Jeanrenaud X, Goy JJ, Kappenberger L (1992) Effects of dual-chamber pacing in hypertrophic obstructive cardiomyopathy. Lancet 339:1318-1323

15. Betocchi S, Losi MA, Piscione F, Boccalatte M, Pace L, Golino P, Perrone-Filardi P, Briguori C, Franculli, F, Pappone C, Salvatore M, Chiariello M (1996) Effects of dual-chamber pacing in hypertrophic cardiomyopathy on left ventricular outflow tract obstruction and on diastolic function. Am J Cardiol 77:498-504
16. Losi MA, Betocchi S, Briguori C, Piscione F, Manganelli F, Ciampi Q, Stabile G, Chiariello M (1998) Dual chamber pacing in hypertrophic cardiomyopathy: influence of atrio-ventricular delay on left ventricular outflow tract obstruction. Cardiology 89:8-13
17. Zile MR, Blaunstein AS, Shimizu G, Gaasch WH (1987) Right ventricular pacing reduces the rate of left ventricular relaxation and filling. J Am Coll Cardiol 10:702-709
18. Betocchi S, Piscione F, Villari B, Pace L, Ciarmiello A, Perrone-Filardi P, Salvatore C, Salvatore M, Chiariello M (1993) Effects of induced asynchrony on left ventricular diastolic function in patients with coronary artery disease. J Am Coll Cardiol 21: 1124-1131
19. Nishimura RA, Hayes DL, Ilstrup DM, Holmes DR, Tajik JA (1996) Effect of dual-chamber pacing on systolic and diastolic function in patients with hypertrophic cardiomyopathy: acute Doppler echocardiographic and catheterization hemodynamic study. J Am Coll Cardiol 27:421-430
20. Gaasch WH, Blaunstein AS, Andrias CW, Donahue RP, Avitall B (1980). Myocardial relaxation. II. Hemodynamic determinants of rate of left ventricular isovolumic pressure decline. Am J Physiol 239:H1-H6
21. Ishida Y, Meisner JS, Tsujoka K, Gallo JI, Yoran C, Frater RWM, Yellin EL (1986) Left ventricular filling dynamics: influence of left ventricular relaxation and left atrial pressure. Circulation 74:187-196
22. Fananapazir L, Epstein ND, Curiel RV, Panza J, Tripodi D, McAreavey D (1994). Long-term results of dual-chamber (DDD) pacing in obstructive hypertrophic cardiomyopathy. Evidence for progressive symptomatic and hemodynamic improvement and reduction of left ventricular hypertrophy. Circulation 90:2731-2742
23. Slade AKB, Sadoul N, Shapiro L, Choinowska L, Simon JP, Saumarez RC, Dodinot B, Camm AJ, McKenna WJ, Aliot E (1996) DDD pacing in hypertrophic cardiomyopathy: a multicentre clinical experience. Heart 75:44-49
24. Rishi F, Hulse JE, Auld DO, McRae G, Kaltman J, Kanter K, Williams W, Campbell RM (1997) Effects of dual-chamber pacing for pediatric patients with hypertrophic cardiomyopathy. J Am Coll Cardiol 29:734-740
25. Posma JL, Blanksma PK, Van der Wall EE, Vaalburg W, Crijins HJ, Lie KI (1996) Effects of permanent dual chamber pacing on myocardial perfusion in symptomatic hypertrophic cardiomyopathy. Heart 76:358-362
26. Betocchi S, Losi MA, Briguori C, Manganelli F, Ciampi Q, Boccalatte M, Gottilla R, Coltorti F, Santomauro M, Chiariello M (1997) Long-term dual-chamber pacing reduces outflow tract obstruction but impairs diastolic function in hypertrophic cardiomyopathy. Eur Heart J 18:604 (abstr)
27. Nishimura RA, Trusty JM, Hayes DL, Ilstrup DM, Larson DR, Hayes SH, Allison TG, Tajik J (1997) Dual-chamber pacing for hypertrophic obstructive cardiomyopathy: a randomized, double-blind crossover trial. J Am Coll Cardiol 29:435-441

Indications and Outcome of Cardiac Surgery for Severely Symptomatic Patients with Hypertrophic Obstructive Cardiomyopathy

F.A. Schoendube

Indication for surgical therapy in patients with hypertrophic cardiomyopathy is still agreed to be restricted to patients with severe symptoms refractory to medical treatment and with significant obstruction to the left ventricular outflow tract (basal gradients > 50 mmHg or > 80 mmHg after provocative manoeuvres) [1,2]. Relevant morbidity (ventricular septal perforation, atrioventricular block) and early mortality represent inherent risks with classical myotomy-myectomy [3], and recognition of subgroups with even elevated risk or with less benefit due to incomplete relief in addition suggests a cautious indication of surgery. A variety of surgical approaches have tried to overcome limitations, but none of them has gained general acceptance. Especially this holds true for mitral valve replacement [4], as notably patients are then faced with the long-term risks of thromboembolism, haemorrhage or other valve related complications. With a modified technique [5-7], which enables better exposure of the basal septum, simplifies myectomy and even allows to extend myectomy to the lateral free wall of the ventricle, attempts were made to obtain safe access to the deeper parts of the ventricle. Transaortic resection of hypertrophied trabeculae and mobilisation or partial excision of papillary muscles become thus feasible and may result in a reliable correction of the patho-anatomic distortions of the subvalvular mitral apparatus in hypertrophic cardiomyopathy.

Patients and Methods

Between 1979 and 1996, 74 severely symptomatic patients, 45 men (60%) and 29 women (40%), age 49 ± 12 years with hypertrophic obstructive cardiomyopathy (HOCM) were operated for relief of significant left ventricular outflow tract gradients. Mean NYHA functional class was 3.1. Most of the patients (95%) were in sinus rhythm, 2 patients had atrial fibrillation and one patient had pre-operatively an implanted permanent pacemaker due to total AV-block. Right or left bundle branch block was present in 15% of the patients. The mean duration of cardiac symptoms was 10.3 ± 6 years, the mean time interval between diagnosis of hypertrophic obstructive cardiomyopathy and operation was 3.3 ± 3 years.

Invasively measured left ventricular outflow tract peak systolic gradients were 85 ± 36 mm Hg at rest and 156 ± 51 mm Hg with provocative manoeuvres. Preoperative echocardiographic studies showed moderate mitral regurgitation in 29% and severe mitral regurgitation in 5% of the patients. All patients had significant systolic anterior motion of the mitral valve (SAM) with prolonged mitral valve-septal contact (3+ – 4+). Concomitant coronary artery disease was present in 16 patients with a history of myocardial infarction in 6 patients. Eleven patients had an indication for simultaneous coronary artery bypass grafting.

Surgical approach to the basal septum was in all patients a low transverse aortotomy [5,6]. After digital palpation of the extent of hypertrophy a sharp triple hook retractor is carefully inserted at the deepest point of the hypertrophied septum, thus defining exactly the intraventricular edge of the bulging muscular tissue. The retractor is pulled forward and longitudinal incisions are placed 2-3 mm underneath the aortic annulus in direction of the prongs of the retractor. This incision can be extended behind the insertion of the mural leaflet of the mitral valve, thus giving access to the deeper structures of the left ventricle. Both papillary muscles are then completely mobilised and all hypertrophied trabeculae as well as hypertrophied parts of the papillary muscles are resected.

Follow-up of the patients included clinical examination and echocardiographic studies for all long-term survivors and was 100% complete. A subgroup of the first 22 consecutive patients was initially followed up with left heart catheterisation; later on, echocardiography became the method of choice for postoperative controls.

Results

The early mortality rate was 1.3%. All other patients surviving the first 30 days [73/74] entered follow-up for a total time interval of 601 patient-years with a mean of 8.1 ± 5.4 years. Peri-operative non-fatal complications included one transient cerebral attack with full recovery during the hospital stay. No heparin anticoagulation was regularly given during hospital stay. Three patients (4%) required permanent pacemaker therapy due to total atrioventricular block after surgery; 2 of them had right bundle-branch block before surgery. There was no ventricular septal perforation in the whole series. The overall linearized mortality rate was 1.9%/patient-year (11/73), 5-year survival rate was 94% and 10-year rate was 86%. The cumulated survival proportion calculated with the Kaplan-Meier method is given in Fig. 1; notably, none of the late deaths occurred suddenly.

Improvement in clinical symptoms, especially in the extent of dyspnea, was the most prominent result in all patients and at long term follow-up 80% of all long-term survivors (49/62) were in NYHA class I or II. Improvement by one or two classes was reported by 84% (52/62) of the long-term survivors. Relief from obstruction was documented in 22 patients, who had left heart catheterization up to 6 months post-op (Fig. 2 and Fig. 3).

Seventy-seven percent of all patients were in sinus rhythm; 14% had a

Survival (%)   Cumulative Survival Proportion

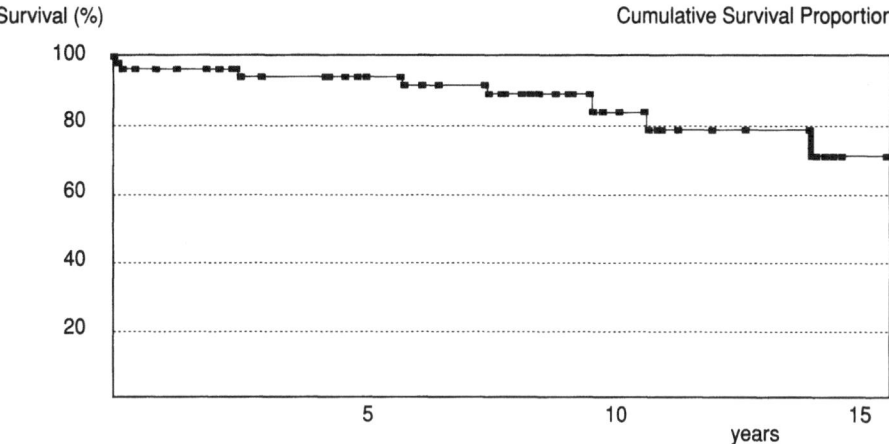

Fig. 1. Plot of cumulative (percent) survival of the whole patient cohort in 16 years calculated with Kaplan-Meier method

permanent pacemaker implanted, seven patients during follow-up, 3 patients directly postoperatively and one patient had his pacemaker already implanted preoperatively. Twenty-two patients had paroxysmal atrial fibrillation and 3 patients had chronic atrial fibrillation. No episodes of ventricular tachycardia were documented early or late.

Echocardiographic studies at long-term follow-up showed a wall thickness of the ventricular septum, which was impressively low (13.4 ± 4 mm) and significantly different from preoperative evaluation (25 ± 5 mm, $p < 0.005$). Measurements of left ventricular end-diastolic diameters (46 ± 6 mm) and end-systolic diameters (32 ± 8 mm) revealed near to normal left ventricular cavity dimensions. None of the patients showed relevant SAM, 8 patients had trivial SAM (1 +). Doppler studies in all patients revealed no flow acceleration at the mid-cavity level or within the outflow tract. No significant mitral regurgitation was detectable, and no aortic regurgitation occurred.

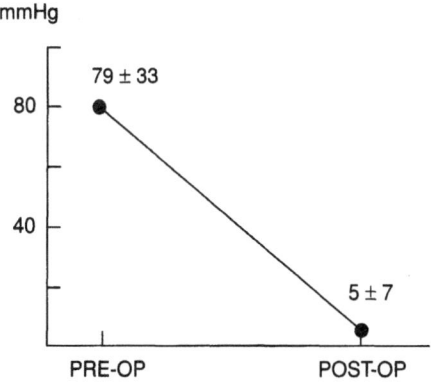

Fig. 2. Left ventricular outflow tract gradients in 22 patients with hypertrophic obstructive cardiomyopathy under basal conditions before (pre-op) and after surgery (post-op)

mmHg

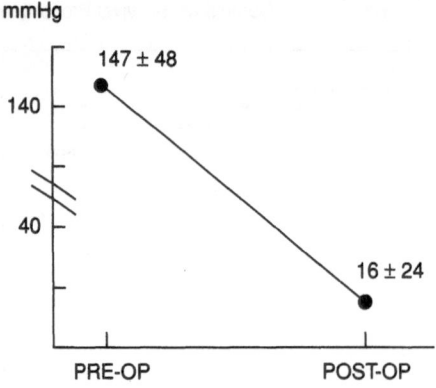

Fig. 3. Left ventricular outflow tract gradients in 22 patients with hypertrophic obstructive cardiomyopathy after provocation (amyl-nitrite inhalation, Valsalva maneouver) before (pre-op) and after surgery

Discussion

Surgical therapy, especially myotomy-myectomy with resection of septal tissue has proven in a number of large series [8-11] to relieve both outflow gradients and symptoms in patients with HOCM. Early mortality rates with myotomy-myectomy are today localised well below 5% and in selected centres, where the most operations are performed, they are even less than 2% [1]. Thus far myotomy-myectomy is still the gold standard for surgical therapy in HOCM patients. Yet, limitations of the classical technique are well recognised, as it includes an inherent risk of creating ventricular septal perforation or, vice versa, resulting in incomplete relief. This dilemma is due to the fact that the tissue identified for resection cannot be exposed completely from a transaortic approach and is therefore not clearly defined. In our experience we obtained a sustained relief in surgically treated HOCM patients without SAM or significant mitral regurgitation at long-term follow-up and with no sudden cardiac death during follow-up. Moreover, no ventricular septal defect was created with this modified technique of septal myectomy.

Several reasons account for these beneficial results. Firstly, insertion of a sharp triple hook retractor simplifies myectomy in that the amount of septal tissue suitable for resection is fixed, and the directions in which incisions are to be performed are clearly defined. Secondly, extension of myectomy behind the insertion of the mural leaflet of the mitral valve creates a trough, which is twice to three times as wide as with classical myectomy and resects a toric muscle bundle, constantly inserting from the lateral wall directly in the mitral annulus. Thirdly, pulling the sharp triple hook retractor forward exposes septal tissue into the view of the surgeon and extends myectomy down to the mid-portions of the left ventricle. In addition, our technique corrects not only the thickened septum but also addresses the changes in papillary muscle morphology which contribute significantly to the pathophysiology of HOCM.

Transaortic extended myectomy and reconstruction of subvalvular mitral apparatus has proven to be a highly effective therapy for patients with severe HOCM. Yet, these favorable results have not prompted extended indications for surgery. We still restrict surgical intervention to severely symptomatic patients, however, there was no more indication for mitral valve replacement during the past 15 years. Continuous follow-up will be necessary to confirm favorable results, nonetheless, application of the presented surgical approach to obstruction may be recommended.

References

1. Spirito P, Seidman, CE, McKenna WJ, Maron BJ (1997) The management of hyper-trophic cardiomyopathy. N Engl J Med 336:775-785
2. McIntosh CI, Maron BJ (1988) Current operative treatment of obstructive hypertrophic cardiomyopathy. Circulation 78:487-495
3. Morrow AG, Reitz BA, Epstein SE, Conkle DM, Itscoitz SB, Redwood DR (1975) Operative treatment in hypertrophic subaortic stenosis. Techniques and the results of pre- and postoperative assessment in 83 patients. Circulation 52:88-102
4. Cooley DA, Leachmann RD, Hallmann GL (1971) IHSS: Surgical treatment including mitral valve replacement. Arch Surg 17:606-612
5. Messmer BJ (1994) Extended myectomy for hypertrophic obstructive cardiomyopathy. Ann Thorac Surg 58:575-577
6. Schoendube, FA, Klues HG, Reith S, Messmer BJ (1994) Surgical correction of hyper-trophic obstructive cardiomyopathy with combined myectomy, mobilisation and partial excision of the papillary muscles. Eur J Cardiothorac Surg 8:603-608
7. Schoendube FA, Klues HG, Reith, S, Flachskampf FA, Hanrath P, Messmer BJ (1995) Long-term clinical and echocardiographic follow-up after surgical correction of hyper-trophic obstructive cardiomyopathy with extended myectomy and reconstruction of the subvalvular mitral apparatus. Circulation 92 (Suppl 2):II-122-127
8. Beahrs MM, Abdul JT, Seward JB, Guiliani ER, McGoon DC (1983) HOCM: 10 to 21 year follow-up after partial septal myectomy. Am J Cardiol 51:1160-1166
9. Seiler C, Hess OM, Schoenbeck M, Turina J, Jenni R, Turina M, Krayenbuehl HP (1991) Long-term follow-up of medical versus surgical therapy for hypertrophic cardiomyopathy: a retrospective study. J Am Coll Cardiol 17:634-642
10. Ten Berg JM, Maarten JS, Knaepen PJ, Ernst SM, Vermeulen FE, Jaarsma W (1994) Hypertrophic obstructive cardiomyopathy: Initial results and long-term follow-up after Morrow septal myectomy. Circulation 90:1781-1785
11. Robbins RC, Stinson EB (1996) Long-term results of left ventricular myotomy and myectomy for obstructive hypertrophic cardiomyopathy. J Thorac Cardiovasc Surg 111:586-594

DILATED CARDIOMYOPATHY
Etiology, Pathophysiology and Clinical Data

Genetic Basis of Dilated Cardiomyopathy

J.A. Towbin, K.R. Bowles, R. Ortiz-Lopez and Q. Wang

Introduction

Dilated cardiomyopathy (DCM) is a disease of the myocardium characterized by dilation and impaired function of the left ventricle or both ventricles in the absence of coronary artery disease, valvular abnormalities, pericardial disease, and specific myocardial inflammatory diseases including myocarditis [1]. In general, systolic dysfunction is the main clinical feature with resultant signs and symptoms of congestive heart failure. Although the cause of DCM is usually not known, familial transmission is found in some cases. In this manuscript, the current understanding of the genetic causes of DCM is described.

Incidence and Prevalence of DCM

DCM is reported to be the most common form of cardiomyopathy with an annual incidence of 2-8 cases per 100,000 in the United States and Europe and an estimated prevalence of 36 affected individuals per 100,000 population [2].

Genetically transmitted DCM, so-called familial DCM (FDCM), appears to occur in up to 20%-30% of cases. Michels et al. [3] and Mestroni et al. [4] initially showed familial transmission in 6%-7% of cases based on history. Later, Michels et al. [5] evaluated relatives of probands by echocardiography and identified 20% of families to be affected, albeit without symptoms in many individuals. More recently, Keeling et al. [6] and Gregori et al. [7] both found up to 30% of cases to be familial. In most cases, autosomal dominant inheritance is identified but autosomal recessive, X-linked, and mitochondrial (maternal) inheritance also occur [8].

Identification of Mendelian and mitochondrial inheritance in DCM suggests that single genes may be responsible for the Mendelian inherited forms of DCM while mitochondrial genome mutations are likely causes of the maternally inherited cases. This speculation has recently led to an explosion of molecular genetic studies focused on the mapping and identification of FDCM-causing genes. Although progress has been only modest thus far, several important advances have been reported and are described below.

Dilated Cardiomyopathy with X-linked Inheritance

Two different forms of X-linked dilated cardiomyopathy have been described. The first type, which most commonly presents in infancy, is associated with neutropenia, skeletal myopathy, abnormal mitochondria, and 3-methylgluta- conic aciduria [9,10,11]. The young boys usually present with congestive heart failure and, in many cases, succumb in infancy or early childhood. This form of DCM, known as Barth syndrome, is often associated with episodes of sepsis. Respiratory chain abnormalities have been identified.

The second form of X-linked DCM (XLCM), first described by Berko and Swift [12], usually presents in teenage boys or young adult males in their twenties and progresses rapidly to death or transplantation. Manifesting fema- le carriers may be diagnosed in the fourth or fifth decade and progression is typically slow. In most cases, creatine kinase (total CK and muscle isoform MM-CK) is significantly elevated but little or no skeletal myopathy is iden- tified.

Significant progress has been made in the molecular genetic study of both Barth syndrome and XLCM. In both cases, gene mapping and identification, along with the discovery of gene mutations, have been reported.

Barth Syndrome: Bolhuis et al. [13] initially mapped the gene for Barth syndrome to the long arm of the X-chromosome at Xq28. Identification of the putative gene came several years later with the cloning of G4.5 by Bione et al. [14]. This gene, which consists of 6234 bp, 11 exons, and is differentially spliced, encodes a novel new family of proteins termed "tafazzins". The protein products range in length from 129-292 amino acids and probably act as structural membrane proteins. Mutations have been described including point mutations and an insertion mutation, all of which introduce a stop codon in the open reading frame of the gene and interfere with translation of the protein. Analysis of the exact function(s) of this gene product is ongoing.

XLCM: Towbin et al. [15] first identified genetic linkage to Xp21 at the dystrophin locus in the family initially described by Berko and Swift [12]. In addition to linkage, immunoblotting identified absence or low abundance of dystrophin protein in the myocardium of these patients using N-terminal and rod region antibody, as well as reduced abundance of the 156kD dystrophin- associated glycoprotein (α-dystroglycan) [16]. Analysis of skeletal muscle dystrophin with these antibodies, however, was normal. Subsequently, Muntoni et al. [17] described a deletion of the muscle promoter and exon 1 in a family with XLCM. Similar mutations were later identified by Yoshida et al. (exon 1 deletion) [18] and Milasin et al. (point mutation which alters the consensus sequence of the splicing site of the first muscle exon-intron junction) [19]. Interestingly, the expression of all major dystrophin mRNA isoforms (from the muscle-, brain-, and Purkinje cell-promoters) is comple- tely abolished in the myocardium, while the brain- and Purkinje cell-isoforms (but not the muscle-promoter isoform) are detectable in skeletal muscle [20], consistent with the immunoblotting studies.

Recently, other mutations in dystrophin have been identified that cause the XLCM phenotype. Our laboratory identified the causative mutation in the original family to be a missense mutation (A to G) in exon 9 [21]. This mutation results in the substitution of the amino acid threonine to alanine at position 279 of the protein, that alters of the secondary structure of dystrophin within the first hinge region (between the N-terminus and rod region), causing a change in the flexibility of the protein and destabilization of the muscle membrane.

Finally, Yoshida et al. [18] described deletion of exon 48 in association with severe DCM and very mild skeletal muscle disease (i.e., mild Becker muscular dystrophy). Whether this mutation can cause a pure cardiac phenotype is currently speculative.

Dilated Cardiomyopathy with Autosomal Dominant Inheritance

This form of FDCM is characterized by systolic dysfunction and ventricular dilation occurring between the late teenage years to early thirties, with progressive congestive heart failure and ventricular arrhythmias [1,2]. Typically, these families exhibit low penetrance of disease, absence of early clinical findings, and premature and unexpected death.

Families with "pure" FDCM and autosomal dominant inheritance have been used to map three genetic loci thus far by the genome-wide screening approach. Krajinovic et al. [22] localized a gene to 9q13-q22 in three families with FDCM, while we successfully mapped FDCM-causing genes to 1q32 in one family [23] and 10q21-q23 in another famil. [24]. In the latter, mitral valve prolapse was also associated. None of these genes have thus far been identified.

Gene mapping studies have also successfully been employed in two large families with DCM and conduction system disease. In this peculiar form of FDCM, the patients present with a variety of types of conduction defects including atrioventricular block and arrhythmias during the second to third decade of life and progresses to DCM with congestive heart failure in the fifth to sixth decade. Kass et al. [25] were the first to identify linkage in a large Ohio family, mapping this gene to the centromere of chromosome 1 (1p1-1q1). Although the connexin 40 gene was considered a good candidate gene, it was later excluded. More recently, Olson and Keating mapped a gene to 3p22-p25 in a Swiss-German family with similar clinical presentation [26]. The genes causing FDCM and conduction system disease have also remained elusive.

Recently, Maeda et al. [27] demonstrated that metavinculin abnormalities may be responsible for FDCM while Fadic et al. [28] showed adhalin abnormalities in another group of patients with DCM. The genes encoding these proteins, and other similar proteins, appear to be excellent candidate genes in FDCM.

Mitochondrial Cardiomyopathies

Dilated cardiomyopathy (or hypertrophic cardiomyopathy), with or without skeletal muscle and neurologic disease, has been shown to occur in families with maternal transmission of disease [29]. Mitochondrial DNA (mtDNA) differs from nuclear genomic DNA in that it has no introns, no protective histones, and no effective DNA repair system; the mutation rate is more than 10-fold that of nuclear DNA. In addition, the presence of normal and mutated mtDNA in the same cell and tissue in variable amount (heteroplasmy) could explain the potential selective involvement of the heart, the variability of penetrance and expression, and the clinical heterogeneity among siblings [29].

Energy generation is dependent on the oxidative phosphorylation mechanism (ox-phos) that takes place in mitochondria, which are found in the cytoplasm of most cell types. Within each mitochondria is a single chromosome that encodes for a number of the enzymes of ox-phos (i.e., encodes for 13 of the 69 proteins required for oxidative metabolism) and the tRNAs and rRNAs required for their translation). The remaining enzymes of the ox-phos pathway are encoded by genes on the nuclear chromosomes and the resultant proteins are transported into the mitochondrion. Genetic defects of ox-phos, therefore, can be due either to gene mutations within the X chromosome or autosomes (i.e., nuclear chromosomes), resulting in diseases that behave as Mendelian recessive traits, or to mitochondrial genome defects that cause diseases with non-Mendelian transmission.

The development of DCM is a common clinical feature of several well-known mitochondrial syndromes including MELAS (*M*itochondrial *M*yopathy, *E*ncephalopathy, *L*actic *A*cidosis, and *S*troke-like episodes), MERRF (*M*yoclonus *E*pilepsy and *R*agged *R*ed *F*ibers), *K*earns-*S*ayre *S*yndrome (KSS), and NADH-Coenzyme Q reductase deficiency, amongst others [8,29,30]. In some cases, a cardiospecific phenotype occurs.

Multiple deletions and point mutations in mtDNA have been described in both sporadic and familial cases of DCM [8,29,30]. In fact, there appear to be certain hot spots of the mitochondrial genome where mutations seem to cause DCM (or HCM). These include mtDNA point mutations A3243G in tRNA(Leu) (UUR) and A8344G in tRNA(Lys) which are commonly seen in MELAS and MERRF, respectively. Deletions are commonly seen in KSS.

FDCM Associated with Muscle Disease

The muscular dystrophies are commonly associated with DCM and this cardiac abnormality may play a significant role in the course of disease and survival. The most common forms of muscular dystrophy with DCM include the X-linked forms Duchenne muscular dystrophy and the allelic and less severe Becker muscular dystrophy, X-linked Emery-Dreifuss muscular dystrophy, autosomal dominant myotonic dystrophy (DM) [8], and autosomal dominant limb-girdle muscular dystrophy with cardiac involvement [31].

Duchenne muscular dystrophy and Becker muscular dystrophy and BMD are due to mutations (usually deletions) within the dystrophin gene at Xp21 [8]. This gene, which also causes XLCM when mutated, is the largest gene known (2.5 Mb; 79 exons; 14 Kb mRNA encoding a 457 kD protein) thus far. Out-of-frame mutations typically cause the more severe form of Duchenne muscular dystrophy in which children become wheelchair-bound before age 11 years; in-frame mutations are most commonly responsible for the less severe BMD where children become wheelchair bound beyond age 16 years [32]. Serum CK, particularly CK-MM, clinically marks the skeletal muscle abnormality. The disease is characterized by progressive, generalized muscle weakness and "pseudohypertrophy" of certain muscle groups, particularly the calf. The incidence of Duchenne muscular dystrophy is estimated to be 1 in 3300 live male births and has a high spontaneous mutation rate. The dystrophin protein is a cytoskeletal protein [33] tightly associated with a large oligomeric complex of sarcolemmal glycoproteins [34] including dystroglycan, which binds laminin, a major protein component of the extracellular matrix, and sarcoglycan, which binds to the dystroglycan complex within the sarcolemma. Mutations in dystrophin appear to uncouple the dystrophin from these complexes. In addition, mutations in the dystroglycan/sarcoglycan genes appear to be responsible for other forms of muscular dystrophy (i.e., limb-girdle) in which DCM can occur.

Emery Dreifuss muscular dystrophy is a relatively rare disorder characterized by weakness in the humeroperoneal distribution, early joint contractures, DCM, and X-linked (or, occasionally, autosomal dominant) inheritance [35]. The onset of disease usually occurs between 2 and 10 years of age, with weakness initially noted in the shoulder girdles and upper extremities. The disease evolves slowly and usually stabilizes in the third decade with most patients remaining ambulatory. DCM is common and atrioventricular block is also frequently seen. The gene responsible for Emery Dreifuss muscular dystrophy was initially mapped to Xq28 before being identified as emerin (or STA) which encodes a serine-rich 254 amino acid protein with uncertain function [36]. This 35 kD nuclear membrane protein is seen in both skeletal and cardiac muscle and has been postulated to have a structural role.

Myotonic dystrophy is the most common form of inherited muscular dystrophy in adults, with an incidence of 1 in 8,000 persons [37]. This autosomal dominant disorder affects multiple organ systems; penetrance varies with age and the disease may affect different tissues at different periods of life. The classic clinical presentation of myotonic dystrophy is that of a young adult with new-onset weakness of hands or mild foot drop. Cardiac conduction abnormalities are common (and may be progressive) and DCM may occur. The gene for myotonic dystrophy was mapped to 19q13 and later identified to be myotonin protein kinase, a serine-threonine protein kinase. The genetic basis for myotonic dystrophy is the presence of long stretches of three bases repeated in tandem and referred to as triplet repeats; the severity of disease appears to relate to the length of the repeat expansion with < 50 repeats associated with no disease, 100-250 repeats causing mild to moderate disease, and > 250 repeats causing a more severe phenotype [38]. Melacini et al. showed overt clinical cardiac symptoms (i.e., syncope) and ECG abnormalities to be directly correlated to the size of the triplet repeat expansion [39].

Conclusion

Progress is currently being made in the genetics of DCM. To date, only a handful of DCM-causing genes have been identified (i.e., dystrophin, G4.5) with several other genetic loci mapped. As has been shown in other cardio-vascular diseases such as familial hypertrophic cardiomyopathy (FHCM) and inherited long QT syndrome, a final common pathway is typically responsible for the clinical cardiac phenotype. For instance, in FHCM, defects in genes encoding sarcomeric proteins produce the clinical features seen echocardiographically [40] while long QT syndrome is caused by mutations in genes encoding ion channels [41]. Using these disorders as prototypes, we can speculate that FDCM genes will likely encode similar protein products. Hence, based on the current information on dystrophin, G4.5, the dystrophin-associated glycoprotein complex, and metavinculin, it is likely that the genes responsible for the FDCM phenotypes will encode cytoskeletal/structural membrane proteins. The answers should be forthcoming.

References

1. Report of the 1995 World Health Organization/International Society and Federation of Cardiology Task Force on the definition and classification of cardiomyopathies (1996) Circulation 93:841-842
2. Manolio TA, Baughman KL, Rodenheffer R, Pearson TA, Bristow JD, Michels VV, Abelman WH, Harlan WR (1992) Prevalence and etiology of idiopathic dilated cardiomyopathy (Summary of a National Heart Lung and Blood Institute Workshop). Am J Cardiol 69:1458-1466
3. Michels VV, Driscoll DJ, Miller FA Jr. (1985) Familial aggregation of idiopathic dilated cardiomyopathy. Am J Cardiol 55:1232-1233
4. Mestroni L, Miani D, DiLenarda A, Silvestri F, Bussani R, Filippi G, Camerini F (1990) Clinical and pathologic study of familial dilated cardiomyopathy. Am J Cardiol 65:1449-1453
5. Michels VV, Moll PP, Miller FA, Tajik AJ, Chu JS, Driscoll DJ, Burnett JC, Rodeheffer RJ, Chesebro JH, Tazelaar HD (1992) The frequency of familial dilated cardiomyopathy in a series of patients with idiopathic dilated cardiomyopathy. N Engl J Med 326:77-82
6. Keeling PJ, Gang Y, Smith G, Seo H, Bent SE, Murday V, Cafario ALP, McKenna WJ (1995) Familial dilated cardiomyopathy in the United Kingdom. Br Heart J 73:417-421
7. Gregori D, Rocco C, di Lenarda A, Sinagra G, Miocic S, Camerini F, Mestroni L (1996) Estimating the frequency of familial dilated cardiomyopathy and the risk of misclassification errors. Circulation 94:1-6
8. Towbin JA (1993) Molecular genetic aspects of cardiomyopathy. Biochem Med Metab Biol 49:285-320
9. Neustein HB, Lurie PR, Dahms B, Takahashi M (1979) An X-linked recessive cardiomyopathy with abnormal mitochondria. Pediatrics 64:24-29
10. Barth PG, Scholte HR, Berden JA, Van der Klei-Van Moorsel JM, Luyt-Houwen IEM, Van 'T Veer-Korthof ETH, Van der Harten JJ, Sobotka-Plojhar MA (1983) An X-linked mitochondrial disease affecting cardiac muscle skeletal muscle and neutrophil leukocytes. J Neurol Sci 62:327-355
11. Kelley RI, Chyeatham JP, Clark BJ, Nigro MA, Powell BR, Sherwood GW, Sladky JT, Swisher WP (1991) X-linked dilated cardiomyopathy with neutropenia, growth retardation, and 3-methyl glutaconic aciduria. J Pediatr 119:738-747
12. Berko BA, Swift M (1987) X-linked dilated cardiomyopathy N Engl J Med 316:1186-1191

13. Bolhuis PA, Hensels GW, Hulsebos TJM, Baas F, Barth PG (1991) Mapping of the locus for X-linked cardioskeletal myopathy with neutropenia and abnormal mitochondria (Barth syndrome) to Xq28. Am J Hum Genet 48:481-485

14. Bione S, D'Adamo P, Maestrini E, Gedeon AK, Bolhuis PA, Toniolo D (1996) A novel X-linked gene, G4.5 is responsible for Barth syndrome. Nature Genet 12:385-389

15. Towbin JA, Hejtmancik JF, Brink P, Gelb BD, Zhu XM, Chamberlain JS, McCabe ERB, Swift M (1993) X-linked dilated cardiomyopathy: molecular genetic evidence of linkage to the Duchenne muscular dystrophy (dystrophin) gene at the Xp21 locus. Circulation 87:1854-1865

16. Towbin JA (1995) Biochemical and molecular characterization of X-linked dilated cardiomyopathy (XLCM). In: Clark EB, Markwald RR, Takao A (eds) Developmental mechanisms of heart disease. Futura Publishing Co. New York, pp 121-132

17. Muntoni F, Cau M, Ganau A, Congiu R, Arvedi G, Mateddu A, Marrosu MG, Cianchetti C, Realdi G, Cao A, Antonietta M (1993) Brief report: Deletion of the dystrophin muscle-promoter region associated with X-linked dilated cardiomyopathy. N Engl J Med 329:921-925

18. Yoshida K, Ikeda S, Nakamura A, Kagoshima M, Takeda S, Shoji S, Yanagisawa N (1993) Molecular analysis of the Duchenne muscular dystrophy gene in patients with Becker muscular dystrophy presenting with dilated cardiomyopathy. Muscle & Nerve 16:1161-1166

19. Milasin J, Muntoni F, Severini GM, Bartoloni L, Vatta M, Krajinovic M, Mateddu A, Angelini C, Camerini F, Falaschi A, Mestroni L, Giacca M (1996) A point mutation in the 5' splice site of the dystrophin gene first intron responsible for X-linked dilated cardiomyopathy. Hum Mol Genet 5:73-79

20. Muntoni F, Wilson L, Marrosu G, Marrosu MG, Cianchetti C, Mestroni L, Ganau A, Dubowitz V, Sewry C (1995) A mutation in the dystrophin gene selectively affecting dystrophin expression in the heart. J Clin Invest 96:693-699

21. Ortiz-Lopez R, Su J, Goytia V, Towbin JA (1997) Evidence for a dystrophin missense mutation as a cause of X-linked dilated cardiomyopathy (XLCM). Circulation 95:2434-2440

22. Krajinovic M, Pinamonti B, Sinagra G, Vatta M, Severini GM, Milasin J, Filaschi A, Camerini F, Giacca M, Mestroni L (1995) Linkage of familial dilated cardiomyopathy to chromosome 9. Am J Hum Genet 57:846-852

23. Durand J-B, Bachinski LL, Bieling L, Czernuszewicz GZ, Abchee AB, Yu QT, Tapscott T, Hill R, Ifegwu J, Marian AJ, Brugada R, Daiger S, Gregoritch JM, Anderson J, Quinones M, Towbin JA, Roberts R (1995) Localization of a gene responsible for familial dilated cardiomyopathy to chromosome 1q32. Circulation 92:3387-3389

24. Bowles KR, Gajarski R, Porter P, Goytia V, Bachinski L, Roberts R, Pignatelli R, Towbin JA (1996) Gene mapping of familial autosomal dominant dilated cardiomyopathy to chromosome 10q21-23. J Clin Invest 98:1355-1360

25. Kass S, MacRae C, Graber HL, Sparks EA, McNamara D, Boudoulas H, Basson CT, Baker PB, Cody RJ, Fishman MC, Cox N, Kong A, Wooley CF, Seidman JG, Seidman CE (1994) A gene defect that causes conduction system disease and dilated cardiomyopathy maps to chromosome 1p1-1q1. Nature Genet 7:546-551

26. Olson TM, Keating MT (1996) Mapping a cardiomyopathy locus to chromosome 3p22-p25. J Clin Invest 97:528-532

27. Maeda M, Holder E, Lowes B, Bies RD (1997) Dilated cardiomyopathy associated with deficiency of the cytoskeletal protein metavinculin. Circulation 95:17-20

28. Fadic R, Sunada Y, Waclawik AJ, Buck S, Lewandoski PJ, Campbell KP, Lotz BP (1996) Brief report : deficiency of a dystrophin-associated glycoprotein (adhalin) in a patient with muscular dystrophy and cardiomyopathy. N Engl J Med 334:362-366

29 Ozawa T (1994) Mitochondrial cardiomyopathy. Herz 19:105-118

30. Johns DR (1996) The other human genome: mitochondrial DNA and disease. Nature Med 2:1065-1067

31. van der Kooi AJ, Ledderhof TM, de Voogt WG, Res CJ, Bouwsma G, Troost D, Busch HF, Becker AE, de Visser M (1996) A newly recognized autosomal dominant limb-girdle muscular dystrophy with cardiac involvement (LGMD1B) to chromosome 1q11-21. Ann Neurol 39:636-642

32. Malhotra SB, Hart KA, Klamut HJ, Thomas NS, Bodrug SE, Burghes AH, Bobrow M, Harper PS, Thompson MW, Ray PN, Worton RG (1988) Frameshift deletions in patients with Duchenne and Becker muscular dystrophy. Science 242:755-759
33. Ahn AH, Kunkel LM (1993) The structural and functional diversity of dystrophin. Nature Genet 3:283-291
34. Ozawa E, Yoshida M, Suzuki A, Mizuno Y, Hagiwara Y, Noguchi S (1995) Dystrophin-associated proteins in muscular dystrophy. Hum Mol Genet 4:1711-1716
35. Emery AE (1987) X-linked muscular dystrophy with early contractures and cardiomyopathy (Emery-Dreifuss Type). Clin Genet 32:360-367
36. Bione S, Maestrini E, Rivella S, Mancini M, Regis S, Romeo G, Toniolo D (1994) Identification of a novel X-linked gene responsible for Emery-Dreifuss muscular dystrophy. Nature Genet 8:323-327
37. Towbin JA, Roberts R (1994) Cardiovascular diseases due to genetic abnormalities. In: Schlant RC, Alexander RW (eds) Hurst's The Heart, Eighth Edition. McGraw-Hill, New York, pp 1725-1759
38. Fu Y-H, Pizzuti A, Fenwick RG, King J, Rajnarayan S, Dunne PW, Dubel J, Nasser GA, Ashizawa T, de Jong P, Wieringa B, Korneluk R, Perryman MB, Epstein HF, Caskey CT (1992) An unstable triplet repeat in a gene related to myotonic muscular dystrophy. Science 255:1256-1258
39. Melacini P, Villanova C, Menegazzo E, Novelli G, Danieli G, Rizzoli G, Fasoli G, Angelini C, Buja G, Miorelli M, Dallapiccola B, Dalla Volta S (1995) Correlation between cardiac involvement and CTG trinucleotide repeat length in myotonic dystrophy. J Am Coll Cardiol 25:239-245
40. Schwartz K, Carrier L, Guicheney P, Komajda M (1995) Molecular basis of familial cardiomyopathies. Circulation 91:532-540
41. Wang Q, Chen Q, Li H, Towbin JA (1997) Molecular genetics of long QT syndrome: from genes to patients Curr Opinion Cardiol 12:310-320

Virus Infection in Cardiomyopathies: Brief Overview, Recent Advances

S. Tracy and N.M. Chapman

Introduction

Viruses are a primary cause of acute inflammatory human heart disease and are believed to contribute significantly as well to the development of dilated cardiomyopathy (DCM) [1-3]. Human enteroviruses seem at present to be the primary viral agents of human viral heart disease. Based upon isolation of virus from diseased human heart tissue, a host of serological studies, and a variety of molecular data, the coxsackie B viruses (CVBs) are the most common enterovirus group implicated as agents of human heart disease [4,5]. However, within the past few years, adenoviruses have also been implicated in pediatric inflammatory heart disease, and it is possible that adenoviruses may be more common agents of heart disease, at least in children, than the enteroviruses [6]. Other viruses (herpesviruses, influenza viruses, HIV) have been implicated as agents of human heart disease but none close to the frequency of either the CVBs or adenoviruses.

At present, there are no vaccines available against any of the human enteroviruses with the exception of the polioviruses. An adenovirus vaccine is available but is not used to protect against heart disease. Neither are vaccines against the CVBs likely to be developed and made available in the near future. Thus, enteroviral heart disease will remain for the foreseeable future an infectious heart disease for which there are neither vaccines nor effective anti-viral pharmaceuticals.

As enteroviral involvement has been noted in about 25% of DCM cases examined [1-3] and as DCM is a primary contributor to the need for heart transplantation, we have asked whether we might be able to employ artificially-attenuated CVB3 constructs to express key immunomodulatory cytokines as one approach to the treatment of the inflammatory response involved in post-transplantation heart rejection processes.

Methods

Previous work from this laboratory has shown that CVB3 may be artificially attenuated for cardiovirulence by at least two separate mechanisms. In one, the replacement of the 5' non-translated region in an infectious cDNA clone of a CVB3 genome with that from another enterovirus, such as a poliovirus, results in a chimeric virus that is attenuated for heart disease when measured in the C3H/HeJ male mouse. In another approach, the mutation of the U residue at position 234 (in the context, 5'-CG*U*UA) in the 5' non-translated region in CVB3 to either C or G results in attenuation of cardiovirulence when measured in mice ([7]; S Tracy, N Chapman, unpublished). Thus, we believe that it should be possible to develop a useful stable of cardiotropic CVB vectors that are also completely attenuated for cardiac disease.

We have constructed an attenuated CVB3 vector that expresses murine interleukin-4 (IL-4). The murine mRNA coding sequence for IL-4 was cloned at the junction of the viral capsid coding proteins and the non-structural protein coding region, P-2. On either side of the murine IL-4 sequence was cloned a sequence that codes for the recognition amino acid sequence of the viral protease P-2A. Upon translation of the viral genome, the protease P-2A autocatalytically cleaves itself from the nascent viral polyprotein, then cleaves the mIL-4 peptide from the capsid protein, P-1D.

Results

The chimeric genome, pCVB3/0-mIL4, is infectious when transfected in HeLa cells or murine heart fibroblasts. Progeny virus, termed CVB3/0-mIL4, replicates well and without significant kinetic difference in HeLa cells from its parental strain, CVB3/0 [8].

That CVB3/0-mIL-4 expresses murine IL-4 in HeLa cells was confirmed by ELISA. Virus was inoculated onto HeLa cells, excess virus removed by washing at one hour post infection, and the cells were refed. At various times post-inoculation, the supernatant was removed and then the cells were frozen in a similar volume of fresh medium. Following freezing and thawing and removal of cell debris by centrifugation, the cell medium samples and the cell fractions were assayed using a commerically available ELISA test for murine IL-4 (BioSource International, Inc.). CVB3/0-mIL-4 produced mIL-4 intracellularly well above the uninfected control background, reaching 300 pg/ml by 6 hours in cultures producing 10^6 TCID$_{50}$ units of virus/ml.

CVB3/0-mIL4 expressed murine IL-4 is also biologically active. HeLa cells were infected with the virus, washed with media, incubated for 6-8 hours, then frozen and thawed. Supernatants cleared of cellular debris were assayed for ability to induce MC/9 mouse mast cells to proliferate using an MTT assay [9] with recombinant mIL-4 as standard. CVB3/0-mIL-4-infected HeLa cultures produced 3 units/ml (equivalent to 250 pg/ml of recombinant mIL-4). This compares favorably with IL-4 levels in coronary sinus blood concentrations in cardiac transplant patients (229 pg/ml; [10]) .

In an initial test of the ability of CVB3/0-mIL-4 to decrease inflammatory disease induced by enteroviruses, we employed a pancreovirulent CVB4 strain (CVB4/V; [11]) as the inducer of inflammatory disease. A different CVB serotype was chosen in these early experiments to obviate the possibility that neutralizing antibodies might reduce the replication of CVB3/0-mIL-

4 in the doubly-infected mouse. The pancreatic disease induced by CVB4 is likely to have an immune component based on the lack of correlation between virulence and virus replication in the pancreas and the dependence upon host genetic background [12].

One or three days following inoculation of mice with CVB4/V, mice were inoculated with CVB3/0-mIL-4. Control mice were inoculated with the parental (without mIL-4 insert and 2A-cleavage site insert) CVB3/0 at the same times or were inoculated either with unsupplemented media without virus or with a single virus (CVB3/0-mIL-4, CVB4/V, or CVB3/0). Mice were sacrificed 10 days post-inoculation, the pancreata fixed in formalin, sectioned, stained with hemotoxylin and eosin, and examined microscopically.

All mice inoculated only with CVB4/V incurred massive pancreatic damage. Mice inoculated first with CVB4/V and then subsequently with CVB3/0-mIL-4 either on day 1 or day 3 demonstrated a significant ablation in the extent of disease. Mice that were inoculated with CVB4/V and subsequently were inoculated with the attenuated parental CVB3 strain, CVB3/0, at either day 1 or 3 demonstrated significantly damaged pancreata that were indistinguishable from the CVB4/V only mice. Although serum IL-4 and virus titers in pancreas were not measured in these first experiments, it may be reasonably inferred that the diminution of pancreatic damage observed in mice that received first pancreovirulent CVB4/V, then CVB3/0-mIL-4 on day 1 or 3, is due to the expression of the mIL-4 in the chimeric CVB3 strain.

Discussion

In this work, we have begun to explore the therapeutic potential inherent in an artificially-attenuated and cardiotropic CVB vector that is able to express one or more immunomodulatory cytokines. Preliminary experiments suggest that the expression of just the single key cytokine, IL-4, is sufficient to significantly suppress pancreatic disease caused by another CVB serotype. Current work is examining the effects of this specific virus against enterovirus-induced murine heart disease and will soon be extended to studying the effects upon allograft survival in a murine model of heart transplantation. We believe this approach holds significant potential for a novel and useful approach to therapy of inflammatory diseases of the heart.

Acknowledgement. This study was supported in part by grants from the National Institutes of Health and the American Heart Association.

References

1. Martino T, Liu P, Petric M, Sole M (1995) Enteroviral myocarditis and dilated cardiomyopathy: a review of clinical and experimental studies. In: Rotbart H (ed) Human Enterovirus Infections. ASM Press, Washington, D.C.
2. Martino T, Liu P, Sole M (1994) Viral infection and the pathogenesis of dilated cardiomyopathy. Circ Res 74:182-188

3. Tracy S, Chapman N, Mahy B (eds) (1997) The Coxsackie B Viruses. Springer-Verlag, Berlin Heidelberg New York
4. Woodruff J (1980) Viral myocarditis. A review. Am J Pathol 101:425-484
5. Friman G, Wesslen L, Fohlman J et al. (1995) The epidemiology of infectious myocarditis, lymphocytic myocarditis and dilated cardiomyopathy. Eur Heart J 16 [Suppl O]:36-41
6. Martin AB, Webber S, Fricker FJ, Jaffe R, Demmier G, Kearney D, Zhang Y_H, Bodurtha J, Gelb B, Ni J, Bricker JT, Towbin JA (1994) Acute myocarditis. Rapid diagnosis by PCR in children. Circulation 90:330-339
7. Tu, Z, Chapman N, Hufnagel G, Tracy S, Romero JR, Barry WH, Zhao L, Currey K, Shapiro B (1995) The cardiovirulent phenotype of coxsackievirus B3 is determined at a single site in the genomic 5' nontranslated region. J Virol 69:4607-4618
8. Chapman N, Tu Z, Tracy S, Gauntt C (1994) An infectious cDNA copy of the genome of a non-cardiovirulent coxsackievirus B3 strain: its complete sequence analysis and comparison to the genomes of cardiovirulent coxsackieviruses. Arch Virol 135:115-130
9. Gieni R, Li Y, HayGlass K (1995) Comparison of [^{3}H] thymidine incorporation with MTT- and MTS-based bioassays for human and murine IL-2 and IL-4 analysis. Tetrazolium assays provide markedly enhanced sensitivity. J Immunol Methods 187:85-93
10. Fyfe A, Daly P, Galligan L, Pirc L, Feindel C, Cardella C (1993) Coronary sinus sampling of cytokines after heart transplantation: evidence for macrophage activation and interleukin-4 production within the graft. J Am Coll Cardiol 21:171-176
11. Ramsingh A, Araki H, Bryant S, Hixson A (1992) Identification of candidate sequences that determine virulence in Coxsackievirus B4. Virus Res 23:281-292
12. Chapman N, Tracy S, Ramsingh A (1997) The genetics of CVB virulence. In: Tracy S, Chapman N, Mahy B (eds) The Coxsackie B Viruses. Current Topics in Microbiology and Immunology vol 223. Springer-Verlag, Berlin Heidelberg New York, pp 227-258

Organ-Specific Cardiac Autoantibodies in Dilated Cardiomyopathy: Pathogenetic Implications

A.L.P. Caforio, J.H. Goldman, A.J. Haven, M.K. Baig and W.J. McKenna

Introduction

In autoimmune conditions, disease- and organ-specific autoantibodies are found in patients and a proportion of their symptom-free relatives [1]. In patients with dilated cardiomyopathy (DCM) circulating autoantibodies to multiple cardiac autoantigens have been described, providing evidence for autoimmune involvement [2-6]. Using indirect immunofluorescence (IFL) and absorption studies, we reported organ- and disease-specific cardiac autoantibodies in one third of distinct patient series from England [7], Poland [8] and Italy [9]. Similar findings have been presented in DCM patients from the United States [10]. Relevant autoantigens recognised by the antibodies detected by IFL include α (atrial) and β (ventricular and slow skeletal) myosin heavy chain [5]. In the majority of other organ-specific autoimmune conditions autoantibodies are not directly involved in myocardial damage, which is T cell-mediated, but represent reliable pathogenetic markers and non-invasive predictors of symptom-free individuals at risk, particularly relatives of affected patients [1]. We will focus upon clinical significance and pathogenetic implications of the organ-specific cardiac antibodies detected by the IFL test in DCM patients and their relatives.

Cardiac Antibodies Detected by IFL: Frequency in Heart Disease

The pooled frequencies of the different cardiac antibody types detected by IFL in DCM and controls are given in Table 1. Clinical and diagnostic features of patients and control subjects have been reported [7-9]. Sera were tested by indirect IFL at 1/10 dilution on 4 μm-thick unfixed fresh frozen cryostat sections of blood group O normal human atrium, ventricle and skeletal muscle, and cardiac antibody IFL staining patterns were classified as described [7-9]. These patterns are illustrated in the original report [7]. Organ-specific cardiac antibodies were more frequently found in patients with DCM (25%) than in those with other cardiac disease (1%; $p = 0.0001$), with ischemic heart failure (1%, $p = 0.0001$) or in normals (2.5%, $p = 0.0001$). These antibodies were detected at a higher frequency compared to normal only in patients with autoimmune polyendocrine diseases [11].

Table 1. Frequency of the cardiac antibodies detected by IFL in DCM, myocarditis and control subjects

	Organ-specific n (%)	Cross-reactive 1 n (%)	Cross-reactive 2 n (%)
DCM (n = 327)	83 (25)*^	35 (11)*^^	3 (1)
Clinical and biopsy proven myocarditis (n = 35)	7 (20)*^	3 (8)	3 (8)
Healthy relatives of DCM patients (n = 342)	68 (20)*^	19 (5.5)	0 (0)
OCD (n = 160)	1 (1)	7 (4)	5 (3)
IHF (n = 141)	1 (1)	1 (1)	8 (6)
Normals (n = 270)	7 (2.5)	8 (3)	9 (3)

Adapted from references 9-12, 25.
DCM, dilated cardiomyopathy; IHF, ischemic heart failure; OCD, other cardiac disease (n = 55 rheumatic heart disease, n = 67 hypertrophic cardiomyopathy, n = 38 congenital defects)
$* p = 0.0001$ vs disease controls; $^p = 0.0001$ and $^^p = 0.0003$ vs normals

Cardiac antibodies of the cross-reactive 1 type, which exhibited partial organ-specificity for heart antigens by absorption [7], were also more frequently detected in DCM than in controls. Conversely, cardiac antibodies of the cross-reactive 2 type, which were entirely skeletal muscle cross-reactive by absorption [7], were found in similar proportions among the study groups.

Cardiac Antibodies in DCM Patients: Relation with Disease Progression

To determine the relation of cardiac autoantibody and disease status, we performed prospective antibody testing, by IFL and by cardiac specific enzyme-linked immunosorbent assay (ELISA), at diagnosis and at follow-up (mean 14±12 months), in 110 consecutive patients with idiopathic DCM [12]. Patients underwent complete evaluation at diagnosis and clinical and non-invasive assessment at follow-up, including exercise testing with maximal oxygen consumption measurements. The frequency of cardiac specific antibodies by IFL was lower at follow-up than at diagnosis (25% vs 10%, $p = 0.002$). Mean antibody levels at follow-up were also lower than at diagnosis. None of the patients negative at diagnosis, by IFL or ELISA, became positive at follow-up. Presence of antibody at diagnosis was associated with milder symptoms and greater exercise capacity at follow-up, persistence of antibody at follow-up with stable disease and milder symptoms at diagnosis. These data indicated that cardiac specific autoantibodies in DCM become undetectable with disease progression; this is a recognized feature of other autoimmune conditions, e.g. Type 1 diabetes mellitus. Thus, we hypothesized that detection of these antibodies might provide a non-invasive marker of early DCM.

Cardiac Antibodies as Risk Markers of Progression to DCM in Symptom-Free Family Members

Organ-specific autoimmune diseases occur as a result of genetic predisposition and environmental influences [1]. The inheritance of susceptibility is usually polygenic, involving both HLA and non-immune-response genes [13-14]. Genetic susceptibility to autoimmunity is responsible for the fact that circulating autoantibodies, as well as other immune abnormalities, are detected in family members even years before the development of disease [1, 15]. DCM is familial in at least 25% of cases, and 9%-21% of asymptomatic relatives have mild left ventricular enlargement associated with preserved systolic function [16-17], which may indicate early disease [18]. To provide evidence for genetic susceptibility to autoimmunity and to identify symptom-free relatives at potential risk of disease development, we performed non-invasive cardiological assessment and cardiac antibody IFL screening test in 342 symptom-free relatives, 177 from 33 pedigrees with familial DCM and 165 from 31 families with only 1 affected member (non-familial DCM) [19]. The frequency of cardiac antibodies was higher among DCM patients (41%) and their relatives (20%) than in controls (3.5%). Antibodies were not detected in genetically unrelated symptom-free individuals from the same household, in particular the patients' spouses. In 37 (58%) of the pedigrees studied cardiac antibodies were found in the proband and/or in at least one family member, and were more common in familial (24%) than in non-familial DCM (15%). In the 27 remaining families no antibodies were found in the index case, or in family members. Although some relatives from these families could develop cardiac antibodies at follow-up, the data might indicate that in the antibody negative families autoimmunity is not involved. Antibody positive relatives were younger and had larger mean echocardiographic left ventricular end-systolic dimension and reduced percent fractional shortening compared to antibody negative relatives [19]. These findings suggested that the antibody could be associated with early disease, but follow-up was needed to determine whether antibody status was predictive of disease susceptibility.

Short-term follow-up (mean 33±60 months) is currently available in 108 symptom-free relatives who had positive antibody test and/or mild echocardiographic abnormalities at baseline [20]. During follow-up disease progressed in 10 of them. The finding of cardiac antibodies at baseline was more common among relatives who progressed (9/10, 90%) compared to those who did not (52/98, 53%, $p = 0.02$). These data suggest that cardiac antibodies may identify symptom-free relatives at risk of progression to DCM, although extended follow-up is warranted.

Cardiac Antibodies in DCM: Pathogenetic Implications

The presence of organ- and disease-specific cardiac antibodies of IgG class detected by more than one group of investigators in DCM patients from different countries [6-10], supports the involvement of autoimmunity in at least one third of patients, regardless of ethnically related differences in immunogenetic backgrounds. The absence of antibodies in the majority of cases at diagnosis could indicate that cell-mediated autoimmune mechanisms are predominant, and/or that autoimmunity is not involved, but it might also relate to reduction of antibody levels with disease progression [1]. Cardiac antibodies at diagnosis were associated with shorter symptom duration (< 2 years), and minor severity (NYHA functional class I-II) [7], as well as with greater exercise capacity [12]. In the majority of patients who were antibody positive at diagnosis these markers became undetectable at follow-up [12]. These findings strongly suggest that cardiac autoantibodies are early markers and raise the issue that autoimmunity might account for a subset of DCM patients greater than one third.

The absence of antibodies in control patients with heart dysfunction not due to DCM and the decrease in antibody titers with disease progression among DCM patients also point out that these markers are not epiphenomena associated with tissue necrosis of various causes, but represent specific markers of immune pathogenesis. This does not imply that the cardiac-specific autoantibodies detected by IFL have a direct cytotoxic role; at present this hypothesis has not been tested. Passive transfer of the myocarditis/DCM phenotype to genetically susceptible animals by patient sera containing the cardiac-specific antibodies is necessary to provide conclusive evidence for antibody-mediated pathogenesis in this condition [1,15]. This does not undermine the role of the antibodies as disease markers or even as predictors for individuals at risk, as the islet cell autoantibodies in type I diabets mellitus [1,15].

The detection of cardiac-specific antibodies in family members of DCM patients, particularly asymptomatic relatives with mild left ventricular enlargement and/or systolic dysfunction on echocardiography, is in keeping with this view [19]. Furthermore, the available short-term follow-up observations suggest that positive antibody status at baseline evaluation may identify relatives at risk of developing DCM [20]. The relatively high proportion of antibody positive relatives who, in the short-term, did not progress is likely to reflect long-latency period and slow progression rate. This emphasizes the importance of extended follow-up, to better define predictive accuracy of the IFL test and possible role of early preventative therapy, in particular ACE-inhibitors and immunosuppression, in antibody-positive relatives. In addition to the IFL markers [7-9, 11], other antibody specificities are found in DCM [2-6]. At present it is unknown whether the antibody types not detected by IFL (e.g. the anti-β adrenergic receptor [4] or the anti-adenine nucleotide translocator antibodies [3]) will represent independent or additional predictors in symptom-free individuals at risk. It is theoretically conceivable that subjects classified as seronegative for one antibody will be positive for another [1,15] and that combined testing may be advantageous. To this end, standardization of nomenclature and protocols for antibody detection and exchange of sera among laboratories currently assessing the individual antibody specificities will be useful.

References

1. Doniach D, Bottazzo GF (Eds) (1987) Endocrine and other organ-oriented autoimmune disorders. In: Bailliere's Clinical Immunology and Allergy vol 1, London
2. Maisch B, Deeg P, Liebau G, Kochsiek K (1983) Diagnostic relevance of humoral and cytotoxic immune reactions in primary and secondary dilated cardiomyopathy. Am J Cardiol 52:1072-1078
3. Schultheiss HP, Bolte HD (1985) Immunological analysis of autoantibodies against the adenine nucleotide translocator in dilated cardiomyopathy. J Mol Cell Cardiol 17:603-617
4. Magnusson Y, Marullo S, Hoyer S, Waagstein F, Andersson B, Vahlne A, Guillet JG, Strosberg AD, Hjalmarson A, Hoebeke J (1990) Mapping of a functional autoimmune epitope on the β-adrenergic receptor in patients with idiopathic dilated cardiomyopathy. J Clin Invest 86:1658-1663
5. Caforio ALP, Grazzini M, Mann JM, Keeling PJ, Bottazzo GF, McKenna WJ, Schiaffino S (1992) Identification of the α and β myosin heavy chain isoforms as major autoantigens in dilated cardiomyopathy. Circulation 85:1734-1742
6. Goldman JH, Keeling PJ, Warraich RS, Redwood S, Baig KM, Elliott PM, Dalla Libera L, Sanderson JE, Caforio ALP, McKenna WJ (1995) Autoimmunity to α-myosin in a subset of patients with idiopathic dilated cardiomyopathy. Br Heart J 74:598-603
7. Caforio ALP, Bonifacio E, Stewart JT, Neglia D, Parodi O, Bottazzo GF, McKenna WJ (1990) Novel organ-specific circulating cardiac autoantibodies in dilated cardiomyopathy. J Am Coll Cardiol 15:1527-1534
8. Bilinska ZT, Caforio ALP, Grzybowski J, Michalak E, Kusmierczyc-Droszcz B, Goldman JH, Haven AJ, Rydlewska-Sadowska W, McKenna WJ, Ruzyllo W (1995). Organ-specific cardiac autoantibodies in dilated cardiomyopathy: frequency and clinical correlates in Polish patients. Eur Heart J 16:1907-1911
9. Caforio ALP, Bauce B, Boffa GM, De Cian F, Angelini A, Melacini P, Razzolini R, Fasoli G, Chioin R, Schiaffino S, Thiene G, Dalla Volta S (1997) Autoimmunity in myocarditis and dilated cardiomyopathy: cardiac autoantibody frequency and clinical correlates in a patient series from Italy. G Ital Cardiol 27:106-112
10. Neumann DA, Burek CL, Baughman KL, Rose NR, Herskowitz A (1990) Circulating heart-reactive antibodies in patients with myocarditis or cardiomyopathy. J Am Coll Cardiol 16:839-846
11. Caforio ALP, Wagner R, Gill JR, Bonifacio E, Bosi E, Miles A, McKenna WJ, Bottazzo GF (1991) Cardiac autoantibodies: new serological markers for systemic hypertension in autoimmune polyendocrinopathy. Lancet 337:1111-1115
12. Caforio ALP, Goldman JH, Baig MK, Haven AJ, Dalla Libera L, Keeling PJ, McKenna WJ (1997) Cardiac autoantibodies in dilated cardiomyopathy become undetectable with disease progression. Heart 77:62-67
13. Theofilopoulos AN (1995) The basis of autoimmunity: part II. Genetic predisposition. Immunol Today 16:150-159
14. Lander E, Kruglyak L (1995) Genetic dissection of complex traits: guidelines for interpreting and reporting linkage results. Nature Genet 11:241-247
15. Rose NR, Bona C (1991) Defining criteria for autoimmune diseases (Witebsky's postulates revisited). Immunol Today 14:426-428
16. Michels VV, Moll PP, Miller FA, Tajik JA, Chu JS, Driscoll DJ, Burnett JC, Rodeheffer RJ, Chesebro JH, Tazelaar HD (1992) The frequency of familial dilated cardiomyopathy in a series of patients with idiopathic dilated cardiomyopathy. N Engl J Med 326:77-82

17. Keeling PJ, Gang Y, Smith G, Seo H, Bent SE, Murday V, Caforio ALP, McKenna WJ
    (1995) Familial dilated cardiomyopathy in the United Kingdom. Br Heart J 73:417-421
18. Baig MK, Goldman JH, Caforio ALP, Coonar AS, Keeling PJ, McKenna WJ (1998)
    Familial dilated cardiomyopathy: cardiac abnormalities are common in asymptomatic
    relatives and may represent early disease. J Am Coll Cardiol 31:195-201
19. Caforio ALP, Keeling PJ, Zachara E, Mestroni L, Camerini F, Mann JM, Bottazzo GF,
    McKenna WJ (1994) Evidence from family studies for autoimmunity in dilated
    cardiomyopathy. Lancet 344:773-777
20. Caforio ALP, Baig KM, Goldman JH, Haven AJ, Reardon K, McKenna WJ (1997).
    Cardiac autoantibodies may identify asymptomatic relatives at risk of dilated
    cardiomyopathy. J Am Coll Cardiol 29 [Suppl A]: 193A

Inflammatory Cardiomyopathy:
Diagnostic and Therapeutical Options

U. Kühl, M. Pauschinger and H.-P. Schultheiss

Introduction

Strategies for immunosuppressive treatment of chronic inflammatory myocardial diseases are still a controversial issue. This dilemma is still unresolved
despite the "American Myocarditis Trial" which, as many other studies before, could not demonstrate any positive therapeutic effects of the immunosuppressive therapy [1]. This, however, is not due to a general unresponsiveness
of cardiac inflammation to immunosuppressive therapy, but rather reflects an
inappropriate study design, that did not select the optimal group of patients
for therapy. Histological diagnosis of the inflammatory process may have
been inaccurate and the study did not take into consideration the spontaneous
course of the disease or a possible viral persistence [2-8]. Though the prerequisites for diagnosing virus-induced myocardial disease have been considerably improved by new diagnostic techniques in recent years, there have not
yet been any prospective randomized therapeutic studies with precisely
characterized patient populations. Ultimately decisive for the development of
adequate therapeutic strategies, however, is a precise clinical evaluation of
the patients to be treated. Besides documenting the clinical status, it is extremely important to differentially analyze the inflammatory reaction and possible viral persistence in the myocardial tissue by histological, immunohistological and molecular-biological techniques [8]. The histological and particularly the immunohistological techniques accurately detect both the acute and
chronic myocardial inflammatory process [9,10]. New highly sensitive molecular-biological methods such as in situ hybridization and the polymerase
chain reaction (PCR) now detect the viral genome (e.g., enteroviruses) even
for latent infection with restricted replication [11-15]. Only these differential
diagnostics enable precise characterization of the disease process, which is
now a prerequisite for the appropriate selection of patients for treatment.

Virus and Autoimmune Hypothesis

An enteroviral infection is regarded as the triggering event in most cases of
human myocarditis [16]. For a long time, the viral etiology was controversial
for some of the inflammatory myocardial diseases, since the standard virolo-

gical methods only detect myocardial viruses in isolated cases. Only the introduction of sensitive and specific molecular-biological methods like slot blot hybridization [11], in situ hybridization [13,17] and the polymerase chain reaction [12,18] in virological diagnostics enabled the demonstration of very small amounts of genomic viral RNA or DNA in infected myocardial tissue. Apart from enteroviruses [19,20], adenoviruses [21], cytomegaloviruses [22], herpes simplex type 2 viruses and hepatitis C viruses [23] could be detected in varying frequencies when examining myocardial biopsies by molecular-biological techniques.

Apart from the question of myocardial virus persistence, the idea of an autoimmune pathogenesis has recently been gaining importance in discussions on the etiology of the disease and its possible progression to dilated cardiomyopathy. These pathophysiological considerations are supported by numerous clinical and experimental animal studies or immunohistochemical findings. These include the immunohistological detection of myocardial inflammation as well as organ-specific autoantibodies to the myocardial membrane [24] and intracellular target structures like the contractile apparatus or the mitochondria [25-27]. Autoantigens identified thus far include myosin [24], the β receptor [28], the ADP/ATP carrier [29-31], the Ca^{2+} channel [32,33], the connexon of the gap junctions [34], the muscarine receptor and structures of the myocardial connective tissue [35].

Moreover, elevated concentrations of various cytokines such as interleukin-1, interleukin-2 or tumor-necrosis factor-alpha in serum of patients with myocarditis or dilated cardiomyopathy are indicative of an activated immunological process [36,37].

Diagnosis of Myocarditis

Besides in situ hybridization, mainly PCR has become an established procedure in the routine clinical diagnostics for virus detection in endomyocardial biopsies. Different frequencies of viral persistence have been reported so far, ranging from 24% to 56% (Table 1). These differences are probably caused by the different molecular-biological methods that were used and due to a different clinical selection of patients. According to our data, PCR detected enteroviral RNA in endomyocardial biopsies from 54/128 patients suffering from myocarditis or dilated cardiomyopathy [38] (Table 1). Moreover, initial findings also suggest the detectability of replicative intermediates in enteroviral infection of the myocardium by a (+/–)-strand-specific analysis (Pauschinger, unpublished results).

In the past, myocarditis diagnostics were based almost exclusively on histomorphological assessment of criteria in compliance with the Dallas Classification [39]. In the meantime, however, numerous studies have pointed out the limited value of information gained by only performing a histomorphological analysis of the myocardial inflammatory process [8,40-42].

Because of the immune markers applied, the immunohistochemical staining techniques are markedly superior to a purely histological analysis, particu-

Table 1. Molecular-biological detection of enteroviral RNA in endomyocardial biopsies of patients with the tentative clinical diagnosis of dilated cardiomyopathy

	in situ hybridization (from [51])	slot-blot technique (from [19])	Polymerase chain-reaction (from [50])	Polymerase chain-reaction (from [18])
Myocarditis	clinically suspected 23/95 (24%)	histology 28/69 (24%)	histology 5/9 (56%)	histology 26/61 (43%)
Dilated Cardiomyopathy	8/47 (17%)	46/130 (35%)	6/24 (25%)	28/67 (42%)
Controls	0/53 (0%)	2/45 (4%)		0/43 (0%)

larly in diagnosing an inflammatory reaction in the post-acute stage. Besides the exact identification, quantification and phenotypic characterization of the infiltrating cells, it is possible by recording further inflammatory parameters, e.g. adhesion molecules and cytokines, to detect the inflammatory process, even in cases of focal cell infiltration, and thus markedly reduce the sampling error [8-10,43] (Fig. 1).

Normal myocardial tissue without immunohistological evidence of a myocardial inflammatory reaction contains less than 1 lymphocyte per high power field (HPF: magnification x400; mean cell counts: 0.65 ± 0.44 cells (n = 890) [44]. Biopsies must already be regarded as irregular if they contain more than 1.5-2.0 CD3-positive lymphocytes/per field at high magnification (x400), corresponding to 7.0 lymphocytes per mm^2 [8]. The concurrence of enhanced histocompatibility antigen expression and several adhesion molecules in conjunction with these low lymphocyte counts already indicates an immunologically active process in the total myocardial tissue (Table 2).

The higher sensitivity and specificity and the enormous information value of the immunohistological analysis of myocardial biopsies were demonstrated by a prospective study in 299 patients biopsied under the tentative clinical diagnosis of dilated cardiomyopathy [8,38,44]. Histologically, 94,4% of the examined tissues did not present increased immunocompetent infiltrates. The immunohistological examination, on the other hand, demonstrated a persistent inflammatory process with increased lymphocytic infiltrates and a concomitantly enhanced expression of adhesion molecules in 43% of the examined myocardial biopsies (Fig. 2).

Classification of Chronic Inflammatory Myocardial Disease

Cardiomyopathies have been reclassified by the World Health Organization based on clinical and experimental knowledge gained in recent years [16]. Apart from idiopathic (etiology unknown) and familial (approx. 20%) cardiomyopathy, this classification includes the relatively large group of

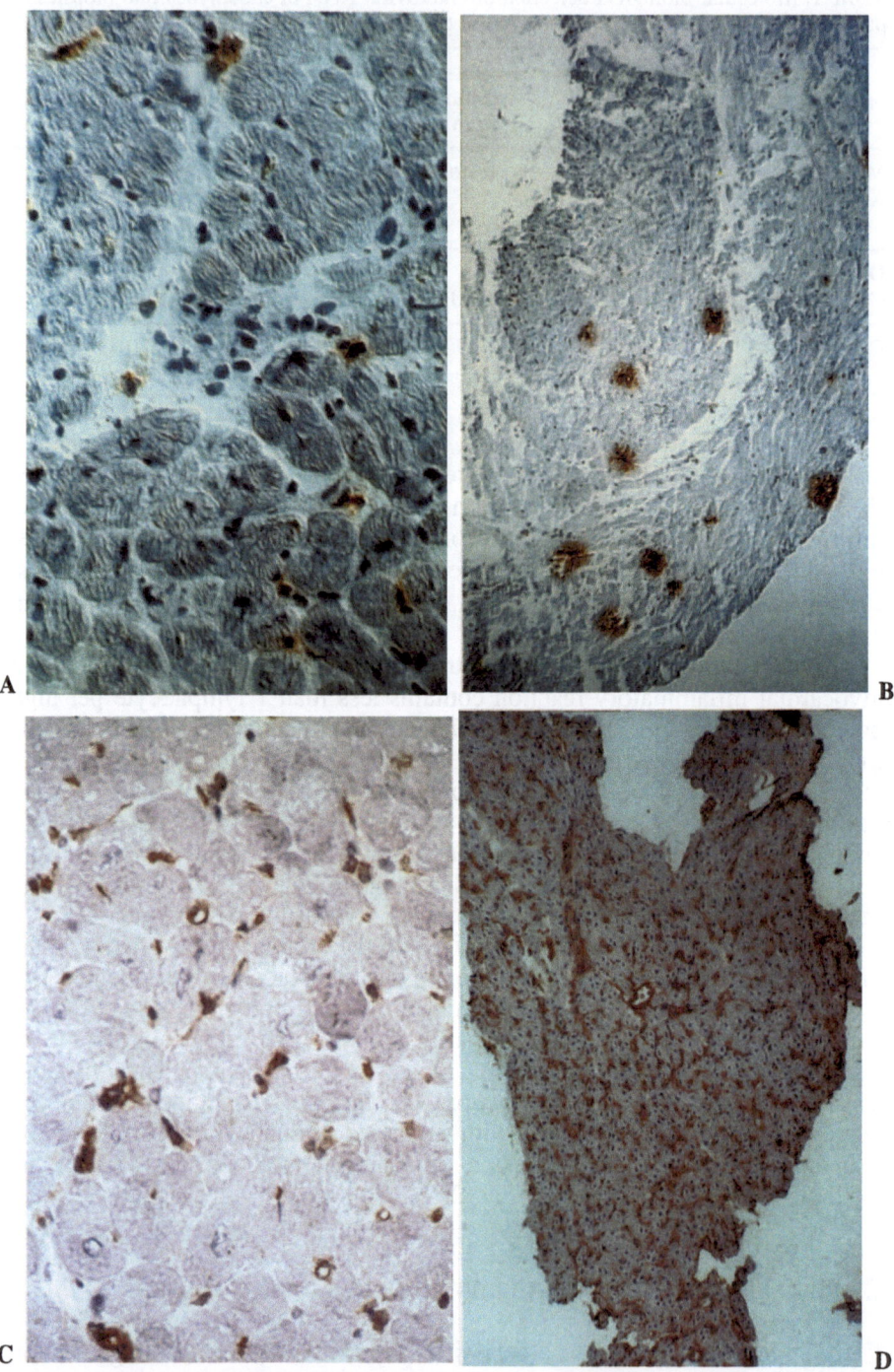

Fig. 1. Immunohistochemical staining of endomyocardial biopsies: anti-CD3 T-lymphocytes (**A**); activated macrophages (**B**); normal (**C**) and enhanced HLA-DR (**D**) staining in cardiac tissue; (magnification: **A-C**: x400, **D**: x40)

Table. 2. Immunohistological definition of cardiac inflammation in patients with inflammatory cardiomyopathy. HPF, high power field, magnification: x 400

Cells/antigens	CD	Definition of pathologically/ positive infiltrating cells
Lymphocytes	CD3	>2,0 cells/HPF (>7,0 cells/mm^2)
Macrophages	27E10/25F9	>2,0 cells/HPF
Lymphocyte - independent markers of inflammation and cell activation		
Interstitial cells	HLA - I/II CD18, CD54	enhanced expression
Endothelium	HLA - I/II CD54, VLA - 4	enhanced expression

inflammatory cardiomyopathies caused by viral and immunological mechanisms as a further significant subgroup [16]. Our investigations now indicate the expediency of dividing dilated cardiomyopathies into at least 4 subgroups based on the described histological, immunohistological and molecular-biological findings from the endomyocardial biopsies [38,44]. These different

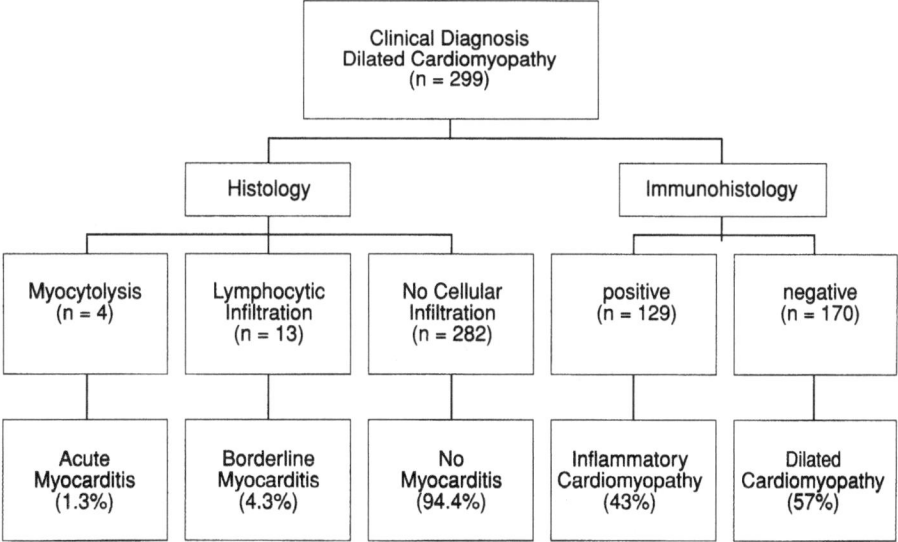

Fig. 2. Comparison of histological and immunohistological analysis of endomyocardial biopsies from 299 patients with a clinical diagnosis of dilated cardiomyopathy

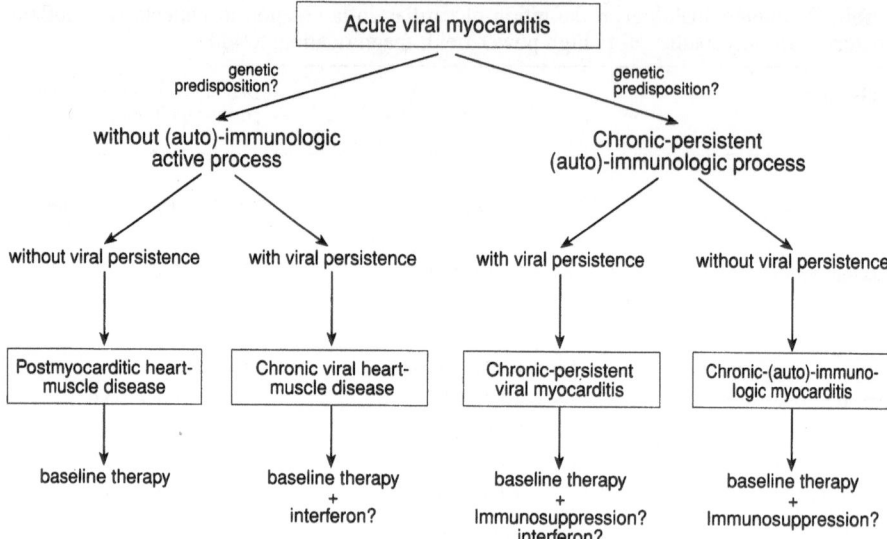

Fig. 3. Immunohistogical and molecular biological classification of inflammatory cardiomyopathy

entities, which can be characterized as disease with or without cardiac inflammation, and within these two groups with or without viral persistance (Fig. 3), markedly influence therapeutic strategies.

Therapeutic Strategies

Acute Myocarditis

Immunosuppressive therapy is not indicated for histologically confirmed acute myocarditis according to the Dallas Classification in view of the negative effects in animal experiments and the high spontaneous healing rate of acute myocarditis [45]. Moreover, studies in mice have demonstrated that early corticoid therapy has fatal consequences in virus-induced myocarditis (Coxsackie-B3) due to delayed virus elimination and extension of the viral replication phase [46]. Suppression of the autoimmune response at this stage of still active viral replication probably promotes a viremia that causes virus-induced myocardial damage (myocytolysis) with subsequent impairment of myocardial function.

Inflammatory Cardiomyopathy

In cases of persistent myocardial inflammation with exclusion of persistent viral replication, immunosuppression is presently under discussion as a suitable causal therapeutic regimen for chronic autoimmune myocarditis. The extremely variable spontaneous course of myocarditis and the inadequate accessibility of the clinical course by single-time observation necessitates a follow-up of the clinical findings and the myocardial inflammatory process at a 3-4 month interval to evaluate the natural course. Provided that persistent inflammation is diagnosed without evidence of improved myocardial function, we recommend immunosuppressive therapy on the basis of our own experience [47,48].

Initial results of our study group suggest that immunohistochemical characterization of chronic autoimmune myocarditis is crucial for the indication of appropriate immunosuppression, leading to significant clinical and hemodynamic improvement in 65%-70% of cases [8,48] (Fig. 4). The clinical and hemodynamic improvement thus achieved lies markedly above the hemodynamic improvement after spontaneous remission of the inflammatory process [8]. Even patients with severely impaired left-ventricular function show significant improvement. It is evident, however, that those with mildly or moderately impaired left-ventricular function and active myocardial inflammation tend to profit more from this anti-inflammatory treatment, since they did not yet develop substantial myocardial damage.

Conclusions

Differential diagnostics are of decisive importance in developing specific strategies for immunosuppressive therapy of inflammatory cardiomyopathy. Thus immunosuppressive therapy is not indicated in the acute phase of inflammatory cardiomyopathy with histologically detectable myocytolysis. On the other hand, the pilot studies available thus far suggest that immunosuppression exerts a favorable influence on the clinical course of patients with chronic

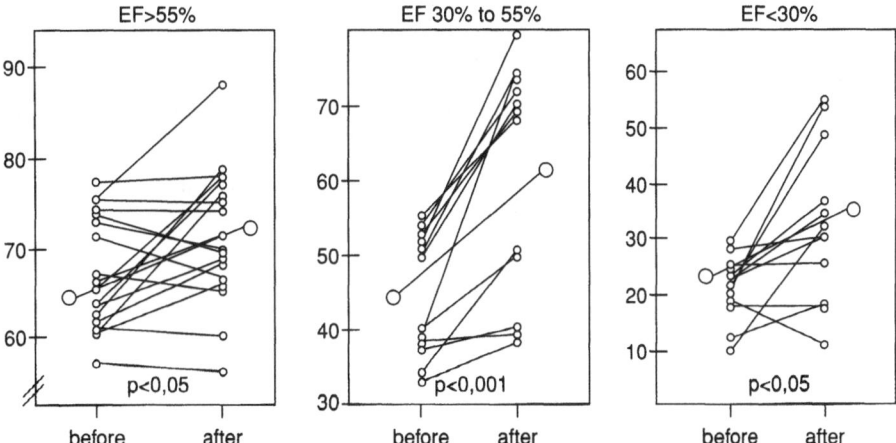

Fig. 4. Hemodynamic improvement after 6 months of immunosuppressive therapy in patients with chronic autoimmune myocarditis, according to ventricular dysfunction

autoimmune myocarditis if cardiac inflammation was characterized by histological, immunohistological and molecular-biological methods [48,49]. However, the general recommendation for this type of treatment is contingent on the results of ongoing randomized studies.

When planning immunosuppressive or virustatic therapy, the time of diagnosis and therapy should be chosen in such a way as to initiate effective treatment before the development of marked myocardial dysfunction. While normalization is rare in cases of severe contraction disturbances, our experience has shown that patients with slightly to moderately impaired myocardial function benefit most from immunosuppressive therapy. Assuming that inflammatory cardiomyopathy clinically manifested as dilated cardiomyopathy is an end-stage disease, it seems paradoxical that immunosuppressive therapy is frequently recommended only for severe ventricular dysfunction, particularly in clinical studies. Our main therapeutic goal should rather be to prevent the progression of such advanced myocardial damage by early therapeutic intervention.

References

1. Mason JW, O'Connell JB, Herskowitz A et al. (1995) A clinical trial of immunosuppressive therapy for myocarditis. N Engl J Med 333:269-275.
2. Hahn EA, Hartz VL, Moon TE, O'Connell JB, Herskowitz A, McManus BM, Mason JW, for the Myocarditis Treatment Trial Investigators (1995): The Myocarditis Treatment Trial: design, methods and patient enrollment. Eur Heart J 16[Suppl 0]:162-167
3. McKenna WJ, Davies MJ (1995) Immunosuppression for myocarditis. N Engl J Med 333:312-313
4. Maisch B, Camerini F, Schultheiss HP (1995a) Immunosuppressive therapy for myocarditis [letter]. N Engl J Med 333:1714
5. Cunnion RE, Parillo JE (1995) Immunosuppression for myocarditis [letter]. N Engl J Med 333: 1713
6. Cooper LT, Shabetai R (1995) Immunosuppression for myocarditis [letter]. N Engl J Med 333:1713-1714
7. Mason JW, O'Connell JB, McManus BM (1995) Immunosuppression for myocarditis N Engl J Med 333: 1714
8. Kuhl U, Noutsias M, Seeberg B, Schultheiss HP (1996) Immunohistological evidence for a chronic intramyocardial inflammatory process in dilated cardiomyopathy. Heart 75:295-300
9. Kuhl U, Noutsias M, Seeberg B, Schannwell M, Welp LB and Schultheiss HP (1994) Chronic inflammation in the myocardium of patients with clinically suspected dilated cardiomyopathy. J Card Failure 1:13-27
10. Kuhl U, Noutsias M, Seeberg B, Schannwell M, Welp LB and Schultheiss H. (1994) Immunohistological evaluation of myocardial biopsies from patients with dilated cardiomyopathy. J Heart Failure 9: 231-245
11. Bowles NE, Richardson PJ, Olson EGJ, Archard LC (1986). Detection of coxsackie-B-virus-specific RNA sequences in myocardial biopsy samples from patients with myocarditis and dilated cardiomyopathy. Lancet 17:1120-1123
12. Jin O, Sole MJ, Butany JW, Chia W-K, McLaughlin PR, Liu P, Liew CC (1990) Detection of enterovirus RNA in myocardial biopsies from patients with myocarditis and cardiomyopathy using gene amplification by polymerase chain reaction. Circulation 82:8-16
13. Kandolf R, Ameis D, Kirschner P, Canu A, Hofschneider PH (1987) In situ detection of enteroviral genomes in myocardial cells by nucleic acid hybridization: an approach to the diagnosis of viral heart diesease. Proc Natl Acad Sci 84:6272-6276

14. Tracy S, Chapmann NM, McManus BM, Pallansch MA, Beck MA, Carstens J (1990) A molecular and serologic evaluation of enteroviral involvement in human myocarditis. J Mol Cell Cardiol 22:403-414
15. Weiss LM, Movahed LA, Billingham ME, Cleary ML (1991) Detection of coxsackievirus B3 RNA in myocardial tissues by the polymerase chain reaction. Am J Pathol 138:497-503
16. WHO (1996) Report of the 1995 World Health Organization/International Society and Federation of Cardiology Task Force on The Definition and Classification of Cardiomyopathies. Circulation 93:841-842
17. Kandolf R, Klingel K, Zell R, Selinka HC, Raab U, Schneider-Brachert W, Bultmann B (1993) Molecular pathogenesis of enterovirus-induced myocarditis: virus persistence and chronic inflammation. Intervirology 35:140-151
18. Pauschinger M, Preis S, Triesch A, Doerner A, Schultheiss H-P (1994) Detection of enteroviral RNA in patients having chronic myocarditis respectively dilated cardiomyopathy. Circulation 90 [Suppl I]:1174
19. Archard LC, Bowles NE, Cunningham L, Freeke CA, Olsen EG, Rose ML, Meany B, Why HJF, Richardson FJ (1991) Molecular probes for detection of persisting enterovirus infection of human heart and their prognostic value. Eur Heart J 12[Suppl D]:56-59
20. Tracy S, Wiegand V, McManus B, Gauntt C, Pallansch M, Beck M, Chapman N (1990) Molecular approaches to enteroviral diagnosis in idiopathic cardiomyopathy and myocarditis. J Am Coll Cardiol 15: 1688-1694
21. Martin AB, Webber S, Fricker FJ, Jaffe R, Demmler G, Kearny D, Zhang Y-H, Bodurtha J, Gelb B, Ni J, Bricker JT, Towbin JA (1994) Acute myocarditis, rapid diagnosis by PCR in children. Circulation 90:330-339
22. Schönian U, Crombach M, Maisch B (1993) Assessment of cytomegalovirus DNA and protein expression in patients with myocarditis. Clin Immunol Immunopathol 68:229-233
23. Matsumori A, Matoba Y, Sasayama S (1995) Dilated cardiomyopathy associated with hepatitis C virus infection. Circulation 92:2519-2525
24. Caforio ALP (1994) Role of autoimmunity in dilated cardiomyopathy. Br Heart J 72: S30-S34
25. Schultheiss HP (1987) The mitochondrium as antigen in inflammatory heart disease. Eur Heart J 8[Suppl J]:203-210
26. Schultheiss HP (1993) Disturbance of the myocardial energy metabolism in dilated cardiomyopathy due to autoimmunological mechanisms. Circulation 87[Suppl 5]:IV43-IV48
27. Schultheiss HP, Schulze K, Schauer R, Witzenbichler B, Strauer BE (1995) Antibody-mediated imbalance of myocardial energy metabolism, a causal factor of cardiac failure. Circ Res 76:64-72
28. Limas CJ, Goldenberg IF, Limas C (1984) Autoantibodies against adrenoceptors in human idiopathic dilated cardiomyopathy. Eur Heart J 5:97-103
29. Schultheiss HP (1992) Dysfunction of the ADP/ATP carrier as a causative factor for the disturbance of the myocardial energy metabolism in dilated cardiomyopathy. Basic Res Cardiol 87:311-320
30. Schultheiss HP, Schulze K, Dorner A (1996) Significance of the adenine nucleotide translocator in the pathogenesis of viral heart disease Molec Cell Biochem 163/164:319-327
31. Schulze K, Becker BF, Schultheiss HP (1989) Antibodies to the ADP/ATP carrier, an autoantigen in myocarditis and dilated cardiomyopathy, penetrate into myocardial cells and disturb energy metabolism in vivo. Circ Res 64:179-253
32. Kuhl U, Melzner B, Schafer B, Schulteiss HP, Strauer BE (1991) The Ca-channel as cardiac autoantigen. Eur Heart J 12:99-104
33. Schultheiss HP, Janda I, Kuhl U, Ulrich G, Morad M (1988) Antibodies against the ADP/ATP carrier interact with the calcium channel and induce cytotoxicity by enhancement of calcium permeability. In: The Calcium Channel: Structure, Function and Implications. Eds.: Morad M, Nayler W, Kazda S, Schramm M. Springer-Verlag, Berlin, Heidelberg, NewYork, pp 619-631

34. Schultheiss, H-P, Kuhl, U, Schulze, K, Schwimmbeck, P, Strauer, BE (1990) Biomolecular changes in dilated cardiomyopathy. In: Baroldi G, Camerini F, Goodwin JF (eds) Advances in Cardiomyopathies. Springer Verlag Berlin, Heidelberg, New York, pp 221-234
35. Wolff P, Kuhl U, Schultheiss HP (1989) Laminin distribution and autoantibodies to laminin in dilated cardiomyopathy and myocarditis. Am Heart J 117:1303-1309
36. Matsumori A, Yamada T, Suzuki H, Matoba Y, Sasayama S (1994) Increased circulating cytokines in patients with myocarditis and cardiomyopathy. Br Heart J 72:561-566
37. Matsumori A (1996) Cytokines in myocarditis and cardiomyopathies. Current Opinion in Cardiol 11:302-309
38. Kuhl U, Pauschinger M, Schultheiss HP (1997) Äthiopathogenetische Differenzierung der entzündlichen Kardiomyopathie. Internist 38:590-601
39. Aretz HT (1987) Myocarditis, the Dallas Criteria. Human Pathol 18:619-624
40. Billingham ME (1987) Acute myocarditis: a diagnostic dilemma. Brit Heart J 58:6-8
41. Hauck AJ, Kearney DL, Edwards WD (1989) Evaluation of postmortem endomyocardial biopsy specimen from 38 patients with lymphocytic myocarditis: Implication for role of sampling error. Mayo Clin Proc 64:1235-1245
42. Shanes JG, Ghali J, Billingham ME, Ferrans VJ, Fenoglio JJ, Edwards WD, Tsai CC, Saffitz JE, Isner J, Furner S, Subramanian R (1987) Interobserver variability in the pathologic interpretation of endomyocardial biopsy results. Circulation 75:401-405
43. Chow LH, Ye Y, Linder J, McManus BM (1989) Phenotypic analysis of infiltrating cells in human myocarditis. Arch Pathol Lab Med 113:1357-1362
44. Kuhl U, Pauschinger M, Schultheiss HP (1997) Neue Konzepte zur Diagnostik der entzündlichen Herzmuskelerkrankung. DMW 122:690-698
45. Kawai C, Matsumori A, Fujiwara H (1987) Myocarditis and dilated cardiomyopathy. Ann Rev Med 38:221-239
46. Tomioka N, Kishimoto C, Matsumori A, Kawai C (1986) Effects of prednisolone on acute viral myocarditis in mice. J Am Coll Cardiol 7:868-872
47. Schultheiss H-P (1992) Immunsuppressive Therapie bei Myokarditis und dilatativer Kardiomyopathie. Internist 33:650-662
48. Kuhl U, Schultheiss H-P, Strauer BE (1994) Methylprednisolone in chronic myocarditis. Postgrad Med J 70 [Suppl 1]:S35-S42
49. Maisch B, Herzum M, Hufnagel G, Bethge C, Schönian U (1995b) Immunosuppressive treatment for myocarditis and dilated cardiomyopathy. Eur Heart J 16 [Suppl O]:153-161
50. Koide H, Kitaura Y, Deguchi H (1992) Genomic detection of enteroviruses in the myocardium-studies on animal hearts with coxsackievirus B3 myocarditis and dilated cardiomyopathy. Jpn Circ J 56:1081-1083
51. Kandolf R, Kirschner P, Ameis D, Canu A, Erdmann E, Schulteiss HP, Kempkes B, Hofschneider PH (1988) Enteroviral heart disease: diagnosis by in situ hybridization. In: Schulteiss H (ed) New Concepts in Viral Heart Disease. Springer-Verlag, Berlin Heidelberg New York, pp 337-348

Mitochondrial DNA Mutations and Cardiomyopathies

E. Arbustini, M. Diegoli, A. Pilotto, R. Fasani, M. Grasso, N. Banchieri, O. Bellini, B. Dal Bello, G. Magrini, P. Morbini, C. Campana, A. Gavazzi and M. Viganò

Introduction

A new field, mitochondrial (mt) DNA-related pathology, was created in 1988 with the report of mtDNA deletions in spontaneous encephalomyopathies and of mtDNA missense mutations in Leber's hereditary optic neuropathy [1-3]. Since then, several multiorgan-system disorders and a few cardiomyopathies have been described as associated with mt DNA defects [4]. New cardiomyopathies have been described as associated with mt DNA defects [4].

Mitochondrial diseases are characterized by faulty oxidative phosphorylation caused by defects, either single or multiple, in the five complexes of the respiratory chain. The mitochondrial respiratory chain forms through complementation of nuclear and mitochondrial genomes. Both genomes contribute in providing subunits of the respiratory complexes. Mitochondrial DNA provides 13 subunits of the respiratory complexes I, III, IV and V, as well as genes (transfer and ribosomal RNA) for mtDNA translation. Nuclear genome provides the entire complex II, subunits of other complexes, as well as enzymes for prosthetic group synthesis and components for mtDNA replication and expression [5].

The diagnosis of mitochondrial diseases largely benefited from complete mtDNA sequencing and from identification of mt DNA mutations [1]. In addition, mtDNA mutations and oxidative phosphorylation defects have been proposed as involved in the pathogenesis of degenerative diseases and in the human aging process [6,7].

Mitochondria

Mitochondria are bacterium-sized organelles present in all mammalian cells. They represent endosymbionts that were captured by the proto-eukariote early in evolution, when the earth's atmosphere changed from a reducing environment, to an oxidizing one [8].

The mitochondria of cardiac myocytes are elongated; they are present in the subsarcolemmal areas, between the myofibrils and in paranuclear position. An outer and an inner membrane delimitate two compartments: the inter-membrane space (outer compartment), and the inner compartment or matrix. The outer membrane is smooth while the inner membrane is folded inwardly into parallel, shelf-like cristae [9]. Stalked particles line the inner surface of the cristae and contain the enzymes of the respiratory chain, while the matrix contains dense granules, mtDNA, mt RNA and proteins. Each mitochondrion contains 5 to 10 DNA molecules which are independent for their replication, from nuclear DNA [10].

The bulk of energy requirements of the heart is met by mitochondrial oxidative phosphorylation; in mitochondria vital functions are finalized to the aerobic oxidation of energy substrates. In the heart, most of the energy required is provided by oxidation of fatty acids through the sequential activity of the oxidation pathways, the Krebs cycle and the respiratory chain. Postmitotic or slowly dividing tissue cells dependent on high aerobic demand, such as cardiac myocytes, are good candidates for being selectively affected by defects of oxidative phosphorylation [11].

Human Mitochondrial DNA

Mitochondrial DNA is a double strand circular molecule which codes for 22 tRNA, 2 rRNA, and 13 subunits of the respiratory chain (Fig.1). Other subunits of the respiratory chain are coded by nuclear genes, synthesized by cytoplasmic ribosomes, and transported into the mitochondria. The mtDNA transcription resembles that of bacterial DNA in that it is polycystronic: the resulting RNA transcript is cleaved in mRNA and other RNA [1].

A series of distinguishing features characterize mitochondrial DNA:
a) The rate of mutation is at least 10 times higher than that of nuclear DNA: the mtDNA molecules are free in the mitochondrial matrix and are exposed to the damage of the free radicals generated during the oxidative phosphorylation.
b) Mitochondrial DNA lacks repair systems and therefore any damage accu-

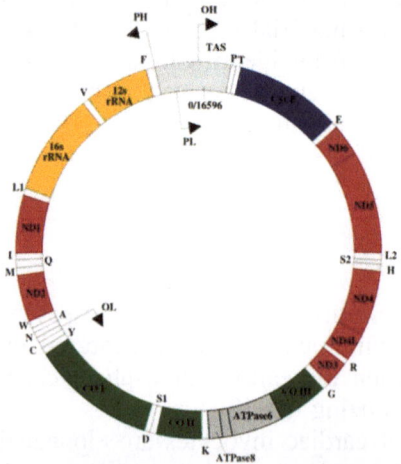

Fig. 1. The human mtDNA map: 2 rRNA (▨ 16s rRNA, 12s rRNA); 22 tRNA (□); 13 subunits of the respiratory chain: NADH Dehydrogenase (■ ND1, ND2, ND3, ND4L, ND4, ND5, ND6), Cytochrome c Oxidase (■ CO I, CO II, CO III) Cytochrome b (■), ATPase (▨ ATPase6, ATPase8), control region (▨)

mulates in the given molecules and is, in turn, transmitted from one generation to the other.

c) Mitochondrial DNA lacks introns, so that any mutation occurs in coding genes or in transfer or ribosomal RNA genes [12].

Mutations may affect part of the DNA molecules for each mitochondrion, part of the mitochondria of a cell, part of the cells of a tissue: given that the amount of mutated mtDNA varies from cell to cell and from tissue to tissue, the percentage of mutated DNA may differ greatly, from a few molecules to the entire mtDNA. The presence of a dual mtDNA population, one mutated and one wild type, is termed heteroplasmia. The presence of more than two mtDNA populations is termed polyplasmia.

Heteroplasmia is considered one of the major criteria for pathogenicity of mtDNA mutations: it indicates that the mutation is recent and that is compatible with life, thanks to the residual amount of wild type mtDNA. Any given mutation has his own threshold value and the degree of heteroplasmia is a major determinant for any related phenotype. In other words, a phenotype associated with the given mutation, becomes clinically or morphologically overt only when the proportion of the corresponding mtDNA reaches this critical value, i.e. its threshold value. In a same family, progeny carrying an mtDNA mutation may be or may be not affected, depending on the amount of mutated DNA in the target organ/tissue, namely on the degree of heteroplasmia. Even gradual changes in mitochondrial genotypes may cause abrupt appearance of the phenotype determined by the threshold value of each given mutation. Furthermore the phenotype also depends on the type of affected mitochondrial DNA gene (whether RNA- or enzyme subunit-coding genes), on the characteristics of the mutation itself, as well as on its functional importance.

Inheritance of Mitochondrial DNA

The most important feature of mtDNA genetics is the maternal, non-mendelian transmission of the mitochondrial genotype. MtDNA is transmitted through the mitochondria of the oocyte. Spermatozoon mitochondria do not enter the oocyte during fertilization. Therefore mitochondria are of exclusive maternal origin. Accordingly, the inheritance follows the population genetic rules rather than the mendelian laws. Males and females can be equally affected by mtDNA-related defects, but only females transmit such mitochondrial diseases [13].

In contrast with nuclear genes, which are represented by 2 alleles (one maternal and one paternal], multiple copies of maternally-inherited mtDNA, and therefore of mitochondrial genes, are present in most cells: since there are hundreds of mitochondria in a cell and each mitochondrion contains several mtDNA molecules, the mitochondrial genotype of each cell is determined by the contribution of thousands of mtDNA molecules [14].

At mitosis, the distribution of mitochondria in progeny follows statistic rather than mendelian laws. Therefore, if the parental cell harbors different DNAs, or heteroplasmic DNA, the proportion of different (wild type and mutated) mitochondria in progeny may vary during subsequent mitotic events (mitotic segregation). This condition is associated with an increased variability of mitochondrial genotypes.

Mitochondrial DNA Defects

They can be classified according to their molecular characteristics and pattern of transmission.

1)Large scale rearrangements, either single mtDNA deletions or, rarely, partial duplications are obligatory heteroplasmic and sporadic in most of the cases. They vary in range from 1.3 to 7.6 Kb (more frequently 5 to 7.4Kb) in length and affect both mRNA and tRNA genes [15]. Slippage and mispairing of the single mtDNA strands during replication have been proposed as the molecular mechanisms causing deletions, because deleted regions are flanked by repeats of variable length [16,17]. Translation activity of mtDNA in affected cells largely depends on the proportion of deleted mtDNA; within a same mitochondrion, translation can still be effective through the complementation of deleted genomes by wild-type ones.

Although several reports have described mtDNA deletions in cardiomyopathies, most studies have been performed using PCR techniques [30,31]. With double controlled PCR and Southern blot assays, we observed a high proportion of mtDNA deletions identified with PCR techniques but not with Southern blot in cardiomyopathy patients. A similar proportion of PCR positive cases was observed in control ischemic and valvular heart disease patients as well as in normal heart samples from donors over 50 years of age. In positive controls, i.e. patients affected by Kearn Sayre syndrome, we identified deletions with Southern blot analysis. At present, we do not attribute unique or specific pathogenic significance to PCR-detected mtDNA deletions in cardiomyopathy hearts.

2)Point mutations of mtDNA and pathogenicity. Several point mutations in mtDNA have been reported as associated with well-defined clinical disorders. These point mutations are maternally inherited and may affect mRNA, tRNA and rRNA. There are rules that must be respected in order to attribute a pathologic significance to mitochondrial DNA point mutations. These rules can be summarized as follows:

– The mutation must have involved a nucleotide that is highly conserved throughout evolution.

– The mutation must be heteroplasmic: if all mitochondrial DNA is mutated (homoplasmic), the mutation is unlikely to play a major pathogenic role. Conversely, if only part of the mitochondrial DNA is mutated (heteroplasmic), then the possibility that the mutation itself plays a role in the pathogenesis of the disease is higher, because some function is likely maintained by the complementation of mutated with wild-type DNA; the amount of mutated DNA seems to be the true determinant of the decrease or loss of function, in some organ rather than in others. To assess heteroplasmia, we need to distinguish wild type from mutated DNA: if the mutation modifies the restriction enzyme map, the given gained or lost enzyme can be simply used to digest PCR product: the mutated DNA will be cut in a different way from the wild type one. A further densitometric analysis will quantify the mutant. If the mutation does not modify the restriction enzyme map, we perform a mispaired PCR with a mismatch primer, namely a primer with one or more base changes that, in combination with the given mutation, gain or loose a restriction enzyme site.

– The mutation should segregate with the phenotype and the percentage of heteroplasmia must be higher in affected than in non-affected subjects: in other words, not the mutation itself, but rather its amount should segregate with the phenotype

– The mutation should be associated with a functional defect such as decrease or loss of a given mitochondrial enzyme activity. However, some of the so-called pathogenic mutations in encephalomyopathies do not respect this rule [18,19].

– The mutation should be absent from healthy controls.

Mitochondrial DNA Mutations in Cardiomyopathies

In the last few years, cardiomyopathies associated with mtDNA defects have been described. These cardiomyopathies can occur as isolated disorders [20-22] or may be associated with peripheral myopathies [23-25] or with multi-system disorders [26-28]. Cardiac involvement in fatal infantile mitochondrial encephalomyopathies has been reported as the major determinant of their poor final outcome [28-29].

Several mtDNA deletions may occur in affected hearts, but the proportion of deleted mtDNA or the threshold value for the given deletions has not been defined [30,31].

Point mutations occur preferentially in tRNA genes (tRNALeu, tRNAIle, tRNALys, tRNAGly) [20-28]. Such tRNA mutations are characteristically heteroplasmic, with higher proportion of mutated DNA in the heart than in blood, and are positioned in regions that are highly conserved through evolution. The cytochrome c oxidase, partly encoded by mtDNA genes, is the enzyme that more frequently resulted affected in patients with mtDNA tRNA mutations [32]. Missense mutations in genes coding for mitochondrial enzyme subunits have also been reported in a MELAS (Mitochondrial Encephalopathy with Lactic Acidosis and Stroke-like episodes) case with cardiac involvement [18] but no isolated cardiomyopathy has been selectively associated with a missense mutation. Other missense mutations in polypeptide-coding genes are associated with milder phenotypes [33,34].

Cardiomyopathy type. Mitochondrial DNA mutations have been reported in patients with hypertrophic cardiomyopathy phenotype and particularly in those who developed congestive heart failure late in the course of the disease [35]. In other cases, the cardiac phenotype is not defined and patients are described as affected by cardiomyopathy with congestive heart failure [21,22,25].

Mitochondrial DNA Mutations in Patients
with Dilated Cardiomyopathy (DCM): The Pavia Experience

Most cardiomyopathies associated with mtDNA point mutations have been described as single case family reports. No systematic analysis of mtDNA has been performed in large cardiomyopathy series.

To date, only patients with clear maternal inheritance or with associated mitochondrial myopathy, have been investigated for mtDNA mutations. Morphologic markers that could guide molecular screening have not been identified; the interpretation of histoenzymatic stain in small endomyocardial biopsy samples can be limited by the numerous artifactitious contraction bands that occur in these small samples. Large myocardial samples from hearts excised at transplantation, provide better results (Fig. 2). Ultrastructural study and immunocytochemistry may provide useful information: abnormal mitochondria with inclusion bodies, concentric, tubular, lamellar, etc cristae and decreased anti-enzyme subunit immunostain, may be used to select cardiomyopathy patients for mtDNA analysis (Fig. 3). Although ultrastructural mitochondrial changes do not represent markers specifically associated with mtDNA defects, they are easily investigated on EMB samples: lacking alternative tools, we approached the screening of our cardiomyopa-

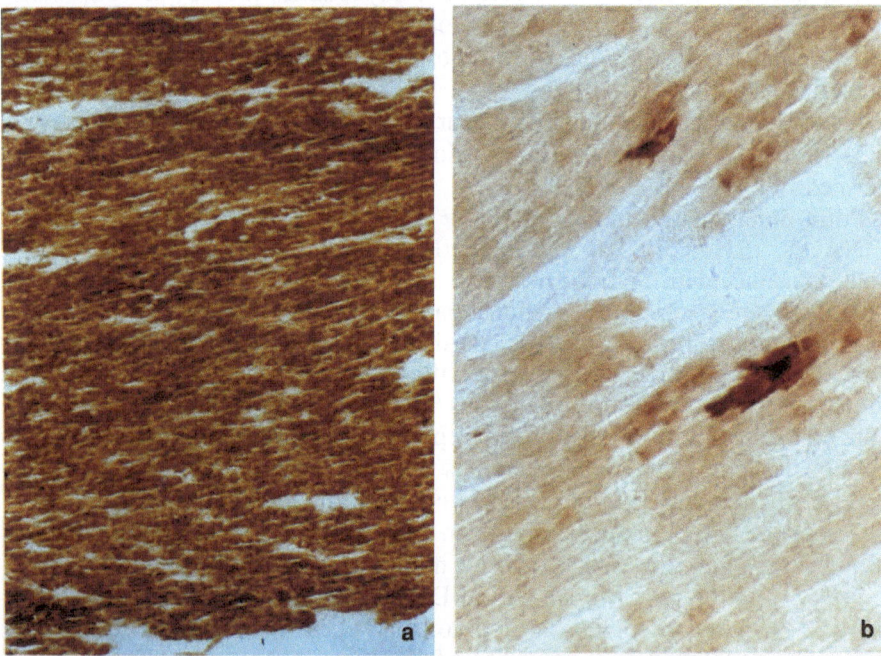

Fig. 2. Light micrographs showing: **a** normal histochemical reaction for cytochrom c oxidase. **b** Severe decrease of stain in most cardiac myocytes in the myocardium of a patient with mitochondrial DNA heteroplasmic point mutation in tRNA^{Ile} (Cox histochemical reaction a:120x; b:180x)

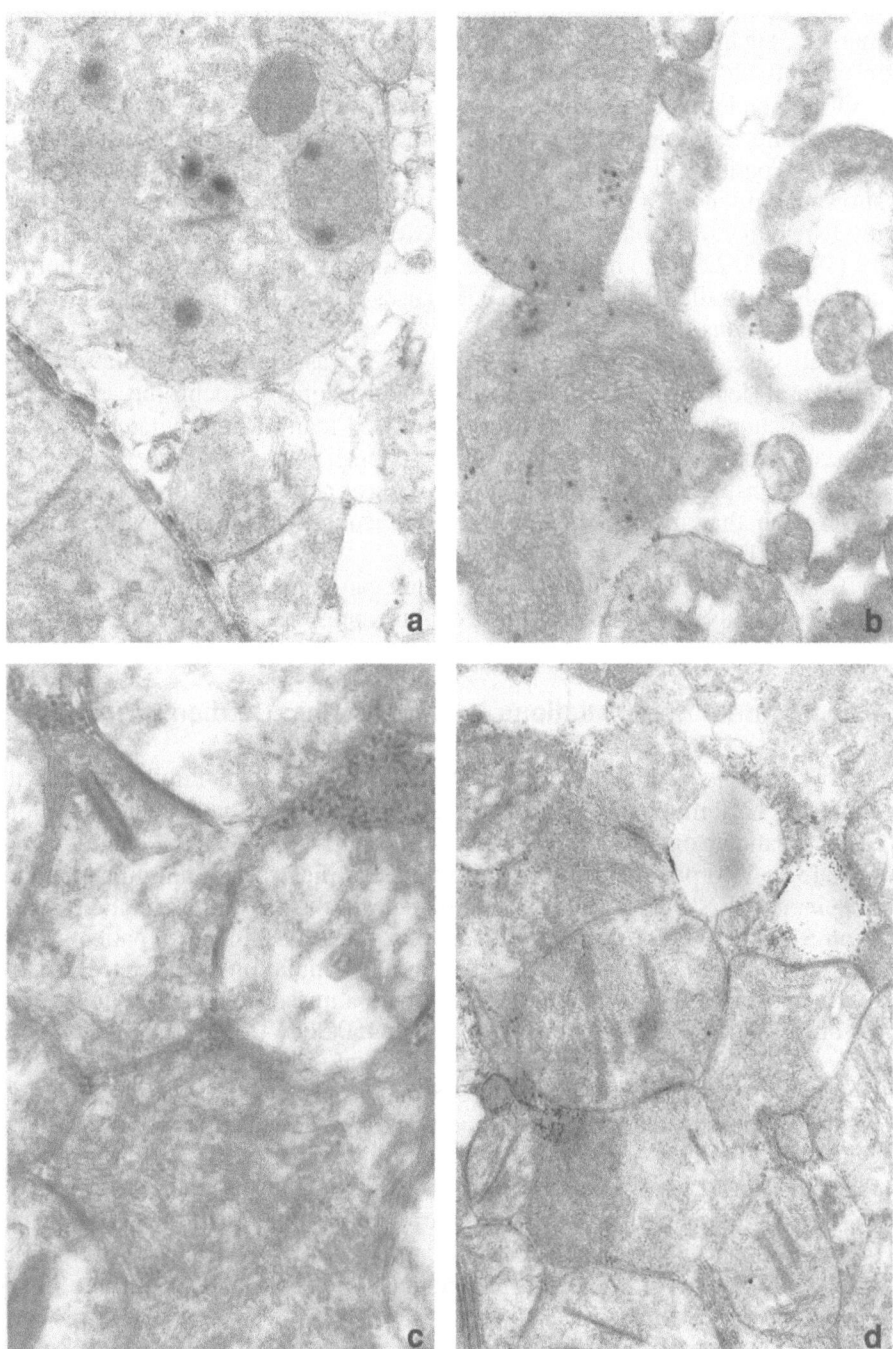

Fig. 3a-d. Electron micrographs showing some of the mitochondrial abnormalities found in the endomyocardial biopsy samples of dilated cardiomyopathy patients with heteroplasmic point mutations in the mitochondrial DNA (**a, b, c, d**: uranyl acetate, lead citrate)

thy patient biopsy using ultrastructural study-derived information. Other markers, such as lactic acidosis or signs of peripheral myopathy, are absent in patients with an isolated cardiomyopathy.

Of 601 endomyocardial biopsy performed from January 1985 to December 1996 at the Cardiology Department of the IRCCS-Policlinico San Matteo of Pavia in patients with DCM presenting with congestive heart failure, 85 showed evidence of mitochondrial changes similar to those reported in mtDNA defect-associated myopathies. MtDNA molecular analysis identified 19 (19 of 85, 22.35%) heteroplasmic mutations that were not found in normal controls. Overall, 19 of the 601 DCM cases (3.16%) showed mtDNA pathogenic mutations.

In all cases the amount of mutated DNA was higher in cardiac than in peripheral leukocyte DNA. Electron microscopy cytochrome c oxidase immuno-stain was markedly lower in mutated than in non-mutated cases; in hearts of patients that, later on in the course of their disease, underwent cardiac transplantation, cytochrome c oxidase activity resulted significantly lower than that measured in the heart of control cardiomyopathy patients without mtDNA mutations [36].

It can be argued that ultrastructural study can guide our investigation in this field, especially in isolated cardiomyopathies presenting as sporadic disorders.

Mitochondrial DNA Mutations in Hypertrophic Cardiomyopathies

In four patients from three different families, two with familial, one with sporadic cardiomyopathy, we identified two potentially pathogenic mutations in each patient: one in the mtDNA, one in the β-myosin heavy chain nuclear gene [37]. Two patients from two different families carried an mtDNA mutation in the tRNAIle (A4300G) combined with a missense mutation in the exon 9 of the β–myosin heavy chain gene (Arg249Gln); two patients from one family, mother and son, carried an mtDNA mutation in the cytochrome c oxidase, subunit III (T9957C) combined with a missense mutation in the exon 14 of the β–myosin heavy chain gene (Lys450Glu). Both mtDNA mutations have been separately reported as disease-causing in one familial hypertrophic cardiomyopathy [21] and in a MELAS patient [18], respectively. Of the two β–myosin heavy chain missense mutations, one has been reported in a large Canadian kindred (Arg249Gln) with familial hypertrophic cardiomyopathy [37], and one (Lys450Glu) is novel [38].

The overall scenario of hypertrophic cardiomyopathy further complicates and more than one gene defect in different genomes (nuclear and mitochondrial) may coexist in the same patients and therefore may contribute in the phenotype of the disease.

Conclusions

The myocardium has all prerequisites for being an ideal candidate for mtDNA-related disorders: it is highly dependent on energy supply, and it is a slowly/non-dividing tissue. If we assume that the major rules that establish pathogenicity of mitochondrial DNA mutations are absence from controls, heteroplasmy, occurrence in conserved region, other than associated decrease of function, then a certain proportion of mutations found in our as well as in other reported cases, are pathogenic. We estimate that mtDNA mutations are involved in the pathogenic mechanisms of about 3% of adult dilated cardiomyopathies. Most cases appear as sporadic, and this is likely related to the malignant effect of the mutant amount and of its accumulation with ageing rather than to the "malignancy" of the mutations themselves.

Mitochondrial DNA defects are also good candidates as cofactors in other cardiac disorders, such as hypertrophic or restrictive cardiomyopathies, even in those cases in whom another mutation has been found: too often in fact we must attribute to the age-related penetrance of any given mutation in nuclear DNA, the lack of disease in mutated but clinically healthy subjects and again, too often mild instrumental signs, such as negative T waves in EKG leads, are reported as the only evidence of the disease. The important message from our experience, is that more than one gene defect may occur in cardiomyopathy patients and that the simple detection of a mutation can not necessarily predict which mutated young subject will develop the disease. Apart from diagnostic implications, integration of multiple information can also provide future therapeutic perspectives.

Acknowledgement. This work was supported by grants RF - IRCCS Policlinico San Matteo, Pavia 1992-1995.

References

1. Anderson S, Bankier AT, Barrell BG, de Bruijn MHL, Coulson AR, Drouin J, Eperon IC, Nierlich DP, Roe BA, Sanger F, Schreier PH, Smith AJH, Staden R, Young IG (1981) Sequence and organization of the human mitochondrial genome. Nature 290:457-465
2. Holt IJ, Harding AE, Morgan-Hughes JA (1988) Deletions of muscle mitochondrial DNA in patients with mitochondrial myopathies. Nature 331:717-719
3. Wallace DC, Singh G, Lott MT, Hodge JE, Schur TG, Lezza AMS, Elsas II LJ, Nikoskelainen EK (1988) Mitochondrial DNA mutation associated with Leber's optic atrophy. Science 242:1427-1430
4. Di Mauro S (1996) Mitochondrial encephalomyopathies. What next? J Inher Metab Dis 19:489-503
5. Wallace DC (1993) Mitochondrial diseases: genotype versus phenotype. TIG 9:128-133
6. Shoffner JM, Brown MD, Torroni A, Lott MT, Cabell MF, Mirra SS, Beal MF, Yang CC, Gearing M, Salvo R, Watts RL, Juncos JL, Hansen LA, Crain BJ, Fayad M, Reckord CL, Wallace DC (1993) Mitochondrial DNA variations observed in Alzheimer disease and Parkinson disease patients. Genomics 17:171-184
7. Ozawa T (1997) Genetic and functional changes in mitochondria associated with ageing. Physiol Rev 77:425-464
8. Di Mauro S, Wallace DC (1993) Mitochondrial DNA in human pathology. Raven Press, New York
9. Barth E, Stammler G, Speiser B, Schaper J (1992). Ultrastructural quantitation of mitochondria and myofilaments in cardiac muscle from 10 different animal species includ-

ing man. J Mol Cell Cardiol 24:669-681

10. Di Mauro S, Moraes CT (1993) Mitochondrial encephalomyopathies. Arch Neurol 50:1197-1208
11. Taegtmeyer H (1994) Energy metabolism of the heart: from basic concepts to clinical applications. Curr Prob Cardiol 19:59-113
12. Wallace DC (1989) Report of the Committee on human mitochondrial DNA. Cytogenet Cell Genet 51:612-621
13. Giles RE, Blanc H, Cann HM, Wallace DC (1980) Maternal inheritance of human mito-chondrial DNA. Proc Natl Acad Sci USA 77:6715-6719
14. Kim H, Kim D, Lee I, Rah B, Sawa Y, Schaper J (1992) Human fetal heart develop-ment after mid-term morphometry and unltrastructural study. J Mol Cell Cardiol 24:949-965
15 Shoffner JM, Lott MT, Voljavec AS, Soueidan SA, Costigan DA, Wallace DC (1989) Spontaneous Kearn-Sayre/chronic external ophtalmoplegia plus syndrome associated with a mitochondrial DNA deletion: a slip replication model and metabolic therapy. Proc Natl Acad Sci USA 86:7952-7956
16. Moraes CT, DiMauro S, Zeviani M (1989) Mitochondrial DNA deletions in progres-sive external ophtalmoplegia and Kearn-Sayre syndrome. N Engl J Med 320:1293-1299
17. Schon EA, Rizzuto R, Moraes CT, Nakase H, Zeviani M, DiMauro S (1989) A direct repeat is a hot spot for large-scale deletions of human mitochondrial DNA. Science 244:346-349
18. Manfredi G, Schon EA, Moraes CT, Bonilla E, Berry GT, Sladky JT, DiMauro S (1995) A new mutation associated with MELAS is located in a mitochondrial DNA polypep-tide-coding gene. Neuromusc Disord 5:391-392
19. Wallace DC (1989) Mitochondrial DNA mutations and neuromuscular disease. Human genetic disease. Trends Genet 5:9-13
20. Merante F, Tein I, Benson L, Robinson BH (1994) Maternally inherited hypertrophic cardiomyopathy due to a novel T-to-C transition at nucleotide 9997 in the mitochondr-ial tRNAGlycine gene. Am J Hum Genet 55:437-446
21. Casali C, Santorelli F, D'Amati G, Bernucci P, DeBiase L, DiMauro S (1995) Novel mtDNA point mutation in maternally inherited cardiomyopathy. Biochem Biophys Res Commun 213:588-593
22. Merante F, Myint T, Tein I, Benson L, Robinson BH (1996) An additional mitochon-drial tRNAIle point mutation (A-to-G at nucleotide 4295) causing hypertrophic cardiomyopathy. Hum Mutat 8:216-222
23. Zeviani M, Cellera C, Antozzi C, Rimoldi M, Morandi L, Villani F, Tiranti V, DiDo-nato S (1991) Maternally inherited myopathy and cardiomyopathy; association with mutation in mitochondrial DNA tRNALeu(UUR). Lancet 338:143-147
24. Silvestri G, Santorelli FM, Shanske SB, Whitley CB, Schimmenti LA, Smith SA, Di Mauro S (1994) A new mitochondrial DNA mutation in the tRNALeu(UUR) gene asso-ciated with maternally inherited cardiomyopathy. Hum Mut 3:37-43
25. Taniike M, Fukushima H, Yanagihara I, Tsukamoto H, Tanak J, Fujimura H, Nagai T, Sano T, Yamaoka K, Inui I, Okada S (1992) Mitochondrial tRNAIle mutation in fatal cardiomyopathy. Biochem Biophys Res Commun 186:47-53
26. Santorelli FM, Mak S, Vazquez-Aceredo M, Gonzalez-Astiazaran A, Ridaura-Sauz C, Gonzalez-Halphen D, DiMauro S (1995) A novel mitochondrial DNA point mutation associated with mitochondrial encephalomyopathy. Biochem Biophys Res Commun 216:835-840
27. Santorelli FM, Mak S, El-Schahawi M, Casali C, Shanske S, Baram TZ, Madrid RE, DiMauro S (1996) Maternally inherited cardiomyopathy and hearing loss associated with a novel mutation in the mitochondrial tRNALys gene (G8363A). Am J Hum Genet 58:933-939
28. Tanaka M, Ino H, Ohno K, Hattori K, Sato W, Ozawa T, Tanaka T, Itoyama S (1990) Mitochondrial mutation in fatal infantile cardiomyopathy. Lancet 2:1452
29. Tanaka M, Ino H, Ohno K, Obayashi T, Ikebe S, Sano T, Ichiki T, Kobayashi M, Wada Y, Ozawa T. Hattori K, Sato,W, Ozawa T (1991) Mitochondrial DNA mutations in mitochondrial myopathy, encephalopathy, lactic acidosis, and stroke-like episodes (MELAS). Biochem Biophys Res Commun 174:861-868

30. Checcarelli N, Prelle A, Moggio M, Comi G, Bresolin N, Papadinitrious A, Fagiolari G, Bordoni A, Scarlato G (1994) Multiple deletions of mitochondrial DNA in sporadic and atypical cases of encephalomyopathy. J Neurol Sci 123:74-79
31. Ozawa T, Tanaka M, Sugiyama S, Hattori K, Ito K, Ohno K, Takahashi A, Sato W, Takada G, Mayumi B. Multiple mitochondrial DNA deletions exist in cardiomyocytes of patients with hypertrophic or dilated cardiomyopathy (1990) Biochem Biophys Res Commun 170:830-836
32. Wallace DC (1992) Diseases of the mitochondrial DNA. Annu Rev Biochem 61:1175-1212
33. Mackey D, Howell N (1992) A variant of Leber hereditary optic neuropathy characterized by recovery of vision and by an unusual mitochondrial genetic etiology. Am J Hum Genet 51:1218-1228
34. Johns DR, Berman J (1991) Alternative, simultaneous complex I mitochondrial DNA mutations in Leber's hereditary optic neuropathy. Biochem Biophys Res Commun 174:1324-1330
35. Obayashi T, Hattori K, Sugiyama S, Tanaka M, Tanaka T, Itoyama S, Deguchi H, Kawamura K, Koga Y, Toshima H, Takeda N, Nagano M, Ito T, Ozawa T (1992) Point mutations in mitochondrial DNA in patients with hypertrophic cardiomyopathy. Am Heart J 124:1263-1269
36. Arbustini E, Diegoli M, Fasani R, Grasso M, Morbini P, Banchieri N, Bellini O, Dal Bello B, Pilotto A, Magrini G, Campana C, Fortina P, Gavazzi A, Narula J, Viganò M (1998) Mitochondrial DNA mutations and mitochondrial abnormalities in dilated cardiomyopathy (submitted)
37. Rosenzweig A, Watkins H, Hwang DS, Miri M, McKenna W, Traill TA, Seidman JG, Seidman CE (1991) Preclinical diagnosis of familial hypertrophic cardiomyopathy by genetic analysis of blood lymphocytes. N Engl J Med 325:1753-1760
38. Arbustini E, Fasani R, Morbini P, Diegoli M, Grasso M, Dal Bello B, Marangoni E, Banfi P, Banchieri N, Bellini O, Comi G, Narula J, Campana C, Gavazzi A, Danesino C, Viganò M (1998) Coexistence of mitochondrial DNA and β-myosin heavy chain mutations in hypertrophic cardiomyopathy with late congestive heart failure. Heart (in press)

Pathophysiologic Role of Coronary Microcirculatory Impairment in Dilated Cardiomyopathy

D. Neglia, M. Gallopin, A. Giorgetti, G. Sambuceti, M. Bartoli, G. Gensini, A. L' Abbate and O. Parodi

Myocardial blood flow (MBF) abnormalities, despite the presence of angiographically normal coronary arteries, have been documented in patients with heart failure due to idiopathic dilated cardiomyopathy (DCM). In particular, a reduction in MBF at rest [1] and/or in response to either metabolic [2] or pharmacologic vasodilating stimuli [3] has been reported. The cause-effect relationship between MBF abnormalities and ventricular dysfunction in DCM, however, is not fully elucidated. An intriguing hypothesis, coming out from the recent recognition of functional abnormalities of the coronary microcirculation in these patients [4-6], points to the relevance of coronary microvascular disease as a primary pathogenetic process leading to progressive ventricular dysfunction. Further testing of this hypothesis implies the demonstration that: 1) in advanced DCM, MBF abnormalities cannot be fully ascribed to the effects of structural and hemodynamic derangement of the myocardium; 2) coronary microvascular dysfunction may be detected also in early stage DCM and may predict progressive deterioration of ventricular function and worse prognosis.

Coronary Blood Flow in Patients with Advanced DCM

Coronary blood flow and myocardial perfusion are reduced in advanced DCM. Theoretically, myocardial perfusion might be blunted at this stage of the disease by the secondary effects of left ventricular dysfunction on coronary circulation, such as reduced oxygen demand due to depressed inotropism and compression of the coronary bed by stressed myocardium. Moreover, myocardial perfusion could be limited by structural or functional abnormalities of the coronary small vessels possibly associated with the disease process.

Evidence that myocardial perfusion can be impaired in DCM patients secondary to hemodynamic derangement has been collected in the last 20 years. Weiss and colleagues [1] assessed MBF with [133]Xenon, while simultaneously measuring the determinants of myocardial oxygen consumption in DCM patients and in control subjects. The authors observed that resting left ventricular (LV) perfusion per unit mass was significantly reduced in DCM, proportionally to the reduction in myocardial performance, and suggested that functional damage of myocytes may down-regulate resting MBF to meet the reduced metabolic needs. Besides the documented abnormality of resting myocardial perfusion, later studies in DCM patients with severe disease clearly showed a limitation in coronary flow reserve apparently dependent on the extent of hemodynamic impairment [3, 7]. Opherk et al. [3] observed depressed coronary blood flow after pharmacological vasodilation with dipy-ridamole in DCM patients with a positive correlation between minimal coro-nary resistance and LV end-diastolic pressure; this finding was mainly ascri-bed to the increased extravascular components of coronary resistance. A simi-lar relation between coronary flow vasodilation after papaverine and LV end-diastolic pressure was also found by Inoue using a Doppler coronary flow velocity estimate [7].

In more recent years, however, evidence that myocardial perfusion can be impaired in DCM patients by abnormalities of the coronary microcirculation has also been collected [4-6]. Since DCM does not cause any morphologic abnormality of the coronary microvessels [3-4, 8] a primary functional distur-bance of the coronary microcirculation was suggested. Nitenberg et al. [9], by using a coronary sinus thermodilution technique, did not confirm the rela-tion between decrease in coronary flow reserve elicited by dipyridamole and elevated LV end-diastolic pressure, suggesting a multifactorial genesis of the observed abnormalities. Treasure et al. [5], by coronary Doppler catheters, demonstrated an impaired relaxation of coronary small vessels in response to the endothelium-dependent vasodilator acetylcholine in DCM patients. In a recent study, Inoue et al [6], using the same technique, demonstrated that the vasodilation of coronary resistance vessels in DCM is impaired in response to both endothelium-independent and endothelium-dependent stimulation by papaverine and acetylcholine, respectively. However, in contrast with papa-verine, the impaired flow response to acetylcholine was not related to deter-minants of extravascular compressive forces resulting from LV dysfunction.

In spite of all these results, the relative role of primary or secondary deter-minants of coronary blood flow in causing myocardial perfusion abnormali-ties in DCM was not fully elucidated. It must be underlined that in the repor-ted studies a correct quantification of absolute regional MBF could not be performed, due to the intrinsic limitations of the flow measurement techni-ques adopted.

Quantitation of MBF in Excised Hearts from Patients with Advanced DCM

The measurement of absolute blood flow in the myocardium is probably the best approach to the study of the pathophysiologic mechanisms causing perfusion abnormalities in DCM. Absolute measurement of MBF, and parti-cularly of its transmural distribution within the myocardial layers, can be accurately obtained by ^{11}Carbon or ^{68}Gallium-labelled human albumin micro-spheres [10-11].

In a study of DCM and ischemic heart disease (IHD), in patients with seve-re cardiac failure undergoing orthotopic heart transplantation, we quantitated absolute regional MBF in the left and right ventricle and evaluated its tran-smural distribution by injecting 99mTechnetium-labeled microspheres into the left atrium during the surgical procedure [12]. The heart transplant model allows direct assay by well counter of tissue tracer radioactivity distribution within the heart, as well as correlation with histologic and biochemical markers of myocardial viability and fibrosis. MBF spatial distribution may furthermore be assessed by gamma-camera imaging to obtain a more precise estimate of the extension of perfusion defects in the whole myocardial slice and their possible histologic correlates [13].

An impairment of LV transmural flow was observed both in DCM and IHD patients (Fig. 1). However, the endocardial to epicardial flow ratio was greater than one in DCM patients, indicating a preferential perfusion of the inner half of the left ventricle with respect to ischemic hearts, where a flow shift towards the epicardium was documented (Fig. 1). Transmural perfusion appeared to be dependent on the severity of hypertrophy in cardiomyopathic hearts; the endocardial to epicardial flow ratio was in fact inversely related to heart weight only in the DCM group. Quantitative determination of fibrosis [14] showed lower transmural fibrosis in DCM than in ischemic patients. When MBF was compared with the extent of fibrosis assessed in the same wedge by biochemical analysis, no correlation was found (Fig. 2) both in DCM and ischemic patients. These findings were also confirmed by gamma camera analysis of an adjacent myocardial slice, which was subsequently processed for histology to determine the percentage of myocardial fibrosis with respect to total slide area from corresponding myocardial regions. In DCM patients, myocardial fibrosis, intermyocellular or microfocal, was uniformly minimal or mild (below 5%) both in the endocardium and in the epicardium, as was also demonstrated in a large series of hearts analyzed by

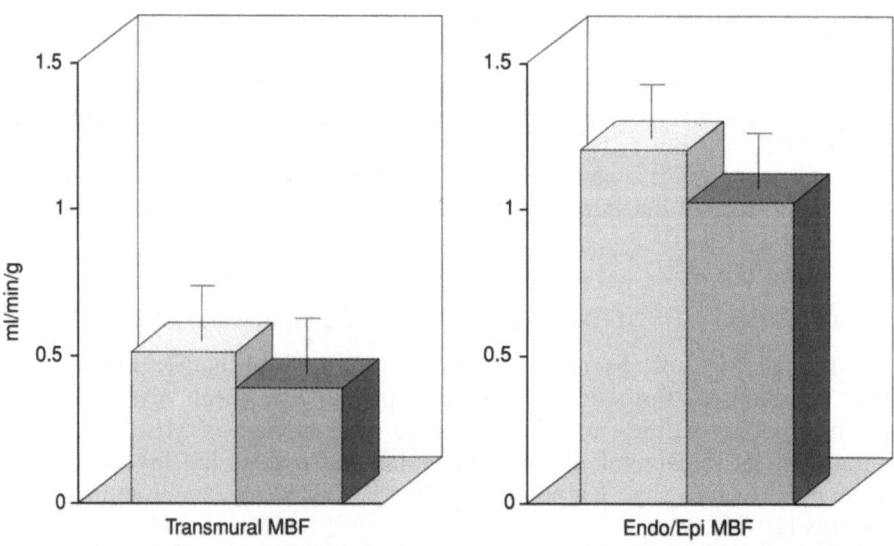

Fig. 1. Mean transmural left ventricular myocardial blood flow (MBF) and endocardial to epicardial flow ratio (endo/epi MBF) in patients with severe heart failure due to dilated cardiomyopathy (dark bars) and ischemic heart disease (light bars) undergoing heart transplantation. See text for details

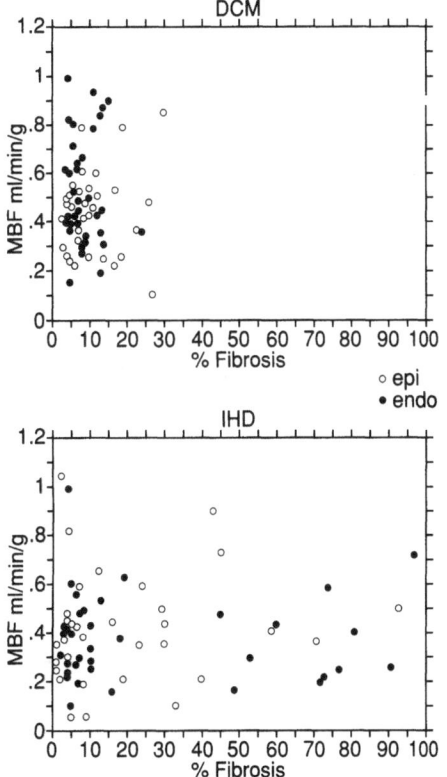

Fig. 2. Correlation between the extent of fibrosis (% Fibrosis) assessed by biochemical analysis and the corresponding myocardial blood flow (MBF) values in dilated cardiomyopathy (DCM) and ischemic heart disease (IHD) patients. Closed and open circles indicate the endocardial and epicardial wedges in which flow and fibrosis were assessed.

light microscopy and special staining techniques [15]. When the extent of fibrosis by histologic criteria was related to the severity of flow impairment assessed in the same territory by gamma camera analysis, again no correlation could be demonstrated.

Thus, in advanced DCM a severe impairment in regional MBF is present, similar to that present in IHD patients, despite the markedly lower degree of fibrosis and lack of flow limiting stenosis in the former group. The absence of correlation between the degree of MBF impairment and extent of myocardial fibrosis underscores that in DCM patients with severe LV dysfunction undergoing heart transplantation, myocardial fibrosis is not the main determinant of globally depressed myocardial perfusion. Moreover, in these patients the endocardium was better perfused than the epicardium in the face of very low perfusion rates and augmented intramyocardial pressures, suggesting that, as postulated from an experimental dog model [16], the autoregulatory mechanism in the coronary microcirculation is not affected by hemodynamic impairment.

Quantitation of MBF in Patients with Early Stage DCM

Studies performed so far included patients with advanced disease characterized by severe LV dysfunction, usually associated with overt heart failure.

Evaluation of MBF at an early stage of the disease might provide a definite clue to the understanding of the relation between flow and function in DCM, since in these patients abnormalities at the microvascular level should not be masked by impaired ventricular hemodynamics.

In patients with mild disease the measurement of absolute blood flow in the myocardium could be non-invasively obtained by position emission tomography (PET) and ^{13}N-ammonia as a flow tracer [17-18] and results have been reported [19]. So far, 34 patients with early DCM have been studied by PET in our laboratory. This population was selected by the presence of electrocardiographic abnormalities (complex ventricular arrhythmias, left bundle branch block) and/or atypical chest pain, NYHA class I-II, reduced LV ejection fraction (< 0.50) and abnormal LV wall motion at radionuclide angiography, angiographically normal coronary arteries and normal or mildly abnormal LV end-diastolic pressure (≤ 20 mmHg) [20]. Results were compared with those obtained in 15 normal subjects with atypical chest pain, angiographically normal epicardial coronary arteries, normal LV function at contrast ventriculography. Regional MBF was measured at rest, during atrial pacing tachycardia and following dipyridamole; MBF was also quantitated during adenosine infusion in a subset of patients. Coronary flow reserve and coronary resistance were calculated.

In DCM patients compared with normal subjects mean MBF at baseline,

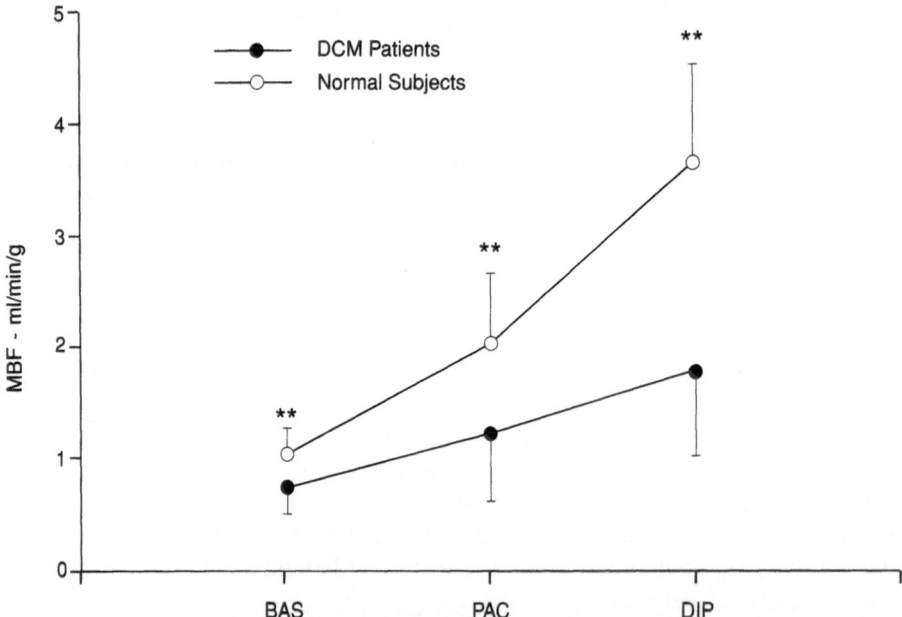

Fig. 3. Mean myocardial blood flow (MBF) in normal subjects and patients with dilated cardiomyopathy (DCM) at baseline (BAS), during atrial pacing (PAC), and after dipyridamole infusion (DIP). Mean MBF was significantly impaired in DCM in all the study conditions. **$p < 0.01$

during pacing and after dipyridamole was reduced (Fig. 3) and mean coronary flow reserve was depressed (2.47 ± 77 vs 3.63 ± 0.96, $p < .01$). In the 10 patients who participated in the PET study during adenosine infusion, mean MBF was similarly impaired during dipyridamole and adenosine (1.67 ± 0.87 vs 1.40 ± 0.72 ml/min/g, ns) (Fig. 4). In the DCM group, individual MBF values were depressed below the range of normal subjects at rest in 37% of patients, during pacing in 74% and after dipyridamole in 79% (Fig. 5). Mean MBF was completely normal in 9% of cases. Regional flow defects, as evaluated by comparing regional flow ratios in DCM and in normal subjects, were present in 20% of patients at baseline, in 26% during pacing and in 17% during dipyridamole. Overall, 34% of cases showed a regional perfusion defect at least in one study condition.

Coronary resistance in DCM patients mirrored the behavior of MBF. However, the analysis of changes in coronary resistance from resting state to dipyridamole induced vasodilation added further information and form the object of an ongoing investigation [21]. The absolute reduction in total coronary resistance elicited by dipyridamole was not significantly different between DCM patients and normal subjects (78 ± 22 vs 68 ± 22 mmHg/ml/min/g, ns) despite a marked reduction in MBF values in the patient group. Moreover, the reduction in coronary resistance after dipyridamole in DCM patients was not different from that induced by exogenous adenosine

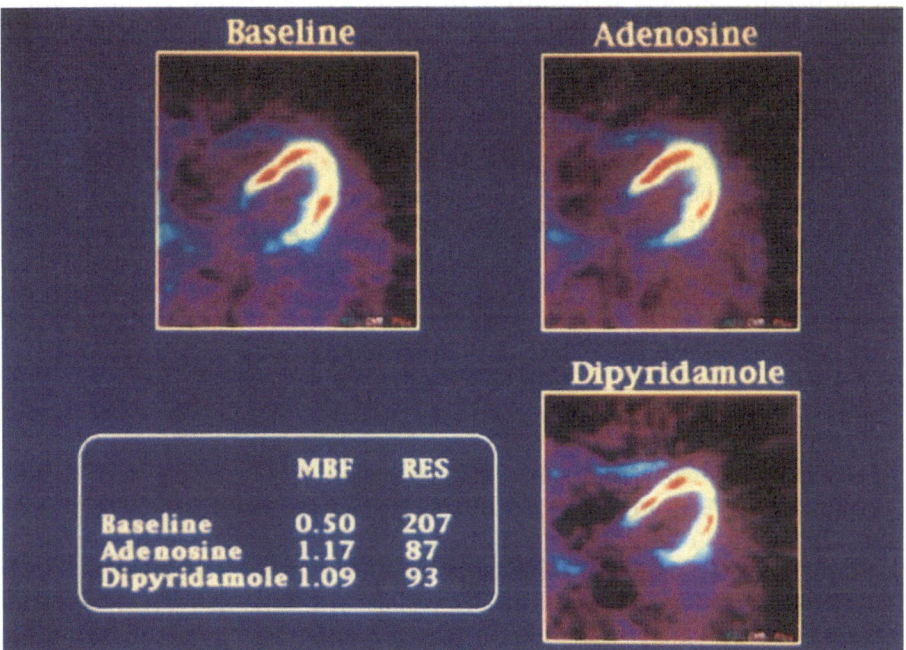

Fig. 4. Positron emission tomography images obtained in the same transaxial plane at baseline, during adenosine infusion (40 μg/Kg in 6'), and after dipyridamole infusion (0.56 mg/Kg in 4') in a representative patient with early stage dilated cardiomyopathy. Mild left ventricular enlargement and perfusion heterogeneities are evident

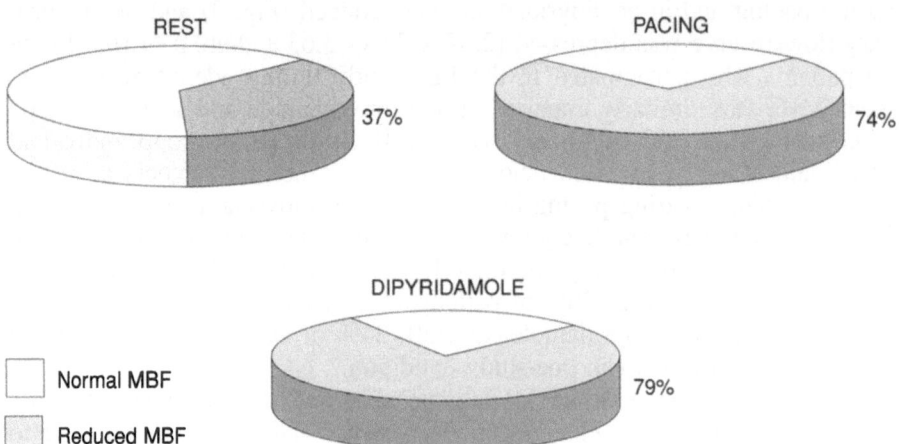

Fig. 5. Frequency of abnormally reduced myocardial blood flow (MBF) in patients with dilated cardiomyopathy

infusion. These observations suggest that: 1) the adenosine-dependent vaso-dilation of the coronary microvessels, as expressed by the ability to reduce resting coronary resistance in response to adenosine-dependent stimulation, is preserved in early DCM; 2) an impaired metabolism of endogenous adenosine in the myocardium is not likely to be the cause of reduced myocardial perfusion; 3) the observed reduction in MBF levels in this population should be linked to the presence of an additional resistance in the coronary microvascular bed not responsive to adenosine.

The results of these non-invasive studies demonstrate that myocardial perfusion is globally impaired in DCM patients, even at an early stage of the disease before the occurrence of the hemodynamic and systemic abnormalities which accompany overt heart failure. Moreover, MBF is reduced in most of these patients (74% - 79%) in response to different vasodilating stimuli and this abnormality is caused by an intrinsic microvascular disease, characterized by the presence of an additional coronary resistor that does not respond to endogenous or exogenous adenosine stimulation.

MBF and Prognosis in Patients with Early Stage DCM

The possible relevance of coronary microvascular disease as a primary pathogenetic process in early stage DCM could be underlined by the demonstration that the extent of MBF abnormalities in these patients may predict progressive deterioration of ventricular function and worse prognosis.

Accordingly, up to now, 29 of the 34 patients with early stage DCM studied by PET completed a clinical and functional follow-up (mean follow-up time of 39.8 ± 21.3 months, range 10-90 months). Adverse events at follow-up were defined as cardiac death, heart transplantation or worsening of left ventricular ejection fraction ($\geq .05$) evaluated at rest or during isometric exercise by equilibrium radionuclide angiography.

At enrolment, mean LV ejection fraction was 39±8% at rest and significantly decreased during isometric exercise to 32±10% ($p < .01$). At follow-up, 16/29 (55%) patients suffered adverse events. In particular, 4 patients died, 3 were transplanted and 9 showed worsening of ejection fraction. When patients with adverse events were compared with patients without adverse events, no significant difference was found at enrolment in LV ejection fraction at rest (0.40±0.09 vs 0.38±0.09; ns) or during isometric exercise (0.34±0.10 vs 0.30±0.9; ns). However, MBF after dipyridamole and MBF reserve at enrolment were significantly lower in patients with adverse events at follow-up compared with patients without adverse events (1.39±0.58 vs 2.15±0.91 ml/min/g, 2.02±0.70 vs 2.83±0.92, respectively; $p < .05$).

These preliminary results in patients with early stage DCM suggest that adverse events at follow-up are associated with a more severe MBF impairment at enrolment, independently of the initial degree of LV dysfunction.

Clinical Implications and Future Directions

The evidence gathered on MBF impairment in DCM might have clinical implications for the early recognition of the disease. Globally depressed ventricular function and angiographically normal epicardial coronary arteries allow identification of patients with advanced DCM. However, in patients with electrical abnormalities or chest pain, without symptoms and signs of heart failure and with moderate impairment of ventricular function, the diagnosis of DCM might be doubtful [20, 22]. As a matter of fact, 82% of patients with this presentation and angiographically normal coronary arteries showed a clear reduction in absolute MBF either at rest or in response to stress when evaluated by PET. Since a globally depressed myocardial perfusion and a blunted flow response to stress are part of the disease process in advanced DCM, similar findings in patients with a doubtful diagnosis would suggest the presence of an underlying myocardial disease. The PET technique is best suited to the recognition of these abnormalities [19], given its unique ability to quantify absolute MBF in different conditions.

It is well known that greater homogeneity of MBF distribution is a distinctive feature of DCM with respect to ischemic cardiomyopathy [23]. However, the findings of our group demonstrate that, together with a high incidence of globally depressed MBF, as many as 34% of patients with early stage DCM may also show regional perfusion defects in keeping with some reports in more advanced disease [12, 24-25]. It is conceivable that regional myocardial perfusion abnormalities may evolve towards a more diffuse flow impairment during the progression of the disease.

The demonstration that a globally and/or regionally altered myocardial perfusion in patients with mild LV dysfunction due to DCM may be linked to a worse prognosis [21] suggests that a careful evaluation and a prolonged follow-up should be carried out in this population. The early recognition of patients at risk of developing heart failure, and the availability of therapeutical strategies targeted at specific pathophysiologic processes might have a major impact on the prognosis of DCM. Prompt therapeutical intervention is probably warranted when signs of LV functional impairment appear. Moreover, it is conceivable that early treatment, with drugs able to influence microvascular vasodilating properties, would be especially useful in selected patients with documented MBF impairment in association with conventional treatment.

References

1. Weiss MB, Ellis K, Sciacca RR, Johnson LL, Schmidt DH, Cannon PJ (1976) Myocardial blood flow in congestive and hypertrophic cardiomyopathy. Relationship to peak wall stress and mean velocity of circumferential fiber shortening. Circulation 54:484-493
2. Pasternac A, Noble J, Streulens Y, Elie R, Henschke C, Bourassa MG (1982) Pathophysiology of chest pain in patients with cardiomyopathies and normal coronary arteries. Circulation 65:778-789
3. Opherk D, Schwartz F, Mall G, Manthey J, Baller D, Kubler W (1983) Coronary dilatory capacity in idiopathic dilated cardiomyopathy: analysis of 16 patients. Am J Cardiol 51:1657-1662
4. Cannon RO, Cunnion RE, Parrillo JE, Palmeri ST, Tucker EE, Schenke WH, Epstein SE (1987) Dynamic limitation of coronary vasodilatory reserve in patients with dilated cardiomyopathy and chest pain. J Am Coll Cardiol 10:1190-1200
5. Treasure CB, Vita JA, Cox DA, Fish RD, Gordon JB, Mudge GH, Colucci WS, StJohn Sutton MG, Selwyn AP, Alexander RW, Ganz P (1990) Endothelium-dependent dilation of the coronary microvasculature is impaired in dilated cardiomyopathy. Circulation 81:772-779
6. Inoue T, Sakai Y, Morooka S, Hayashi T, Takayanagi K, Yamaguchi H, Kakoi H, Takabatake Y (1994) Vasodilatory capacity of coronary resistance vessels in dilated cardiomyopathy. Am Heart J 127:376-381
7. Inoue T, Sakai Y, Morooka S, Hayashi T, Takayanagi K, Yamanaka T, Kakoi H, Takabatake Y (1993) Coronary flow reserve in patients with dilated cardiomypathy. Am Heart J 125:93-98
8. Johnson RA, Palacious I (1982) Dilated cardiomyopathies of the adult. N Engl J Med 307:1051-1058
9. Nitenberg A, Foult J, Blanchet F, Zouioueche S (1985) Multifactorial determinants of reduced coronary flow reserve after dipyridamole in dilated cardiomyopathy. Am J Cardiol 55:748-754
10. Wilson RA, Shea MJ, De Landsheere CM, Turton D, Brady F, Deanfield JE, Selwyn AP (1984) Validation of quantitation of regional myocardial blood flow in vivo with ^{11}C-labeled human albumin microspheres and positron emission tomography. Circulation 70:717-723
11. Selwyn AP, Shea MJ., Foale R, Deanfield JE, Wilson R, De Landsheere CM, Turton DL, Brady F, Pike VW, Brookes DI (1986) Regional myocardial and organ blood flow after myocardial infarction: application of the microsphere principle in man. Circulation 73:433-443
12. Parodi O, De Maria R, Oltrona L, Testa R, Sambuceti G, Roghi A, Merli M, Berlinghieri L, Accinni R, Spinelli F, Pellegrini A, Baroldi G (1993) Myocardial blood flow distribution in patients with ischemic heart disease or dilated cardiomyopathy undergoing heart transplantation. Circulation 88:509-522
13. De Maria R, Parodi O, Baroldi G, Sambuceti G, Testa R, Oltrona L, Grassi M, Parolini M, Barberis M, Sara R, De Vita C, Pellegrini A (1996) Morphological bases for thallium-201 uptake in cardiac imaging and correlates with myocardial blood flow distribution. Eur Heart J 17:951-961
14. Accinni R, Belingheri L, Giglioni A, Micelli G, Quaranta M, Wei J, Lucarelli C (1992) Quantitation of collagen/total protein ratio in biological samples by isocratic high performance liquid chromatography 4-hydroxyproline assay. Giorn It Chim Clin 17:27-33

15. Baroldi G, De Maria R, Silver MD (1996) Pathology of dilated cardiomyopathy of unknown cause. Heart Failure 12:102-110
16. Kjekshus JK (1973) Mechanism for flow distribution in normal and ischemic myocardium during increased ventricular preload in the dog. Circ Res 33:490-499
17. Bergmann SR, Fox KAA, Rand AL, McElvany KD, Welch MJ, Markham MJ, Sobel BE (1984) Quantification of regional myocardial blood flow with $H_2{}^{15}O$. Circulation 70:724-733
18. Bellina CR, Parodi O, Camici P, Salvadori PA, Taddei L, Fusani L, Guzzardi R, Klassen GA, L'Abbate A, Donato L (1990) Simultaneous in vitro and in vivo validation of ^{13}N-Ammonia for the assessment of regional myocardial blood flow. J Nucl Med 31: 1335-1343
19. Neglia D, Parodi O, Gallopin M, Sambuceti G, Giorgetti A, Pratali L, Salvadori P, Michelassi C, Lunardi M, Pelosi G, Marzilli M, L'Abbate A (1995) Myocardial blood flow response to pacing tachycardia and to dipyridamole infusion in patients with dilated cardiomyopathy without overt heart failure. A quantitative assessment by positron emission tomography. Circulation 92:796-804
20. Neglia D, Levorato D, Berti S, Marzilli M, Pelosi G, Marcassa C, Bongiorni MG, L'Abbate A, Contini C (1987) Diagnosi e caratterizzazione funzionale di iniziale danno miocardico in pazienti con aritmie cardiache. Cardiologia 32:713-719
21. Neglia D, Gallopin M, Giorgetti A, Sambuceti G, Schneider-Eicke J, Salvadori P, Simonetti I, L'Abbate A, Parodi P (1997) Function of the adenosine sensitive coronary resistance in patients with mild dilated cardiomyopathy. J Am Coll Cardiol 29:394A (abstr)
22. Keren A, Popp RL (1992) Assignment of patients into the classification of cardiomyopathies. Circulation 86:1622-1633
23. Vaghaiwalla Mody F, Brunken RC, Stevenson LW, Nienaber CA, Phelps ME, Schelbert HR (1991) Differentiating cardiomyopathy of coronary artery disease from nonischemic dilated cardiomyopathy utilizing positron emission tomography. J Am Coll Cardiol 17:373-383
24. Wallis DE, O'Connel JB, Henkin RE, Costanzo-Nordin MR, Scanlon PJ (1984) Segmental wall motion abnormalities in dilated cardiomyopathy: a common finding and good prognostic sign. J Am Coll Cardiol 4:674-679
25. Yamaguchi S, Tsuiki K, Hayasaka M, Yasui S (1987) Segmental wall motion abnormalities in dilated cardiomyopathy: hemodynamic characteristics and comparison with thallium-201 myocardial scintigraphy. Am Heart J 113:1123-1128

Myocardial Catecholamines and Inotropic Response in Heart Muscle Disease

P.M. Seferović, R. Maksimović, A. Ristić, S. Stepanović, M. Ostojić, V. Kanjuh, D. Seferović, S. Simeunović and J.D. Vasilević

Introduction

It is widely accepted that both humoral and tissue alterations of sympathetic nervous system activity exist in various heart muscle diseases, including in idiopathic dilated (IDC) and hypertrophic cardiomyopathy (HCM). In particular, there is increasing evidence that myocardial catecholamines may be important determinants of natural history, pathophysiology and prognosis of these patients.

In 31 patients with IDC, Schoefer et al. [1], using iodine-123 meta-iodobenzylguanidine scintigraphy, disclosed a significant positive correlation between myocardial norepinephrine concentration and left ventricular ejection fraction. Moreover, patients with diffusely reduced or no visible myocardial uptake, suggesting myocardial adrenergic disintegrity, had the lowest left ventricular ejection fraction. Catecholamine depletion appears to be a marker of heart failure severity, rather than a specific feature of IDC: Regitz et al. [2, 3] and De Maria et al. [4] demonstrated comparable myocardial norepinephrine levels in IDC and in coronary or valvular heart disease; in both groups norepinephrine levels were significantly reduced in patients with a left ventricular ejection fraction below 30%.

There is also evidence suggesting a link between HCM and abnormal catecholamine metabolism: in a small group of HCM patients, the neuronal uptake of norepinephrine was decreased and the cardiac artero-venous difference was significantly larger than in controls [5]. Furthermore, recent studies emphasize the etiopathogenetic and prognostic importance of elevated myocardial norepinephrine and epinephrine in HCM [6].

Although data on myocardial catecholamines in other heart muscle diseases are only infrequently reported [7], left ventricular functional impairment seems to be associated with reduced myocardial catecholamine synthesis and re-uptake.

The purpose of this study was to explore myocardial catecholamine distribution and its correlation with hemodynamic parameters in biopsy-proven myocarditis, IDC, and HCM.

Methods

Eighty-six patients were included in the study: twenty (80% males, mean age

36±13 years) had biopsy-proven myocarditis, 32 (75% males, mean age 47±12 years) had IDC and 34 (64% males, mean age 43±14 years) had HCM.

Clinical and Laboratory Assessment

The diagnosis of heart muscle disease was established after a complete work-up that included a medical history, clinical evaluation, echocardiography, right and left heart catheterization, hemodynamic measurements, and coronary arteriography. For the echocardiographic diagnosis of HCM, asymmetric septal hypertrophy or apical hypertrophy, with or without systolic anterior motion of the mitral valve, were required. Echocardiographic diagnosis of IDC was based on left ventricular dilatation (end-diastolic left ventricular diameter > 55 mm) and dysfunction (fractional shortening < 25%). Endomyocardial biopsy was performed by femoral approach, using King's bioptome and long sheath technique. The procedure was started only after one-hour rest in a recumbent position and 15 minutes after the last contrast injection, with no pre-medication except local anesthesia. In all patients, three to six pieces were sampled from the left ventricular apex or free wall. Left ventricular myocardial samples (wet weight ranging from 2 to 4 mg) were split into two halves: one for histology and the other for catecholamine measurements.

Myocardial Catecholamine Assay

One half of the bioptic sample was immediately weighed, frozen in liquid nitrogen, and stored at $-80°$ C. At the time of analysis, the specimens were immersed in cold ($4°$ C) 0.1N $HClO_4$ (0.3 mg of tissue per 30 ml of 0.1N $HClO_4$). The tissue was than centrifugated at 10000 rotations per minute, for 15 minutes, and the clear supernatant (30 ml) was used for the analysis. Myocardial catecholamines were measured without knowledge of the clinical diagnosis using the modified Catechol-O-Methyl-Transferase (COMT) radioenzymatic method of Da Prada and Zürcher (1976), Weise and Kopin (1976) and Peuler and Johnson (1977) [8-10], a fast, highly specific, reliable, and reproducible method. Myocardial catecholamines were converted into the corresponding O-methyl derivates by means of purified COMT in the presence of S-adenosyl-l-(3H-methyl)-methionine (Amersham). The O-methyl derivatives were extracted and oxidized into ³H-vanillin, and the activity of this substance was measured using a liquid beta scintillation counter (Packard). COMT was prepared according to the method of Axelrod and Tomchik (1958). Two samples were analyzed for each patient and the mean value was reported.

Histologic Study

The other half of bioptic samples was fixed in 10% buffered formalin, processed in the usual manner, and embedded in paraffin. Paraffin blocks were cut into 4 mm serial sections by microtome and then stained with hematoxylin-eosin, elastic-van Gieson, and Masson's trichrome. The degree of fibrosis was evaluated and classified into three grades from zero to two. Grade 0 indicated no evident fibrosis, grade 1 focal and minimal fibrosis, and grade 2 moderate or severe fibrosis occupying nearly 30% to 50% of the entire specimen. Only specimens with grade 0 to 1 fibrosis were used for myocardial catecholamine measurement.

The diagnosis of biopsy-proven myocarditis was exclusively histological and required evidence of myocyte necrosis; at least five lymphocytes per high-power microscopic field had to be found in close proximity to necrotic myocytes. Light microscopy findings in IDC consisted of hypertrophied as well as attenuated myocytes, variation of myofiber size, different degrees of fibrosis, and occasional mononuclear cells in the interstitium. The histologic support for diagnosis of HCM was based on the finding of hypertrophied myofibrils (>25 nm in diameter), irregularly shaped nuclei, perinuclear halo, "short runs" of myofibrils, disarray, and interstitial fibrosis.

Statistical Analysis

Continuous variables were expressed as mean ± standard deviation. Frequency and percentage were reported for each non-continuous variable. Differences between two groups were assessed by Student's unpaired t test, with probability less than 0.05 in a two-tailed distribution being statistically significant. One-way analysis of variance (ANOVA) was used for comparison among the three groups.

Results

Clinical, hemodynamic, and angiographic data of the three patient groups are summarized in Table 1. Patients with biopsy-proven myocarditis were younger, had a higher incidence of recent viral infection, but showed less arrhythmias than the IDC and HCM groups. They also developed congestive heart failure more rarely than IDC patients. From the hemodynamic point of view, myocarditis patients had a significantly higher heart rate, but only a moderate decline in left ventricular function. IDC patients were found to have the most severe pump dysfunction, while in the HCM group left ventricular systolic parameters were above the normal range.

The average myocardial concentrations of norepinephrine, epinephrine and dopamine in the three groups are shown in Table 2. Head to head comparison between the groups revealed significant differences for norepinephrine and epinephrine ($p < 0.01$), but not for dopamine. The highest myocardial concentration of norepinephrine and epinephrine was found in HCM, intermediate values in myocarditis patients, and the lowest in IDC. Mean dopamine values were similar in all three groups ($p > 0.05$).

The correlations between myocardial catecholamine concentration and hemodynamic parameters in the three groups are shown in Table 3. In patients with biopsy-proven myocarditis, no significant correlation between myocardial catecholamines and hemodynamic parameters was found. In patients with

Table 1. Clinical, hemodynamic, and angiographic data of patients with biopsy-proven myocarditis, dilated cardiomyopathy and hypertrophic cardiomyopathy

Parameters	Biopsy-proven myocarditis	IDC	HCM
CLINICAL			
Number	20	32	34
Age (yrs)	36±13	47±12	43±14
Sex (% male)	80%	75%	64%
Recent viral infection	50% (9/20)	21.8% (7/32)	14.7% (5/34)
Arrhythmia	35.0% (7/20)	56.3% (18/32)	61.7% (21/34)
Congestive heart failure	20.0% (4/20)	37.5% (12/32)	5.8% (2/34)
HEMODYNAMIC AND ANGIOGRAPHIC			
HR (b/min)	118.4±8.2	82.1±8.3	106.6±18.2
PCWP (mmHg)	18.2±3.6	28.8±2.7	9.9±1.6
LVEDP (mmHg)	19.9±4.3	30.9±2.7	12.3±1.4
LV max dp/dt (mmHg* s-1)	1142.3±166.3	559.0±151.4	2054.9±404.7
LVEF (%)	39.9±4.7	25.1±4.2	75.4±10.4
MAP (mmHg)	89.6±9.3	61.1±10.9	82.4±8.3

IDC, idiopathic dilated cardiomyopathy; HCM, hypertrophic cardiomyopathy; HR, heart rate; PCWP, pulmonary capillary wedge pressure; LVEDP, left ventricular end-diastolic pressure; LV dp/dt max, maximal rate of change of pressure during isovolumetric contraction; LVEF, left ventricular ejection fraction; MAP, mean arterial pressure Results are shown as mean ± SEM

IDC, myocardial concentrations of both norepinephrine and epinephrine, but not dopamine, demonstrated a significant positive correlation with left ventricular dp/dt max and ejection fraction ($p < 0.01$), and a significant negative correlation with pulmonary capillary wedge pressure and left ventricular end-diastolic pressure ($p < 0.01$). In the HCM group, a significant ($p < 0.01$) correlation was observed between myocardial concentrations of both norepinephrine and epinephrine, but not dopamine, and heart rate, left ventricular dp/dt max and ejection fraction.

Table 2. Myocardial catecholamine concentration in heart muscle disease

Myocardial concentration	Biopsy-proven myocarditis	IDC	HCM
Norepinephrine (ng/g)	415.4±71.1 *	262.6±68.9 #	781.9±125.8 +#
Epinephrine (ng/g)	57.3±4.8 *	35.8±6.2 #	91.6±13.9 +#
Dopamine (ng/g)	76.6±9.2	70.1±11.8	76.1±8.3

* $p < 0.01$ (Biopsy -proven myocarditis vs.IDC); + $p < 0.01$ (HCM vs.Biopsy-proven myocarditis); # $p < 0.01$ (HCM vs.IDC)

Table 3. The correlation of myocardial catecholamine concentration and related hemodynamic variables in the three study groups

Hemodynamic parameter	HCM			IDC			Biopsy proven myocarditis		
	NE	E	D	NE	E	D	NE	E	D
HR (b/min)	0.74^{**}	0.73^{**}	0.06	0.35	0.49	0.09	-0.16	-0.29	-0.27
PCWP mean (mmHg)	0.02	-0.03	0.17	-0.83^{**}	-0.76^{**}	-0.07	-0.22	0.17	-0.16
LVEDP (mmHg)	0.16	0.05	0.31	-0.79^{**}	-0.75^{**}	-0.11	-0.09	-0.13	-0.23
LV dp/dt max (mmHg x s^{-1})	0.80^{**}	0.77^{**}	0.07	0.87^{**}	0.74	0.07	0.33	-0.18	-0.09
LVEF (%)	0.71^{**}	0.80^{**}	0.12	0.89^{**}	0.86^{**}	0.02	0.34	0.08	-0.02
MAP (mmHg)	0.13	0.01	-0.30	-0.01	0.17	-0.08	0.12	0.26	0.01

D, dopamine; E, epinephrine; HR, heart rate; NE, norepinephrine; PCWP, pulmonary capillary wedge pressure; LVEDP, left ventricular end-diastolic pressure; LV dp/dt max, maximal rate of change of pressure during isovolumetric contraction; LVEF, left ventricular ejection fraction; MAP, mean arterial pressure
** $p < 0.01$

Discussion

We have previously observed significantly higher myocardial concentrations of both norepinephrine and epinephrine in HCM than in IDC patients [11, 12]. This finding is confirmed in the present investigation; myocardial norepinephrine and epinephrine concentrations were also higher in patients with biopsy-proven mycarditis than in those with IDC, in whom the lowest concentrations were found. Furthermore, myocardial catacholamine levels correlated significantly to left ventricular functional parameters.

Several lines of evidence suggest that both humoral and myocardial sympathetic activity may play an important role in HCM: beta-adrenergic blocking agents can lead to regression of myocardial hypertrophy and have a beneficial therapeutic effect in patients with HCM [13]; catecholamines have been used experimentally to induce myocardial hypertrophy [14]. Almost two decades ago, Perloff [15] speculated that disturbances of the interaction between immature, supersensitive myocardial adrenergic receptors and extracardiac catecholamines were the most important etiopathogenetic link responsible for the development of HCM. Despite substantial evidence suggesting a link between HCM and catecholamine, considerable controversy still exists concerning the role of plasma and myocardial catecholamines in this disorder.

Reports on plasmatic catecholamine levels in patients with HCM are sporadic. While Dargie et al. [16] demonstrated increased plasma norepinephrine at rest or standing in patients with HCM, Sugishita et al. [17] reported no difference in rest and peak exercise plasmatic measurements between

HCM patients and controls. In an exquisite study Maisel et al. [18] confirmed that plasma norepinephrine is high in HCM patients; to explain this finding, they speculated that either intrasynaptic inactivation of norepinephrine after its release from the synaptic nerve was impaired or transport of norepinephrine from the neuronal synapse in the blood was improved.

Myocardial release of norepinephrine in a HCM patient was not elevated in the study by Haneda et al. [19]. Toshima and Koga. [20] showed increased left ventricular inotropic activity and overall cardiovascular response to epinephrine infusion in patients with HCM. Reports on myocardial tissue catecholamines in HCM patients are also infrequent. Pearse [21] reported increased myocardial norepineprine and sympathetic innervation in septal myectomy specimens from patients with obstructive HCM, but this observation was not confirmed by others [22, 23]. Kawai et al. [24], who employed a methodology similar to the one of the present study, found remarkably high mycardial norepineprhine levels in the majority of their HCM patients, although mean values were not significantly different from controls with various heart diseases. Whether high catecholamine concentrations in the present HCM group may have a pathophysiological significance is unclear: hypothetically, these results might be due to the impaired neuronal uptake, harbouring further morphologic and functional consequences [25]. The correlation found in HCM between myocardial catecholamines and indices of left ventricular systolic function (ejection fraction and dp/dt max) suggests the importance of local sympathetic activity in the natural history and, most likely, in the clinical manifestation of the disease and may have long-term prognostic significance [6].

In the present study left ventricular systolic function, as assessed by ejection fraction, was normal in HCM, moderately impaired in myocarditis patients and severely depressed in IDC. These differences in left ventricular inotropism paralleled myocardial catcholamine levels in the three groups. Depressed systolic function and a parallel decrease in myocardial norepinephrine content have been previosuly described [26]. Anderson et al. [27] found myocardial norepinephrine and neuropeptide Y depletion in 30 IDC patients. Decreased norepinephrine stores correlated weakly with beta$_1$-adrenergic receptor down-regulation, suggesting that norepinephrine depletion occurs in response to increased adrenergic drive. In the apical left ventricular myocardium of 42 patients with chronic Chagas' disease, severe LV dysfunction and overt heart failure, Correa-Arraujo et al. [7] observed at autopsy a significant depletion of norepinephrine. In another study in IDC [28], myocardial norepineprhine concentration correlated significantly with left ventricular ejection fraction but only weakly with right ventricular ejection fraction. Norepinephrine depletion may be caused by increased adrenergic stimulation, an inherent feature in heart failure, which consequently produces catecholamine overflow and exhaustion of resynthesis.

Some limitations should be kept in mind when analysing the present findings. Although recently most of the methodological controversies on the accuracy of tissue biochemical measurements, including myocardial catecholamine concentrations, seem to be resolved, some dilemmas still exist.

The major drawbacks include the reproducibility of the method and the lack of normal reference range in human myocardium. Reproducibility is a inherent problem of every biopsy procedure, and is more apparent with high sensitivity assays. We tried to overcome this methodological problem by averaging myocardial catcholamine measurements from two samples of each patient. Good reproducibility of catecholamine assay in endomyocardial biopsy samples is supported by previous studies [2, 3, 24, 29]. Kawai et al. [24] demonstrated a significant correlation between repeated measurements (n = 10) in the two assays for both norepinephrine and epinephrine, while Regitz et al. [3] confirmed a high reproducibility, showing that variance between paired biopsies was below 17%.

In the present study lack of information on myocardial catecholamine concentration in normal myocardium, due to obvious ethical and safety reasons, precludes the comparison of the values in the three study groups with healthy controls: only the differences among patients with myocarditis, IDC and HCM could be analyzed. One of the infrequent studies addressing this issue reported in 10 healthy controls average values of 10.3 ± 2.9 pg/μg of non-collagenous proteins for norepinephrine, 0.36 ± 0.51 pg/μg for epinephrine, and 0.52 ± 0.40 pg/μg for dopamine [29]; although methodological differences limit effective comparison, these values appear far higher than those reported in bioptic samples from our three groups of patients.

Summary

In patients with biopsy-proven myocarditis, IDC and HCM myocardial norepinephrine and epinephrine concentrations were significantly different. Left ventricular inotropic conditions paralleled myocardial catecholmaine concentrations, which were highest in HCM and lowest in IDC, while no differences in dopamine content were found.

In biopsy-proven myocarditis no significant correlations were found among catecholamine levels and hemodynamic parameters. Patients with IDC showed depressed left ventricular systolic function and a corresponding decrease in both myocardial norepinephrine and epinephrine, which were positively related to left ventricular dP/dt max and ejection fraction. Furthermore, patients with HCM demonstrated normal left venticular function which correlated significantly with both myocardial norepinephrine and epinephrine, a finding that supports a role for catecholamines in the clinical manifestation and long term outcome of the disease. However, no significant correlation was noticed between myocardial dopamine and hemodynamics.

References

1. Schofer J, Spielmann R, Schuchert A, Weber K, Schluter M (1988) Iodine-123 meta-iodobenzylguanidine scintigraphy: a noninvasive method to demonstrate myocardial adrenergic nervous system disintegrity in patients with idiopathic dilated cardiomyopathy. J Am Coll Cardiol 12:1252-1258

2. Regitz V, Fleck E (1992) Myocardial adenine nucleotide concentrations and myocardial norepinephrine content in patients with heart failure secondary to idiopathic dilated or ischemic cardiomyopathy. Am J Cardiol 69:1574-1580
3. Regitz V, Leuchs B, Bossaller C, Sehested J, Rappolder M, Fleck E (1991) Myocardial catecholamine concentrations in dilated cardiomyopathy and heart failure of different origins. Eur Heart J 12 [Suppl. D]:171-174
4. De Maria R, Accinni R, Baroldi G, Repossini A, Garino-Cannia G, Caroli A, Vago T, Bevilacqua M, Pellegrini A (1990) Catecholamines, beta receptors and morphology in dilated cardiomyopathy: a preliminary report. In: Baroldi G, Camerini F, Goodwin JF (eds) Advances in cardiomyopathies. Springer, Berlin Heidelberg New York, pp 257-265
5. Brush JE Jr, Eisenhofer G, Garty M, Stull R, Maron BJ, Cannon R (1989) Cardiac norepinephrine kinetics in hypertrophic cardiomyopathy. Circulation 79:836-844
6. Seferovič PM, Stepanovič S, Maksimovič R, et al. (1997) Long-term prognosis in hypertrophic and idiopathic dilated cardiomyopathy: the role of myocardial catecholamine. Eur Heart J 18 [Suppl. A]:P3725
7. Correa-Araujo R, Oliveira JS, Ricciardi-Cruz A (1991) Cardiac levels of norepinephrine, dopamine, serotonin and histamine in Chagas' disease. Int J Cardiol 31:329-36
8. Da Prada M, Zürcher G (1976) Simultaneous radioenzymatic determination of plasma and tissue adrenaline, noradrenaline and dopamine within the femtomole range. Life Sci 19: 1161-1174
9. Weise VK, Kopin IJ (1976) Assay of catecholamines in human plasma. Studies of a single isotope radioenzymatic technique. Life Sci 19:1673-1686
10. Pauler JD, Johnson GA (1977) Simultaneous single isotope radioenzymatic assay of plasma norepinephrine, epinephrine and dopamine. Life Sci 21:625-636
11. Seferovič PM, Stepanovič S, Maksimovič R et al. (1995) Myocardial catecholamine in primary heart muscle diseases: Fact or fancy? Eur Heart J 16 [Suppl.O]: 124-127
12. Seferovič PM, Stepanovič S, Maksimovič R, et al. (1997) Does myocardial catecholamine concentration reflect left ventricular function in heart muscle disease? J Am Coll Cardiol:796
13. Gilbert EM, Olsen SL, Renlund DG, Bristow MR (1993) Beta-adrenergic receptor regulation and left ventricular function in idiopathic dilated cardiomyopathy. Am J Cardiol 71:23-29
14. Himura Y, Felten SY, Kashiki M, Lewandowski TJ, Delehanty JM, Liang CS (1993) Cardiac noradrenergic nerve terminal abnormalities in dogs with experimental congestive heart failure. Circulation 88:1299-1309
15. Perloff JK (1981) Pathogenesis of hypertrophic cardiomyopathy: hypothesis and speculations. Am Heart J 101:219-220
16. Dargie H, Boschetti E, Reid J, Goodwin JF (1980) Autonomic function in hypertrophic cardiomyopathy. Circulation 2 [Suppl. III]: III-301
17. Sugishita Y, Iida K, Matsuda M, et al. (1983) Plasma norepinephrine concentration during exercise in patients with different types of hypertrophic cardiomyopathy. Annual Report of the Idiopathic Cardiomyopathy Research Committee, The Ministry of Health and Welfare of Japan Publication, Tokyo, pp 168-171
18. Maisel AS, Wright M, Wilner KD, Ziegler MG (1988) Norepinephrine kinetics in hypertrophic cardiomyopathy. In: Toshima H, Maron BJ (eds) Hypertrophic Cardiomyopathy. University of Tokyo Press, Tokyo, pp 129-139
19. Haneda T, Miura Y, Miyazawa K, et al. (1978) Plasma norepinephrine concentration in the coronary sinus in cardiomyopathies. Cath Cardiovasc Diag 4:399-405
20. Toshima H, Koga Y (1988) Norepinephrine kinetics in hypertrophic cardiomyopathy. In: Toshima H, Maron BJ (eds) Hypertrophic Cardiomyopathy. University of Tokyo Press, Tokyo, pp 141-153
21. Pearse AGE (1964) The histochemistry and electron microscopy of obstructive cardiomyopathy. In: Wolstenhome GEW, O'Connor M (eds) Cardiomyopathies. G&A Churchill, London, pp 132-164
22. McCallister BD, Brown AL (1967) A fine-structure study of idiopathic hypertrophic subaortic stenosis. Am J Cardiol 19:142-154
23. Van Noorden S, Olsen EGJ, Pearse AGE (1971) Hypertrophic obstructive cardiomy-

opathy, a histological, histochemical and ultrastructural study of biopsy material. Cardiovasc Res 5: 118-131
24. Kawai C, Yui Y, Hoshono T, Sasayama S, Matsumori A (1983) Myocardial catecholamine in hypertrophic and dilated (congestive) cardiomyopathy: a biopsy study. J Am Coll Cardiol 2:834-840
25. Beau SL, Saffitz JE (1994) Transmural heterogeneity of norepinephrine uptake in failing human hearts. J Am Coll Cardiol 23:579-585
26. Schofer J, Tews A, Langes K, Bleifeld W, Reimitz PE, Mathey DG (1987) Relationship between myocardial norepinephrine content and left ventricular function - an endomyocardial biopsy study. Eur Heart J 8:748-753
27. Anderson FL, Port D, Reid BB, Larrabee P, Hanson G, Bristow MR (1992) Myocardial catecholamine and neuropeptide Y depletion in failing ventricles of patients with idiopathic dilated cardiomyopathy. Correlation with beta adrenergic receptor downregulation. Circulation 85:46-53
28. Schofer J, Bleifeld W (1987) Sympathetic activity in idiopathic dilated cardiomyopathy. Influence of captopril and hydralazine. Cardiovasc Drugs Ther 1:177-181
29. Regitz V, Bossaller C, Strasser R, Schuler S, Hetzer R, Fleck E (1990) Myocardial catecholamine content after heart transplantation. Circulation 82:620-623

Molecular Biology of Heart Failure

B. Swynghedauw

Myocardial dysfunction is no more functional in nature and recent progress in molecular biology have allowed a better understanding of the process. The new myocardial phenotype is not only quantitatively, but also qualitatively different from the normal heart. The first evidence that qualitative changes occur after chronic overload was published by our laboratory in 1979 [1]. We were indeed able to show in the rat ventricles, after aortic stenosis or aortic insufficiency, an isomyosin shift resulting in the reexpression of a foetal isoform with a low ATPase specific activity. Further investigations in the rat and in other animal species, have shown that such a shift was responsible for the diminution of the shortening velocity and, partly, for the improvement of the economy of contraction [2,3]. Several other changes in genetic expression were further reported, including those encoding sarcomeric proteins, membrane proteins, receptors, proteins responsible for energy metabolism and also several pathways in charge of the transduction process [4]. The puzzle is now more or less complete and it is now possible to establish a rational link between the aforementioned modifications and the well-documented physiological alterations which characterise the failing myocardium.

The Two Major Biologic Determinants of Myocardial Dysfunction

Myocardial dysfunction depends on only two groups of independently regulated biologic determinants, namely the deleterious consequence of the adaptional process and fibrosis. Only one of these two components can cause cardiac failure, for example pure volume overload is not associated with fibrosis and failure in this particular case depends only on the negative aspects of cardiac adaptation. Nevertheless, the two components are usually associated with each other as in the most common type of cardiac failure, i.e. cardiac failure occurring in the elderly having both coronary disease and arterial hypertension.

The Deleterious Aspects of the Adaptational Process

The adaptational process is a random process. The overloaded heart, like the overloaded skeletal muscle, has to modify its thermodynamic status which is no longer adapted to the new environmental requirements. To modify the phenotype accordingly, it utilises another genetic programme, the only one which is in fact available, the foetal programme. Such a programme is likely to be transcriptionally regulated, although there is some indirect evidence in favour of additional translational mechanisms. The trigger and pathways responsible for such modifications of the genetic expression are probably not unique. Stretch, through stretch receptors, plays certainly a crucial role, nevertheless the corresponding receptors are still not isolated [5]. Local hormone or peptide production, such as the myocardial renin-angiotensin system, endothelin or nitric oxide, may modulate the stretch effects, and even, in certain conditions, be major determinants of changes in genetic expression.

The Growth Process is Reactivated

In adults, cardiocytes never divide, but they hypertrophy, either along the longitudinal axis of the cell in case of volume overload, or on the longitudinal and transversal axis in case of pressure overload. Cardiac hypertrophy can be homogeneous as after valve disease, or heterogeneous as a response to heterogeneous stress induced by multiple areas of necrosis or fibrosis. Such a quantitative adaptation is beneficial for two reasons: it multiplies the number of contractile units available, and lowers wall stress according to the Laplace law. Non-muscle cells, including fibroblasts, endothelial cells, macrophages, both hypertrophy and multiply by mitosis. Several genes participate in the growth process, such as the genes encoding the calcium channel subunits whose concentration parallels the cardiac mass [6].

Several Foetal Genes Are Also Either Reactivated or Blunted

The process is species and tissue specific (it is not the same in ventricles and in atria), nevertheless it is not specific for a given type of overload. The modifications have been reported both in pressure and volume overload: the changes in genetic expression occur usually later after producing aortic incompetence rather than after banding the aorta, and the role of the pressure component in aortic insufficiency is still debatable [7]. The process occurs also during hypothyroidism.

– Specific foetal isoforms, such as the creatine kinase B subunit [8], the $\alpha3$-subunit of the Na^+, K^+-ATPase [9] or the isomyosin form V3 [1], are reexpressed while the corresponding adult forms (the M subunit for creatine kinase, the $\alpha1$-subunit of the Na^+, K^+-ATPase, the isomyosin V1) are blunted.

– There are also genes whose expression is absent during the foetal life. Such genes are not activated by mechanical overload, hence the corresponding product, namely the protein, is diluted in the already hypertrophied cardiocyte and its concentration drops down. Two good examples are the Ca^{2+} ATPase of the Sarcoplasmic Reticulum (SR) and the $\beta1$-adrenergic receptor [10,11].

– A third group of modifications includes transcripts whose concentration is augmented. A good example is the gene of the Atrial Natriuretic Peptides

(ANP). The gene is normally only expressed in atria. Its ventricular expression is triggered by mechanical overload [12].

Each of these changes in genetic expression is a part of a puzzle. The entire puzzle is responsible for myocardial function and dysfunction as explained below. The major point is in fact that most of the molecular modifications have simultaneously a short-term adaptational and beneficial effect, and a long-term deleterious counterpart. A good example is the calcium transient. The duration of the transient depends on several calcium-regulating proteins, including external membrane proteins and proteins from the sarcoplasmic reticulum. Both levels possess enzymes or channels capable of either releasing calcium into the cytoplasm, or transferring the divalent cation into the extracellular space or internal stores. The calcium transient is slowed in compensatory hypertrophy in parallel with a slow shortening velocity. Hence such a slowing initially participates in the adaptational process. Nevertheless simultaneously the increased duration of the calcium transient enhances automaticity, and is a potential cause of arrhythmogenicity. What we presently know concerning the calcium-regulating proteins in cardiac overload suggests that the determinant of the increased duration of the calcium transient is an unbalance between the concentration of the active calcium channels, which is maintained during compensatory hypertrophy, and the system responsible for the release of calcium in the external space (the Na^+/Ca^{2+} exchanger and the Na^+, K^+-ATPase) which is modified.

Fibrosis

Ventricular fibrosis is a major risk factor for cardiac function. Autopsy studies have evidenced a strong clinical link between cardiac performance and the degree of ventricular fibrosis [13], and fibrosis is likely to be a major prognostic factor in aged persons or during myocardial ischaemia. One of the best experimental models of cardiac failure is the 18-month-old Spontaneously Hypertensive Rat (the SHR Okamoto strain). It has recently been suggested that collagen should be the only molecular marker of cardiac failure, i.e. the only probe that is able to establish a difference between 16-month-old SHR with a compensatory cardiac hypertrophy and 18-month-old animals which are in the failing stage of the disease [14]. From a prognostic point of view fibrosis participates in diastolic dysfunction as a major determinant of ventricular stiffness, in systolic dysfunction by creating myocardial heterogeneity, and in arrhythmogenicity by inducing reentry circuits.

Collagen is a normal constituent of ventricular tissue, and allows the myocytes to contract in parallel. An increased collagen mass participates in the adaptational process, and in fact collagen synthesis is one of the first events which follow acute pressure overload [15]. Fibrosis is not only a modification of the mass, but also an increased concentration, whether it is reparative as a scar after myocardial infarction, or diffuse, as during senescence. In both cases fibrosis creates heterogeneity and, because of the stiffness of the collagen fibres, renders the tissue more rigid.

Fibrosis is a mutifactorial process: reparative fibrosis occurs after necrosis or wound healing, reactive fibrosis is linked to inflammatory processes and there are several conditions with lone fibrosis. Ventricular fibrosis is in fact linked to particularities of the epidemiology of cardiac failure. Cardiac failure is a disease of senescence, the main cause of cardiac failure in our countries is myocardial ischaemia (which is not true in Brasil for example, where Chagas disease is more important), diabetes favours coronary disease and causes myocardial fibrosis. An additional source of complexity is the role played by several hormones or peptides, such as catecholamines, angiotensin II, endothelin, aldosterone: each of these components can produce fibrosis although by different mechanisms. For example, an elevated plasma aldosterone level can be at the origin of cardiac hypertrophy, it may also be a consequence of either an activation of the renin-angiotensin system, or of haemodynamic stress. A continuous infusion of aldosterone itself can produce left ventricular hypertrophy and fibrosis within two weeks [16]. The mechanism by which aldosterone creates fibrosis is rather complex and involves a direct effect of the hormone, indirect effects through an upregulation of angiotensin receptors [unpublished data from this laboratory] and an activation of the endothelin system.

Genetic Susceptibility to Cardiac Failure

Whether or not patients having the same degree of mechanical overload are equally suceptible to fall into decompensation is a new and interesting problem. Molecular genetics have indeed already demonstrated that several mutations located into genes encoding various contractile proteins including myosin, tropomyosin or troponin are responsible for the development of Familial Hypertrophic Cardiomyopathy. Although the link between genotype and phenotype is not entirely elucidated, there is at least one point which is for the moment perfectly clear, i.e. the fact that the genetic disorders cause cardiac hypertrophy, and the hypertrophic process plays a compensatory role [17]. The disease is obviously multiallelic, and we need epidemiologic studies to better appreciate the incidence of such mutations in a large population and consequently its potential role as a determinant cofactor of cardiac failure. It is easy to predict that soon the same rationale should apply to problems such as apoptosis [18] or the capacity of cardiocytes to react to an ischemic stress [19].

The Different Cellular Levels

The two fundamental mechanisms described above act simultaneously and modify the entire myocardial phenotype. Such structural modifications form what is more commonly called the myocardial remodelling. Cardiac remodelling was initially described after a myocardial infarction, but it is equally observed in cardiomyopathies. The only difference is symmetry. Structural remodelling is asymmetric after myocardial infarction and associated with infarct expansion and major changes in the geometry of the ventricle. Cardiomyopathies, or hypertensive cardiopathy, usually (but there are several known exceptions) cause symmetric remodelling and concentric hypertrophy. Nevertheless in both cases the molecular basis of cardiac remodelling remains basically the same (Table 1). In contrast, molecular remodelling is very different from one animal species to the other.

Contractile Proteins

A change in the shortening velocity can result from a slowing of the intracellular calcium transient or a modification in the contractile protein apparatus which is the final target for calcium. In the ventricle of animal species such as rats, the maximum shortening velocity of the overloaded fresh cardiac fibres decreases. The same diminution is also observed when the cardiac fibres have been skinned, i.e. when all membrane structures responsible for the intracellular calcium transient have been removed [3]. A shift in the expression of the two isogenes encoding cardiac myosin heavy chains has been demonstrated: from the α chain, which is the main component of the V1 type, the fast isoenzyme, to the β chain which belongs to the V3 type, the

Table 1. Myocardial biological determinants of cardiac remodelling in cardiac failure

Dysfunction	Biological determinants
Diastolic Dysfunction	
Slow active relaxation	SR Ca^{2+} ATPase, Na^+/Ca^{2+} exchanger.
⇑ atrial contractility	isomyosin change to slow myosin.
⇑ ventricular stiffness and heterogeneity	fibrosis
Systolic dysfunction (ventricle)	
⇓ max shortening velocity	⇑ Ca^{2+} transient duration
⇓ sensitivity to catechol. :	⇓ β-AR & ⇑ G_{ai2}
⇓ cardiac output	see above
	+ tissue heterogeneity due to fibrosis
	+ cell loss (necrosis+apoptosis)
Arrhythmias and heart rate	
Benign and severe arrhythmias	
– Re-entry	Fibrosis
– Automaticity	⇓ capacity of the cardiocyte to buffer changes in $[Ca^{2+}]i$
	+ ventricular expression of sinus node markers
– Triggered activity	⇑ action potential duration
⇓ Heart Rate Variability	
– ⇑ catechol	neural damage: ⇓ baroreflexes sensitivity
	⇓ β-AR and ⇑G_{ai2} (homologous regulation)
– adaptation	⇓ β-AR + ⇓ M_2-R
QT	
length	action potential duration (K+ channel)
dispersion	fibrosis
variability	see above

SR, sarcoplasmic reticulum; AR, adrenergic receptor; M_2-R, muscarinic receptor slow isomyosin. V3 has a slow ATPase and also is the myosin of the slow red skeletal muscle [20]. The shift correlates with the shortening velocity, nevertheless thermodynamic studies have evidenced an additional role of calcium movements and calcium regulating membrane proteins [2].

The situation is different in the ventricles of guinea pig [3] and very likely also of humans [21]. In these cases, the shortening velocity of the skinned fiber is unchanged by mechanical overloading, in sharp contrast with the measurements of the contractile velocity made on fresh papillary muscles. The shift in isomyosin composition does not exist in the human ventricle which is already almost 100% V3 [1,20]. Hence the variations of shortening velocity cannot be explained by phenotypic modifications at this level.

In atria from every mammalian species, the atrial myosin composition differs from that of ventricles. Human atria contains almost 100% V1, the fast isoform of myosin: this isoform is an $\alpha\alpha$ myosin heavy chain isoform which is in fact slightly different from the ventricular V1 because it contains specific myosin light chains. Conversely the ventricles in humans are nearly 100% V3, the slow isoform of the enzyme. During mechanical overload of the heart the isomyosin composition of the ventricle remains unchanged, whereas that of the atria is modified. It has been shown by several laboratories including ours [22] that, in human atria, chronic cardiac overloading results in a shift from V1 to V3. This shift is correlated with the degree of atrial hypertrophy as quantitated by echocardiography [22] and can reasonably be interpreted as an adaptational process which allows atria to compensate for the deficit in early ventricular filling in diastolic dysfunction.

Calcium Movements and Membrane Proteins

One of the first applicable results of molecular biology in cardiology was the demonstration, in several different laboratories including ours [10,23], that chronic cardiac overload, in experimental models as well as in humans whatever the mechanism, is constantly associated with a reduction in the concentration of the functionally active Ca^{2+} ATPase molecules of the Sarcoplasmic Reticulum (SR). Data from our laboratory also show that the ryanodine receptor density (this channel is the biological support of the calcium-induced calcium-release) is diminished in parallel [24]. Hence the balance between calcium input and calcium release is maintained at the level of the SR. In contrast both the total number of calcium channels and the calcium inward current per cell increase proportionally with the degree of hypertrophy; however, even though the number of channels increases, their density remains constant since the cardiocytes are larger [6]. Changes in the (Na^+, K^+)-ATPase, the enzyme which is responsible for the Na^+-K^+ homeostasis, are more complex and certainly species-specific. The (Na^+, K^+)-ATPase is functionally coupled with the Na^+/Ca^{2+} exchanger: it maintains the sodium gradient and by so doing allows the exchanger to release calcium in physiological conditions. In the rat there is a shift from the isoform having a high affinity for sodium to a form with low affinity for calcium [9]. In parallel the Na^+/Ca^{2+} exchanger becomes less active in the rat [25], nevertheless the situation is again species-specific and it has been shown that the density of the exchanger is increased in cardiac overload in humans [26].

The calcium transient is prolonged in human cardiac hypertrophy as well as in rats and rabbits. The overall picture is then as follows. At the sarco-lemmal level the elements responsible for calcium input, namely the calcium channels are normal in density. By contrast, those which are supposed to release calcium out of the cell are modified, and we can conclude that there is an imbalance of calcium homeostasis at this level. In the SR, calcium homeostasis is maintained since the density of both the Ca^{2+} ATPase and ryanodine receptors is decreased. In consequence the hypertrophied myocytes is in a fragile equilibrium in terms of calcium homeostasis, and the transient is prolonged.

Ionic Channels

The most consistent change linked to chronic mechanical overload is a lengthening of the action potential duration [reviewed in 27] which, in part, explains the increase in QT interval on the ECG, which has a prognostic value. The action potential duration itself depends on the activity of several ionic channels and can increase both when an outward current is depressed or when an inward current is enhanced [4]. Its determinants are likely to be both species and tissue-specific.

(i) Voltage-sensitive calcium channels are responsible for the slow inward current I_{CaL}, contribute to the plateau phase and could be involved in lengthening the action potential. It has been demonstrated that both the current density and total number of calcium channels are unchanged [6].

(ii) Potassium currents are outward currents which accelerate the repolarisation. A major non-species-specific and reproducible defect in cardiac hypertrophy and failure is a pronounced depression of the early transient outward current I_{to} [28]. Modifications concerning other K^+ currents have been reported for the moment these alterations are controversial. Recent investigations using probes specific for the K^+ channels subunit are in favour of a transcriptional regulation of such a process.

(iii) Three currents or proteins specific for both the sinus node and foetal programme have been evidenced in overloaded ventricles: I_f, the main current responsible for the spontaneous depolarisation of the pace-maker [29], I_{CaT}, a calcium channel specific for the sinus node [30], and the α3-isoform of the sodium pump [9], which is likely to be a marker of the conductive system. The appearance of pacemaker-like molecular structures may constitute an additional factor favouring automaticity.

The Autonomous Nervous System

Cardiac failure is characterised by a sustained enhancement of plasma catecholamines, which is proportional to myocardial dysfunction and to the severity of the disease. The concentration of this hormone has a prognostic significance, it also causes neural damages at the level of the autonomic nervous system (ANS) [31]. One of the consequences of this neural disease is a blunting of the variability of heart rate. Both the low and high frequency oscillations of the sinus rate disappear indicating that the two components of the autonomic nervous system have been simultaneously altered [32]. In addition the sensitivity to both isoproterenol and forskolin of the failing cardiac myofiber is attenuated [33]. Major recent findings at the level of the myocardial tissue itself were a diminution of the density of the β1-adrenergic receptors as a result of a homologous down-regulation, and an increased level of $G_{i\alpha2}$, the inhibitory subunit of the G protein. Such an increase is a direct consequence of the elevated plasma catecholamines [34].

The mechanism of the down-regulation of the adrenergic receptors is more complex and includes an additional phenomenon. Indeed it has been shown that the density of both the β1-adrenergic and M2 muscarinic receptors is diminished in compensated cardiac hypertrophy. Molecular biology data indicate that in fact the genes encoding these two groups of receptors were not activated by the hemodynamic stress and belong to the same family of genes that the SR calcium ATPase. In this family the diminution of the density of the corresponding mRNAs and proteins is due to a dilution into an already hypertrophied cardiocyte [11].

Energy Metabolism

Economy, in biology as well as in politics, is the energy output/energy input ratio. In terms of mechanics, as well as in muscular physiology, the economy of a machine, or the economy of a muscle is optimal for a given velocity and the economy/velocity curve has a bell shape. Another slightly different finding coming from phylogenic studies is that slow muscles have a better economy than the fast ones [20]. When cardiac fibres are suddenly overloaded, they instantaneously contract at a slower speed than normal and the immediate consequence is a diminution in the economy of the system, with the muscle using more oxygen per gramme of developed tension than normal. A normal heart during exercise contracts at a velocity that corresponds to an optimum economy, at the top of the bell-shape curve. At rest, contraction is already less economic, and during overload, the velocity is even slower and is responsible for a drop in economy, i.e. to a diminished energy utilisation/energy production ratio.

Direct quantitation of energy flux has been performed on the failing heart or in compensated cardiac hypertrophy both in experimental models and humans [2]. In both cases it has been shown that economy is improved with less energy utilised per gram of tension produced. The normal aged heart has the same heart weight/body weight ratio than the adult, nevertheless cardiocytes from the left ventricle are hypertrophied, indicating a certain degree of mechanical overload due to the changes in the characteristic impedance of big vessels. Economy has been determined on this model by measuring the curvature of the Hill's force/velocity relationships and is equally improved. In both cases such an improved economy was obtained thanks to changes in genetic expression which allow the contraction velocity to be slower. Heat production measurements allow distinction of tension-dependent heat (the heat produced by the sliding process), tension-independent heat (the heat produced by calcium movements), resting heat (the heat produced by synthesis and ionic homeostasis) and recovery heat (the heat produced by mitochondria). Recovery heat is unchanged in compensated hypertrophy, in contrast both tension-dependent and tension-independent heats are reduced [2]. Hence search for changes in genetic expression responsible for the adaptational process has to focus on contractile proteins or calcium regulating proteins more than on mitochondria. Such a strategy was followed during the last past ten years by most of the laboratories.

Mechanical studies comparing the properties of fresh myofibers to that of fibers without any membrane structure (skinned fibers) from pressure overloaded rats or guinea pigs allowed also another major distinction [3]. The turn over of cross-bridge cycling is indeed modified in rat ventricle, not in guinea pig. Further on, molecular biological studies have confirmed that there are indeed animal species or tissues in which the adaptational process is due to changes at both the membrane and the sarcomere levels, such as rat ventricle or mammalian atria, and species or tissue, such as human, guinea pig, dog ventricles in which the adaptation is only caused by modifications of the calcium transient and corresponding calcium regulating proteins.

Extracellular Matrix

As explained above, fibrosis, i.e. an increased concentration in collagen, does not participate in the adaptational process and has multifactorial origins, but an increased collagen content of the heart with an unmodified concentration is an important component of the adaptation. The collagen network plays a major role in allowing a homogeneous contraction of the heart and maintaining a parallel organisation of the cardiac myofibers. Indeed the activation of collagen synthesis is a very early process occurring within one hour after a sudden mechanical overload [15]. In every model the collagen content increases commensurably with the growth process. In models such as volume-overload or infra-renal aortic stenosis the concentration is unchanged, even though some modifications in the network organisation have been reported [35]. As explained above, fibrosis is differentially regulated.

Determinants of Myocardial Dysfunction

Myocardial dysfunction includes systolic dysfunction, diastolic dysfunction and arrhythmias (Table 1). New concepts concerning cardiac failure arise from large clinical trials and have emphasised the role of cardiac remodelling. Several vasoactive drugs, including isorbide dinitrate, hydralazine and converting enzyme inhibitor, and several β-adrenergic blockers, including carvedilol and bucindolol, are indeed able, not only to prevent, but also to reverse structural remodelling and by so doing, to improve the ejection fraction, which means that such drugs not only act through their haemodynamic effect but that they also have a direct trophic effect.

Diastole

The diastolic properties of the left ventricle are the first to be modified during hypertensive cardiopathy and these changes occur long before there is any sign of systolic failure. Diastole, for the clinician but not for the physiologist, encompasses three different events, namely active relaxation, diastasis and atrial contraction. Clinical investigations provide global data and cannot easily distinguish the various determinants of ventricular filling, i.e. the passive properties of the ventricular myocardium, but also the ventricular filling dynamics resulting from active relaxation and the atrial contraction-relaxation cycle.

A major, if not unique biological determinant of the passive properties of the ventricle, i.e. diastolic stiffness (or passive compliance), is fibrosis. Myocardial stiffness correlates to the myocardial concentration in collagen [35]. As explained above, fibrosis does not necessarily accompany cardiac hypertrophy and several clinical settings have been able to separate patients with the same degree of cardiac hypertrophy due to valvular disease into two groups, one with a normal muscle stiffness, the other with a significant shift of the stress-strain relationship [36].

Active relaxation velocity parallels the shortening velocity in most of the experimental settings and as such is also impaired during cardiac hypertrophy. Such a component is not easy to measure with noninvasive techniques in man. Alterations of the load-dependence of relaxation, an essential property of the SR, are apparently species-specific. They have been reported during cardiac overload both in humans and guinea pig, nevertheless they do not exist in rats.

During diastolic dysfunction, atrial contraction plays a major role to compensate for the impairment of early passive filling. From a biological point of view the adaptation is due to an isomyosin shift, as described above. Such a mechanism is possible in humans only in atria, not in ventricles, because human atria normally contain a fast myosin isoform, and because the shift to be thermodynamically efficient has to increase the amount of the slow isomyosin, as already explained.

Systole

Alterations in systolic function occur later on during the course of hypertensive cardiopathy. Initially the slowing of the shortening velocity of the hypertrophied fiber plays an adaptational role, and the process allows the myofiber to produce force at a lower velocity and with a normal efficiency in terms of moles of ATP per gram of tension. Nevertheless obviously it simultaneously participates in the alteration of cardiac output.

From a biological point of view, systolic dysfunction depends upon three factors, namely contractile proteins, membrane proteins responsible for the calcium transient and tissue homogeneity. As already explained, in human ventricles the main determinants of systolic dysfunction are the membrane proteins responsible for calcium movements. In contrast the determinants of systolic function in human atria are contractile proteins. Myocardial heterogeneity is also an important source of systolic dysfunction. Heterogeneity is generated by fibrotic tissue, as scars or diffuse fibrosis, like in the senescent myocardium or in the border zone around a scar.

Arrhythmogenicity

Arrhythmias in compensated cardiac hypertrophy are related to cardiac remodelling. Two biological modifications – fibrosis and changes in the membrane proteins composition – play a determining role. Three basic mechanisms may be involved in the genesis of benign or severe arrhythmias, namely re-entry, abnormal automaticity and triggered activity.

Re-entry is a mechanism of maintenance of arrhythmias and is directly linked to fibrosis. The propagated impulse may recycle through an abnormal alternative pathway. Re-entry requires an additional conduction block in the normal conductive pathway together with slowed conduction, so that the conduction time in the re-entry circuit exceeds the refractory period of the conducting tissue. Fibrosis can create the alternative pathway and conduction block, and could slow conduction.

Two different biological substrates may explain the increased automaticity of ventricular cells in cardiac failure or hypertrophy. The first is a slowing of the calcium transient as explained above. The other mechanism involves the expression of ionic channels, such as I_f, which normally initiate slow depolarisation in the sinus node [29].

Abnormal activity can be triggered by impulse generation due to early or delayed after-depolarisation. Early after-depolarisation is facilitated by the increased duration of action potential, and, in turn, may result from changes in the expression of various ionic channel genes. Finally myocardial heterogeneity will in turn enhance the propensity of the hypertrophied myocyte to develop triggered activity and automaticity.

References

1. Lompré AM, Schwartz K, Albis A, Lacombe G, Thiem NV, Swynghedauw B (1979) Myosin isozymes redistribution in chronic heart overloading. Nature 282:105-107
2. Alpert NR, Mulieri LA, Hasenfuss G (1992) Myocardial chemo-mechanical energy transduction. In: Fozzard (ed) The heart and cardiovascular system", Raven Press, New York, pp 111-128
3. Clapier-Ventura R, Mekhfi H, Oliviero P, Swynghedauw B (1988) Pressure overload changes cardiac skinned fibers mechanics in rats, but not in guinea pigs. Am J Physiol 254:H517
4. Swynghedauw B (1995) Molecular Cardiology for the Cardiologists. Kluwer, Boston
5. Yamazaki T, Komuro I, Nagai R, Yazaki Y (1996) Stretching, the evidence in case of cardiac growth. Cardiovasc Res 31:493
6. Mayoux E, Callens F, Swynghedauw B, Charlemagne D (1988) Adaptational process

of the cardiac Ca2+ channels to pressure overload: biochemical and physiological properties of the dihydropyridines receptors in normal and hypertrophied rat hearts. J Cardiovasc Pharmacol 12:390-396
7. Mercadier JJ, Lompre AM, Wisnewsky C, Samuel JL, Bercovici J, Swynghedauw B, Schwartz K (1981) Myosin isoenzymic changes in several models of rat cardiac hypertrophy. Circ Res 49:525-532
8. Younes A, Schneider JM, Bercovici J, Swynghedauw B (1985) Creatine kinase isoenzymes redistribution in chronically overloaded myocardium. Cardiovasc Res 19:15-19
9. Charlemagne D, Orlowski J, Oliviero P, Rannou F, Sainte-Beuve C, Swynghedauw B, Lane LK (1994) Alteration of Na, K-ATPase subunit mRNA and protein levels in hypertrophied heart. J Biol Chem 269:1541-1547
10. de la Bastie D, Levitsky D, Rappaport L, Mercadier J.J, Marotte F, Wisnewsky C, Brokovich V, Schwartz K Lompre AM (1990) Function of the sarcoplasmic reticulum and expression of its Ca ATPase gene in pressure overload-induced cardiac hypertrophy in the rat. Circ Res 66:554-564
11. Mondry A, Bourgeois F, Carré F, Swynghedauw B, Moalic JM (1995) Decrease in β_1-adrenergic and M2-muscarinic receptor mRNA levels and unchanged accumulation of mRNAs coding for G_{ai-2} and G_{as} proteins in rat cardiac hypertrophy. J Mol Cell Cardiol 27:2287-2294
12. Mercadier JJ, Lompré AM, De la Bastie D, Wisnewsky C, Schwartz K (1987) Accumulation de l'acide ribonucléique messager du facteur atrial natriurétique dans le ventricule gauche du rat à la phase d'hypertrophie compensée d'une surcharge de pression. C R Acad Sci (Paris) 305:79-82
13. Weber KT (1995) Wound healing in cardiovascular disease. Futura Pub., Armonk, USA
14. Bolyut MO, O'Neill L, Meredith AL, Bing OHL, Brooks WW, Conrad CH, Crow MT, Lakatta EG (1994) Alterations in cardiac gene expression during transition from stable hypertrophy to heart failure. Circ Res 75:23
15. Skosey JL, Zak R, Martin AF, Aschenbrenner V, Rabinowitz M (1972) Biochemical correlates of cardias hypertrophy. V. Labeling of collagen, myosin and nuclear DNA during experimental myocardial hypertrophy in the rat. Circ Res 31:145-157
16. Robert V, Thiem NV, Cheav SL, Mouas C, Swynghedauw B, Delcayre C (1994) Increased cardiac collagens (I) and (III) mRNAs in aldosterone-salt hypertension. Hypertension 24:30-36
17. Schwartz K, Carrier L, Guicheney P, Komajda M (1995) Molecular basis of familial cardiomyopathies. Circulation, 91:532-540
18. Bing OHL (1994) Hypothesis : apoptosis may be a mechanism for the transition to heart failure with chronic pressure overload. J Mol Cell Cardiol 26:943-948
19. Assayag P, Charlemagne D, de Leiris J, Boucher F, Valère PE, Lortet S, Swynghedauw B, Besse S (1997) Senescent heart as compared to pressure overload induced hypertrophy. Hypertension, 29:15-21
20. Swynghedauw B. (1986). Developmental and functional adaptation of contractile proteins in cardiac and skeletal muscles. Physiol Rev 66:710-771
21. Hasenfuss G, Holubarsch, C, Just H, Alpert NR (eds) (1992) Cellular and molecular alterations in the failing human heart. Steinkopff Verlag, Darmstadt
22. Mercadier JJ, de la Bastie D, Ménasché P, N'Guyen Van Cao A, Bouveret P, Lorente P, Piwnica A, Slama R, Schwartz K (1987) Alpha-myosin heavy chain isoform and atrial size in patients with various types of mitral valve dysfunction: a quantitative study. J Am Coll Cardiol 9:1024-1030
23. Nagai R, Zarain-Herzberg A, Brandl C, Fuji J, Tada M, Mac Lennan DH, Alpert N, Periassamy M (1989) Regulation of myocardial Ca^{2+}-ATPase and phospholamban mRNA expression in response to pressure overload and thyroid hormone. Proc Natl Acad Sci USA 86:2966-2970
24. Rannou F, C Sainte-Beuve, P Oliviero, E Do, P Trouvé, D. Charlemagne (1995) The effects of compensated cardiac hypertrophy on dihydropyridine and ryanodine receptors in rat, ferret and guinea pigs hearts. J Mol Cell Cardiol 27:1225-1234
25. Hanf R, Drubaix I, Lelièvre L (1988) Rat cardiac hypertrophy: altered sodium-calcium exchange activity in sarcolemmal vesicles. FEBS Letters 236:145-149
26. Studer R, Reinecke H, Bilger J, Eschenhagen T, Bohm M, Hasenfuss G, Just H, Holtz

J, Drexler H (1994) Gene expression of the cardiac Na$^+$/Ca^{2+} exchanger in end-stage human heart failure. Circ Res 75:443-453

27. Swynghedauw B, Coraboeuf E (1994) Cardiac Hypertrophy and Failure. In: Cardiovascular medicine. 4 Basic Aspects of Myocardial Function, Growth, and Development, JT Willerson and JN Cohn (eds) Churchill Livingstone pub, New York, p 771-789

28. Coulombe A, Montaza A, Richer P, Swynghedauw B, Coraboeuf E (1994) Reduction of calcium-independent transient outward current density in DOCA-salt hypertrophied rat ventricular myocytes. Pflugers Arch 427:47-55

29. Cerbai E, Barbieri M, LI Q, Mugelli A (1994) Ionic basis of action potential prolongation of hypertrophied cardiac myocytes isolated from hypertensive rats of different ages. Cardiovasc Res 28:1180-1187

30. Nuss HB, Houser SR (1993) T-Type Ca^{2+} current is expressed in hypertrophied adult feline left ventricular myocytes. Circ Res 73:777-782

31. La Rovere MT, Mortara A, Pinna GD, Bernardi L (1995) Baroreflex sensitivity and heart rate variability in the assessment of the autonomic status. In: Heart Rate Variability, Malik M, Camm AJ (eds), Futura Pub, Armonk, NY, pp 189-205

32. Task force of the European Society of Cardiology and the North American Society of Pacing and Electrophysiology. Heart rate variability (1996) Standards of measurement, physiological interpretation, and clinical use. Eur Heart J 17:354

33. Brodde O (1991) β_1-β_2-adrenoceptors in the human heart: properties, function, and alterations in chronic heart failure Pharmacol Rev 43:203-241

34. Eschenagen T, Mende U, Nose M, Schmitz W, Scholz H, Haverich A, Hirt S, Döring V, Kalmar P, Höppner W, Seitz HJ (1992) Increased messenger RNA level of the inhibitory G protein a subunit Giα2 in human end stage heart failure. Circ Res 70: 688-696

35. Brilla CG, Pick R, Tan LB, Janicki JS and Weber KT. (1990). Remodelling of the right and left ventricles in experimental hypertension. Circ Res 67:1355-1364

36. Gaasch WH, Apstein CS and Levine HJ (1985) Diastolic properties of the left ventricle. In: Levine HS,Gaasch WH (eds) The ventricle, basic and clinical aspect, Martin Nijhoff, Boston, pp 143-170

Dilated Cardiomyopathy: Does Etiological Heterogeneity Portend Clinical Heterogeneity?

L. Mestroni, C. Rocco, S. Miocic, A. Di Lenarda, G. Sinagra, D. Gregori, M. Vatta, M. Matulic, T. Zerjal, A. Falaschi, F. Camerini and M. Giacca

Etiology of Dilated Cardiomyopathy

The etiology of dilated cardiomyopathy (DC), a disease of the myocardium characterized by dilatation and impaired contraction of the left ventricle or both ventricles, has been actively investigated for several decades. Unfortunately, the cause of DC is still mostly unknown and the diagnosis mainly based on the exclusion of any *specific* heart muscle disease, that is any disease associated with known cardiac or systemic disorders. However, it is expected that with the increasing understanding of the etiology and the pathogenesis of DC, the difference between a true primary cardiomyopathy and specific heart muscle diseases will become indistinguishable in the future [1].

Due to the scarce knowledge, the classification of the etiologic factors is still tentative [1] and, with the exclusion of toxic agents, alcohol and other cardiovascular diseases associated with or mimicking DC, autoimmune disease, persistent viral infection and genetic factors are still considered to be the main causes, as in most of human diseases of unknown etiology. It is hypothesized that DC could represent the final common pathway of a heterogeneous group of disorders. Molecular genetic studies on *specific* cardiomyopathies, which demonstrate that both metabolic and structural defects of myocytes can lead to a common phenotype of myocardial dilatation and dysfunction, support this hypothesis.

Furthermore, very little is known about the clinical implications of the etiological heterogeneity. In other words, does etiological heterogeneity portend clinical heterogeneity? The following discussion will review the present knowledge about the different causes of DC and their clinical correlates. In particular, DC due to inflammatory (infective and autoimmune) and genetic disorders will be discussed.

Infective Agents

The hypothesis of an inflammatory process of the myocardium with chronic damage and development of heart failure has long been considered one of the main causes of DC [2], and the trigger of myocarditis is believed to be a viral infection, with subsequent viral persistence. However, myocarditis, defined as a pathologic process characterized by an inflammatory infiltrate of the myocardium with necrosis or degeneration [3] is usually indistinguishable from other inflammatory non-viral heart diseases, and remains in most cases of unknown origin.

Over the past decade, extensive investigative efforts have addressed the role of enteroviruses, in particular group B coxsackie viruses, in the pathogenesis of DC and myocarditis using molecular biology techniques. However, in spite of the high sensitivity of these techniques, the frequency of positive enteroviral genomes in myocardial tissue of patients with DC was very variable, ranging from 0% to over 40% [4-8]. Therefore, the role of viral, in particular enteroviral, persistence as a cause for DC is still controversial.

Accordingly, the clinical features of patients positive for the presence of enteroviral genomes appear to be very variable. In the study of Why et al [9], patients found positive for enteroviral genome did not differ significantly in age, sex, symptomatic presentation or hemodynamic characteristics from those who were enterovirus-negative. Only the duration of symptoms was significantly shorter in patients with enteroviral RNA (7.8 ± 9.6 versus 14.9 ± 19.0 months). Also, this group of patients had an increased mortality compared with the group negative for viral RNA (25% versus 4%) during a mean follow-up of 25 months.

On the contrary, in another study [10] the enterovirus-negative status correlated with a negative prognosis. These cases showed a deterioration of left ventricular function compared to the enterovirus-positive patients, and an adverse cardiac event rate. Moreover, based on histomorphometric analysis, structural disintegrity was more pronounced in the enterovirus-negative than in the positive group. Except for atrial fibrillation, which occurred more frequently in enterovirus-positive patients, no clinical or hemodynamic feature could predict enteroviral persistence [10]. Accordingly, also in our patient population, there were no significant differences in the clinical features between patients positive and negative for enteroviral genomes, respectively [8].

In contrast with the adult patient population, in the pediatric population, the role of a viral infection in causing DC and myocarditis is more convincing. Martin et al. [11] found viral genomes in 68% of myocardial samples of children (age 1 day to 19 years) with acute onset of left ventricular dilatation and dysfunction. However, other viruses were detected other than enteroviruses (30%), with a prevalence of adenoviruses (58%) followed by herpesvirus (8%) and cytomegalovirus (4%). Histopathology was consistent with myocarditis in about 50% of these patients.

In summary, whereas the pathogenetic role of enteroviral persistence in the chronic disease seen in adults is questionable, studies on the pediatric population indicate that, in the clinical context of acute severe ventricular dilation and dysfunction, age as well as other viruses can be pathologically relevant, and that their role should be investigated in the future.

Immune Abnormalities

Several abnormalities of cell-mediated immunity have been reported in DC, such as a deficit in the function of T suppressor lymphocytes [12,13] and a reduced or absent natural killer activity [14, 15]. It has been hypothesized that a lower T suppressor activity could lead to an altered production of autoantibodies by B lymphocytes in a subset of patients. Nevertheless, these alterations of the immune system are not cardiospecific and cannot be considered as a causal factor for the disease. On the other hand, considering the complexity of cell-mediated immunity, this aspect has not been sufficiently evaluated in DC to draw any conclusions.

Humoral immunity has been more extensively studied. The presence of cardiac organ-specific autoantibodies has been reported, such as anti-cardiac mitochondria, anti-myosin, anti-actin, anti-myolemma, and, finally, anti α- and β-myosin heavy chain, the latter characterized by a high specificity for the heart muscle and intercalated disks [15,16]. Antibodies against the ADP-ATP carrier of the mitochondrial membrane [17] were also described, which seem to interfere with the normal function of membrane calcium channels, and present some homologies with coxsackie virus RNA sequences. These antibodies could alter cardiac metabolism and function by calcium overload and by the reduction of the available ATP.

Studies on anti-β_1-receptor and anti-M2-muscarinic acetylcholine receptor antibodies suggest that these autoantibodies could have a functional role, in particular a positive chronotropic effect [18,19]. As they are not strictly organ-specific, their significance in the pathogenesis of DC is unclear.

The immune response is regulated by the major histocompatibility complex (MHC). A major role of MHC in the pathogenesis of many autoimmune diseases is largely accepted. Accordingly, an association between MHC class II antigens (in particular DR4) and DC has also been hypothesized [20]. However, other studies on selected patient populations with genetically determined DC excluded any association between MHC genes and the disease [21, 22].

In spite of the large number of studies, the significance of immune activation in DC is still unclear, and whether the described alterations represent a consequence or a causal factor has still to be established. Nowadays, clinical markers able to distinguish DC patients with autoimmune activation are not known. Caforio et al. [23] suggested that cardiac organ-specific autoantibodies were associated with the early phase of the disease and with a better prognosis. However, follow-up studies are required to show if organ-specific autoantibodies could play a role in evaluating the stage and the prognosis of the disease.

Interestingly, however, cardiac organ-specific autoantibodies [24] were found to be more frequent in familial dilated cardiomyopathy, both in affected and unaffected relatives. This is an indirect indication that the presence of these antibodies is under genetic control and that the genetic background could play a role in the pathogenesis of the disease.

Genetic Factors

Important advances for the understanding of the etiology of DC have been made by clinical genetic and molecular genetic studies. Firstly, a systematic screening of families of DC patients has recently demonstrated that genetic factors, previously considered to be very rare, have a major role in the pathogenesis of the disease. The occurrence of a genetic transmission (familial DC or FDC) in controlled studies is detectable in at least one third of patients with DC [25-27], as a prevalent autosomal dominant trait. However, these data certainly underestimate the real frequency of FDC, due to the possibility of missing affected individuals, particularly when the pedigrees are small, to the unwillingness of the families to undergo screening when the history of disease is not evident, or to the absence of early markers of disease, or to the reduced penetrance (that is the proportion of carriers of the disease gene who manifest a clinical phenotype). As in FDC the penetrance is age-related, the disease can be clinically not apparent, in particular in young family members. Furthermore, the risk of disease was estimated to be approximately 20% in first degree relatives of DC patients [26] and, in absence of a clinical examination, the risk of missing a familial trait is about 20% [27].

Studies based on systematic family screening could not detect any significant difference between patients with FDC and those with sporadic DC [25,26]. On the other hand, studies on the clinical and genetic characteristics of the inherited form clearly indicate the existence of several different subtypes [28]: autosomal dominant FDC (the most frequent form), autosomal recessive FDC, conduction defects with later development of dilated cardiomyopathy (CDDC), X-linked dilated cardiomyopathy (XLDC), and mitochondrial DC.

Autosomal dominant FDC is characterized by development of ventricular dilation and systolic dysfunction in the second to third decade of life, with progressive heart failure and ventricular arrhythmias. This form is usually characterized by a low penetrance of the disease. Whereas the search for candidate genes (genes encoding proteins which are relevant for myocardial function, such as contractile proteins, proteins involved in the metabolic pathways, or in immune regulation) has been unsuccessful [22,29,30], recently, using a whole-genome random screening, several loci have been mapped. In a large Italian kindred and in two smaller families, a first FDC disease locus was identified on chromosome 9 [31], while in a Utah family with similar clinical features, a second locus was localized on chromosome 1q32 [32]. Finally, another locus has been reported on the short arm of chromosome 10 (10q21-23) [33] in one large kindred, characterized by the association of DC with mitral valve prolapse and by high penetrance.

Another peculiar and rare form of familial DC is a dominant cardiac conduction system disease with later development of dilated cardiomyopathy, named CDDC [34,35]. The affected family members manifest arrhythmias and atrioventricular block in the second to third decade of life, and a progressive cardiomegaly and heart failure in the fifth to sixth decade. In a large Ohio family, a first locus containing the disease gene was mapped in the centromere of chromosome 1 (1p1-1q1) [36]. Recently, in another CDDC family of Swiss-German ancestry, linkage was found with the short arm of chromosome 3 (3p22-p25) [37].

So far, the only known disease gene responsible for dilated cardiomyopathy is the dystrophin gene (Fig. 1), and the knowledge about the molecular bases of this form enables us to fully understand some of the clinical correlates of the disease. The dystrophin gene is the largest gene of the human genome, spanning about 2.5 Mb and having 79 exons [38]. The encoded product, dystrophin, is a 427 kDa cytoskeletal protein, with a key role for membrane stability, force transduction and the organization of membrane specializations in skeletal and cardiac myocytes [38]. Mutations or deletions of this gene cause the Duchenne and Becker muscular dystrophies as well as the X-linked dilated cardiomyopathy (XLDC or XLCM) [39,40]. XLDC is a rapidly progressive DC, presenting generally in young males as congestive heart failure, in the absence of clinical signs of skeletal myopathy. Affected family members can have a mild increase of muscle creatine kinase (MM-CK). Manifesting female carriers have later onset of the disease, as well as a slower progression. This condition is characterized by the transmission of DC with the X chromosome (no male-to-male transmission), in a dominant fashion [41]. The identification of deletions in the region containing the muscle promoter - first muscle exon in two XLDC families [40,42] suggested a critical role of the 5' end of the gene for the expression of dystrophin in the heart. This hypothesis was supported by the subsequent findings of two different point mutations in the same region of the gene in two further XLDC fami-

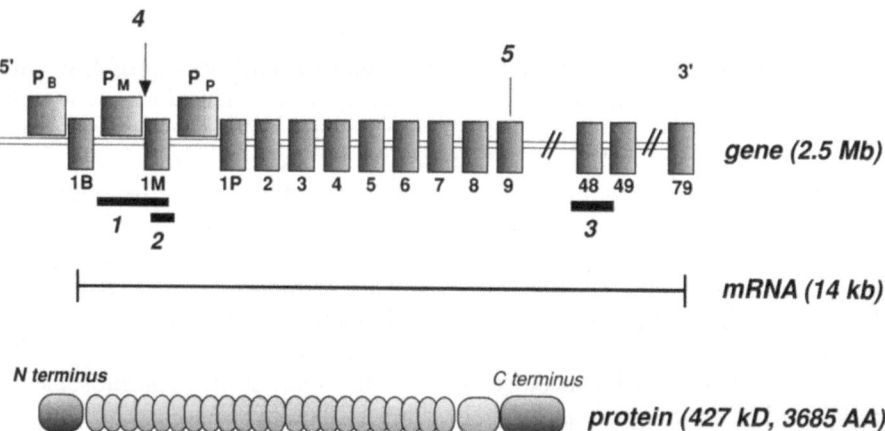

Fig. 1. Dystrophin gene mutations in XLDC (from [55] with permission). The schematic diagrams of dystrophin gene, mRNA and protein are shown. P_B, P_M, and P_P indicate the brain-, muscle- and Purkinje cell-promoters, respectively; 1B, 1M and 1P represent the first exons of the brain-, muscle- and Purkinje cell-isoforms, respectively. The dystrophin gene mutations which have been identified in XLDC are shown: the black bars 1 [40], 2 [42], and 3 [46,47] indicate the deletions; the arrow 4, the splice junction mutation [43], and the line 5 the missense mutation in exon 9 [45]

lies. The first mutation, a G→T substitution, alters the consensus sequence of the splicing site at the first muscle exon - intron junction [43] and abolishes the production of the muscle isoform of the gene. The immunocytochemical study with anti-dystrophin antibodies showed a reduced quantity but normal distribution of the protein in the skeletal muscle, while it was undetectable in the cardiac muscle [43,44] (Fig. 2). This is related to the absence of expression of all major dystrophin mRNA isoforms (from the muscle-, brain- and Purkinje cell-promoters) in the myocardium, while the brain- and Purkinje cell- (but not the muscle-) isoforms are still detectable in the skeletal muscle [43,44]. These findings provide an explanation for the XLDC phenotype, which is characterized by isolated myocardial disease.

The second point mutation recently identified is a missense mutation A→G in exon 9, resulting in the substitution of the amino acid threonine to alanine at position 279 of the protein. The substitution occurs in the first hinge region of the dystrophin protein and is believed to alter the flexibility of the membrane-associated network of dystrophin [45].

Finally, in-frame deletions in the region of exon 48 of the dystrophin gene, previously described in patients with Becker muscle dystrophy associated with DC [46], can also lead to a typical XLDC phenotype [47].

It is therefore possible that different defects both within critical functional regions of the dystrophin protein, or in the regulation of the expression of the dystrophin mRNA could lead to the XLDC phenotype.

By analogy with dystrophin, other cytoskeletal proteins appear to be potential candidates for causing dilated cardiomyopathy. Deficiency of adhalin, a dystrophin-associated glycoprotein, has recently been described in a patient with DC associated with signs of muscle dystrophy [48]. A deficiency of transcription of meta-vinculin (the cardiac isoform of vinculin) has been shown in a patient with FDC [49]. Moreover, δ-sarcoglycan has been found to be the cause of the Syrian hamster cardiomyopathy [50]. Preliminary data from our family studies suggest the existence of a subgroup of families with subclinical skeletal muscle involvement resembling the one seen in XLDC, but with an autosomal dominant pattern of transmission [47]: an altered protein of the cytoskeletal network can be hypothesized also in these cases.

Finally, the possibility that mitochondrial DNA (mtDNA) defects may underlie DC has long been considered, in particular in families with suspected matrilineal transmission of the disease [51]. The development of cardiomyopathy with dilatation, dysfunction with or without hypertrophy, is a common clinical feature of several mitochondrial syndromes [52,53], in which there is invariably a multi-organ involvement and a wide clinical variability due to heteroplasmy. If the causal role of deletions in DC is controversial, and seems to be related rather to the severity of myocardial dysfunction and to age, on the other hand, point mutations of the mtDNA could have a pathogenetic role in a subset of cases with isolated DC [54]. These aspects are discussed more in detail by Arbustini et al., elsewhere in this book.

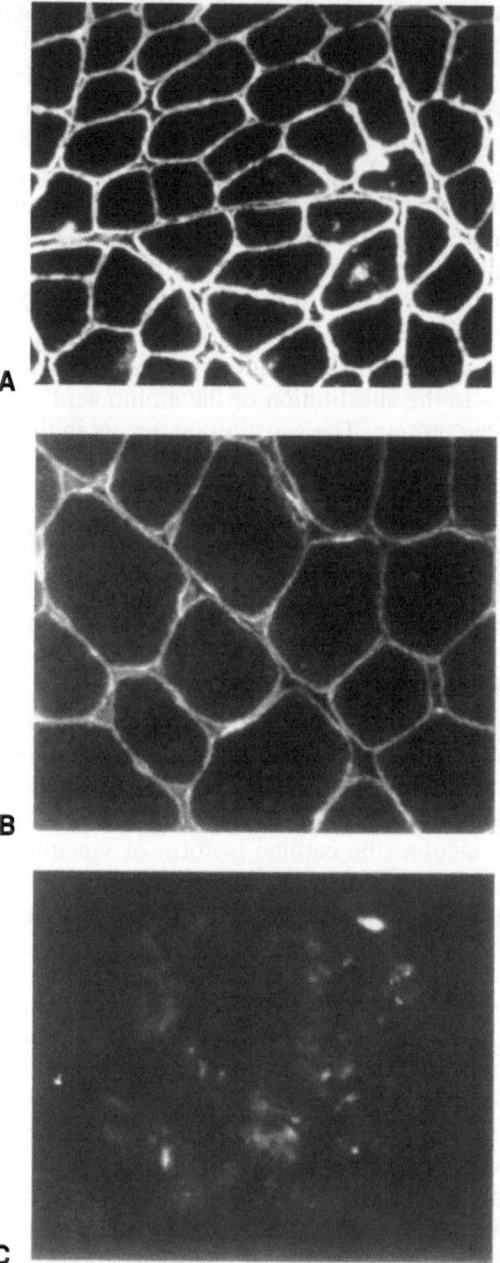

Fig. 2. Immunocytochemistry of skeletal and heart muscle in XLDC (from Milasin et al [43] modified). **A** cryostat section of skeletal muscle from a normal individual immunolabelled with antibodies to the C - terminal region of dystrophin. **B** cryostat sections of the skeletal muscle of an affected member of the family XLDC1, labeled with antibodies against the N- terminus: these antibodies show reduced but structurally preserved staining of the muscle of the patient as compared to that of the normal control (x180). **C** the cryostat section of the cardiac muscle from the patient immunostained with antibodies to the N-terminal showing complete absence of dystrophin (x250)

Conclusions

While the studies on DC due to viral myocarditis and autoimmune DC do not allow the definition of any clinical markers able to discriminate these forms, more promising data come from the study of inherited DC, which demonstrates clinical and genetic heterogeneity. Molecular genetics has offered a powerful tool for the identification of the disease loci. However, any substantial advancement in the understanding of the molecular correlates of most forms of DC must await the identification of the actual disease genes and of their mutations. By analogy with other heart diseases, such as hypertrophic cardiomyopathy and the long QT syndrome, it can be expected that the understanding of the molecular basis of DC will offer clinical benefits, including the possibility of correlating specific mutations to different prognosis, of performing the diagnosis in asymptomatic or border-line patients, and of giving genetic counseling to family members of affected individuals. Moreover, the notion that DC is very frequently an inheritable genetic disorder should be taken into account in clinical practice, by systematically screening at least the first degree relatives of DC patients. If a familial trait is confirmed, the pattern of transmission must be carefully analyzed, to identify in particular families X-linked, or maternal transmission. The detection of an increased serum CK can address the diagnosis toward a dystrophin alteration or another muscle disease, and muscle and endomyocardial biopsies can give another important contribution to the diagnosis. Moreover, family studies and linkage analysis can be used in specific families for the detection of family members at risk of disease.

With the exact understanding of the molecular defects underlying DC, it is expected that, in the future, this disease will become diagnosed and prevented by molecular techniques, not differently from most of other genetically-determined disorders. It is also expected that the rapid advances in the field of molecular medicine will eventually offer the possibility of new treatments able to correct the molecular defects.

Acknowledgment. Francesco Muntoni, MD (Royal Postgraduate Medical School, Hammersmith Hospital, London, UK) is acknowledged for his contributions to the studies on DC with skeletal muscle involvement. The grants of the Associazione Amici del Cuore of Trieste, of the National Research Council (CNR 96.00940.CT04), and of Telethon-Italy (Grant No.E.1024) are gratefully acknowledged.

References

1. Report of the 1995 World Health Organization/International Society and Federation of Cardiolgy Task Force on the Definition and Classification of Cardiomyopathies (1996) Circulation 93:841-842
2. Kasper ED, Agema WRP, Hutchins GM, Deckers JW, Hare JM, Baughman KL (1994) The causes of dilated cardiomyopathy:A clinicopathologic review of 673 consecutive patients. J Am Coll Cardiol 23:586-590
3. Aretz H, Billingham M, Edwards W, Factor S, Fallon J, Fenoglio J, Olsen E, Schoen F (1986) Myocarditis: a histopathologic definition and classification. Am J Cardiovasc Pathol 1:3-14

4. Grasso M, Arbustini E, Silini E, Diegoli M, Percivalle E, Ratti G, Bramerio M, Gavazzi A, Vigano M, Milanesi G (1992) Search for coxsackievirus B3 RNA in idiopathic dilated cardiomyopathy using gene amplification by polymerase chain reaction. Am J Cardiol 69:658-664
5. Jin O, Sole MJ, Butany JW, Chia W-K, McLaughlin PR, Liu P, Liew C-C (1990) Detection of enterovirus RNA in myocardial biopsies from patients with myocarditis and cardiomyopathy using gene amplification by polymerase chain reaction. Circulation 82: 8-16
6. Weiss LM, Liu X-F, Chang KL, Billingham ME (1992) Detection of eneteroviral RNA in idiopathic dilated cardiomyopathy and other human cardiac tissues. J Clin Invest 90: 156-159
7. Bowles N, Rose M, Taylor P, Banner N, Morgan-Capner P, Cunningham L, Archard L, Yacoub M (1989) End-stage dilated cardiomyopathy: persistence of enterovirus RNA in myocardium et cardiac transplantation and lack of immune response. Circulation 80: 1128-1136
8. Giacca M, Severini GM, Mestroni L, Salvi A, Lardieri G, Falaschi A, Camerini F (1994) Low frequency of detection by nested polymerase chain reaction of enterovirus ribonucleic acid in endomyocardial tissue of patients with idiopathic dilated cardiomyopathy. J Am Coll Cardiol 24:1033-1040
9. Why JF, Meany BT, Richardson PJ, Olsen E, Bowles NE, Cunningham L, Freeke CA, Archard LC (1994) Clinical and prognostic significance of detection of enteroviral RNA in the myocardium of patients with myocarditis or dilated cardiomyopathy. Circulation 89:2582-2588
10. Figulla H, Stille-Siegener M, Mall G, Heim A, Kreuzer H (1995) Myocardial enterovirus infection with left ventricular dysfunction: a benign disease compared with idiopathic dilated cardiomyopathy. J Am Coll Cardiol 25:1170-1175
11. Martin A, Webber S, Fricker F, Jaffe R, Demmler G, Kearney D, Zhang Y, Bodurtha J, Gelb B, Ni J, Bricker T, Towbin J (1994) Acute myocarditis: rapid diagnosis by PCR in children. Circulation 90:330-339
12. Fowles RE, Bieber CR, Stinson EB (1979) Defective in vitro suppressor cell function in idiopathic dilated cardiomyopathy. Circulation 59:483-491
13. Eckstein R, Mempel W, Bolte HD (1982) Reduced suppressor cell activity in congestive cardiomyopathy. Circulation 65:1224-1229
14. Anderson JL, Carlquist JF, Higashikubo R (1985) Quantitation of lymphocyte subset by immunofluorescence flow cytometry in idiopathic dilated cardiomyopathy. Am J Cardiol 55:1550-1554
15. Maisch B, Bauer E, Herzum M, Hufnagel G, Izumi T, Nunoda S, Schönian U (1990) Humoral and cell-mediated immunity: pathogenetic mechanisms in dilated cardiomyopathy. In: Baroldi G, Camerini F, Goodwin JF (eds) Advances in cardiomyopathies. Springer-Verlag,Berlin Heidelberg New York, pp 209-220
16. Caforio ALP, Grazzini M, Mann JM, Keeling PJ, Bottazzo GF, McKenna WJ, Schiaffino S (1992) Identification of α and β-cardiac myosin heavy chain isoforms as major autoantigens in dilated cardiomyopathy. Circulation 85:1734-1742
17. Schulze K, Becker BF, Schauer R, Schultheiss HP (1990) Antibodies to ADP-ATP carrier - an autoantigen in myocarditis and dilated cardiomyopathy - impair cardiac function. Circulation 81:959-969
18. Magnusson Y, Wallukat G, Waagstein F, Hjalmarson A, Hoebeke J (1994) Characterization of antibodies against the beta1-adrenoreceptor with positive chronotropic effect. Circulation 89:2760-2767
19. Fu L-X, Magnusson Y, Bergh C-H, Liljeqvist JÅ, Waagstein F, Hjalmarson Å, Hoebeke J (1993) Localization of a functional autoimmune epitope on the muscarinic acetylcholine receptor-2 in patients with idiopathic dilated cardiomyopathy. J Clin Invest 91: 1964-1968
20. Carlquist JF, Menlove RL, Murray MB, O'Connell JB, Anderson JL (1991) HLA class II (DR and DQ) antigen associations in idiopathic dilated cardiomyopathy. Validation study and meta-anlysis of published HLA association studies. Circulation 83:515-522
21. Mestroni L, Martinetti M, Cappello N, Misefari V, Giacca M, Camerini F (1992) HLA linkage analysis in familial dilated cardiomyopathy and right ventricular dysplasia. Circulation 86:I-794

22. Olson TM, Thibodeau SN, Lundquist PA, Schaid DJ, Michels VV (1995) Exclusion of a primary gene defect at the HLA locus in familial idiopathic dilated cardiomyopathy. J Med Genet 32:876-880
23. Caforio ALP, Bonifacio E, Stewart JT, Neglia D, Parodi O, Bottazzo F, McKenna W (1990) Novel organ-specific circulating cardiac autoantibodies in dilated cardiomyopathy. J Am Coll Cardiol 15:1527-1534
24. Caforio ALP, Keeling PJ, Zachara E, Mestroni L, Camerini F, Mann JM, Bottazzo GF, McKenna WJ (1994) Evidence from family studies for autoimmunity in dilated cardiomyopathy. Lancet 344:773-777
25. Michels VV, Moll PP, Miller FA, Tajik AJ, Chu JS, Driscoll DJ, Burnett JC, Rodeheffer RJ, Chesebro JH, Tazelaar H (1992) The frequency of familial dilated cardiomyopathy in a series of patients with idiopathic dilated cardiomyopathy. N Engl J Med 326: 77-82
26. Keeling PJ, Gang G, Smith G, Seo H, Bent SE, Murday V, Caforio ALP, McKenna WJ (1995) Familial dilated cardiomyopathy in the United Kingdom. Br Heart J 73: 417-421
27. Gregori D, Rocco C, Di Lenarda A, Sinagra G, Miocic S, Camerini F, Mestroni L (1996) Estimating the frequency of familial dilated cardiomyopathy, and the risk of misclassification errors. Circulation 94:1-270
28. Mestroni L, Milasin J, Vatta M, Pinamonti B, Sinagra G, Rocco C, Matulic M, Falaschi A, Giacca M, Camerini F (1996) Genetic factors in dilated cardiomyopathy. Arch Mal Coeur 89(II):15-20
29. Krajinovic M, Mestroni L, Severini GM, Pinamonti B, Camerini F, Falaschi A, Giacca M (1994) Absence of linkage between idiopathic dilated cardiomyopathy and candidate genes involved in the immune function in a large Italian pedigree. J Med Genet 31: 766-771
30. Mestroni L, Krajinovic M, Severini GM, Falaschi A, Giacca M, Camerini F (1994) Molecular genetics of dilated cardiomyopathy. Herz 19:97-104
31. Krajinovic M, Pinamonti B, Sinagra G, Vatta M, Severini GM, Milasin J, Falaschi A, Camerini F, Giacca M, Mestroni L (1995) Linkage of familial dilated cardiomyopathy to chromosome 9. Am J Hum Genet 57:846-852
32. Durand J-B, Bachinski LL, Bieling LC, Czernuszewicz GZ, Abchee AB, Yu QT, Tapscott T, Hill R, Ifegwu J, Marian AJ, Brugada R, Daiger S, Gregoritch JM, Anderson JL, Quiñones M, Towbin J, Roberts R (1995) Localization of a gene responsible for familial dilated cardiomyopathy to chromosome 1q32. Circulation 92:3387-3389
33. Bowles KL, Gajarski R, Porter P, Goytia V, Bachinski L, Roberts R, Pignatelli R (1996) Gene mapping of familial autosomal dominant dilated cardiomyopathy to chromosome 10q21-23. J Clin Invest 98:1355-1360
34. Graber HL, Unverferth DV, Baker PB, Rayan JM, Baba N, Wooley CF (1986) Evolution of a hereditery cardiac conduction and muscle disorder: a study involving a family with six generations affected. Circulation 74:325-327
35. Mestroni L, Miani D, Di Lenarda A, Silvestri F, Bussani R, Filippi G, Camerini F (1990) Clinical and pathologic study of familial dilated cardiomyopathy. Am J Cardiol 65:1449-1453
36. Kass S, MacRae C, Graber HL, Sparks EA, McNamara D, Boudoulas H, Basson CT, Baker III PB, Cody RJ, Fishman MC, Cox N, Kong A, Wooley CF, Seidman JG, Seidman CE (1994) A gene defect that causes conduction system disease and dilated cardiomyopathy maps to chromosome 1p1-1q1. Nature Genet 7:546-551
37. Olson TM, Keating MT (1996) Mapping a cardiomyopathy locus to chromosome 3p22-p25. J Clin Invest 97:528-532
38. Ahn AH, Kunkel LM (1993) The structural and functional diversity of dystrophin. Nature Genet 3:283-291
39. Towbin JA, Hejtmancik F, Brink P, Gelb BD, Zhu XM, Chamberlain JS, McCabe ERB, Swift M (1993) X-linked cardiomyopathy (XLCM): molecular genetic evidence of linkage to the Duchenne muscular dystrophy (dystrophin) gene at the Xp21 locus. Circulation 87:1854-1865
40. Muntoni F, Cau M, Ganau A, Congiu R, Arvedi G, Mateddu A, Morrosu MG, Cianchetti C, Realdi G, Cao A, Melis MA (1993) Deletion of the dystrophin muscle-promoter region associated with X-linked dilated cardiomyopathy. N Engl J Med 329:921-925

41. Berko B, Swift M (1987) X-linked dilated cardiomyopathy. N Engl J Med 316:1186-1191
42. Yoshida K, Ikeda SI, Nakamura A, Kagoshima M, Takeda S, Shoji S, Yanagisawa N (1993) Molecular analysis of the Duchenne muscular dystrophy gene in patients with Becker muscular dystrophy presenting with dilated cardiomyopathy. Muscle & Nerve 16:1161-1166
43. Milasin J, Muntoni F, Severini GM, Bartoloni L, Vatta M, Krajinovic M, Mateddu A, Angelini C, Camerini F, Falaschi A, Mestroni L, Giacca M (1996) A point mutation in the 5' splice site of the dystrophin gene first intron responsible for X-linked dilated cardiomyopathy. Hum Mol Genet 5:73-79
44. Muntoni F, Wilson L, Marrosu MG, Cianchetti C, Mestroni L, Ganau A, Dubowitz V, Sewry C (1995) A mutation in the dystrophin gene selectively affecting dystrophin expression in the heart. J Clin Invest 96:693-699
45. Ortiz-Lopez R, Li H, Su J, Goytia V, Towbin JA (1997) Evidence for a dystrophin missense mutation as a cause of X-linked dilated cardiomyopathy (XLCM). Circulation 95:2434-2440
46. Melacini P, Fanin M, Danieli GA, Fasoli G, Villanova C, Angelini C, Vitiello L, Miorelli M, Buja GF, Mostacciuolo ML, Pegoraro E, Dalla Volta S (1993) Cardiac involvement in Becker muscular dystrophy. J Am Coll Cardiol 22:1927-1934
47. Mestroni L, Muntoni F, Milasin J, Di Lenarda A, Sinagra G, Rocco C, Vatta M, Matulic M, Falaschi A, Camerini F, Giacca M (1996) Familial dilated cardiomyopathy with subclinical skeletal muscle involvement. Circulation 94:I-271
48. Fadic R, Sunada Y, Waclawik AJ, Buck S, Lewandoski PJ, Campbell KP, Lotz BP (1996) Brief report: deficiency of a dystrophin-associated glycoprotein (adhalin) in a patient with muscular dystrophy and cardiomyopathy. N Engl J Med 334:362-366
49. Maeda M, Holder E, Lowes B, Valent S, Bies RD (1997) Dilated cardiomyopathy associated with deficiency of the cytoskeletal protein metavinculin. Circulation 95:17-20
50. Nigro V, Okazaki Y, Belsito A, Piluso G, Matsuda Y, Politano L, Nigro G, Ventura C, Abbondanza C, Molinari AM, Acampora D, Nishimura M, Hayashizaki Y, Puca GA (1997) Identification of the Syrian Hamster cardiomyopathy gene. Hum Mol Genet 6:601-607
51. Suomalainen A, Paetau A, Leinonen H, Majander A, Peltonen L, Somer H (1992) Inherited dilated cardiomyopathy with multiple deletions of mitochondrial DNA. Lancet 340:1319-1320
52. Santorelli FM, Mak S-C, El-Schahawi M, Casali C, Shanske S, Baram TZ, Madrid RE, DiMauro S (1996) Maternally inherited cardiomyopathy associated with a novel mutation in the mitochondrial tRNA Lys gene (G8363A). Am J Hum Genet 58:933-939
53. Zeviani M, Gellera C, Antozzi C, Rimoldi M, Morandi L, Villani F, Tiranti V, DiDonato S (1991) Maternally inherited myopathy and cardiomyopathy: association with mutation in mitochondrial DNA tRNA Leu(UUR). Lancet 338:143-147
54. Grasso M, Fasani R, Diegoli M, Bianchieri N, Porcu E, Concardi M, Pilotto A, Fortina P, Surrey S, Vigano' M, Arbustini E (1995) Mitochondrial DNA base changes in sporadic and familial dilated cardiomyopathy (DCM) and in controls. J Mol Med 73:A28
55. Mestroni L, Giacca M (1997) Molecular genetics of dilated cardiomyopathy. Curr Op Cardiol 12:303-309

Recent Advances in Etiopathogenesis of Dilated Cardiomyopathy: Which Relevance for the Clinical Cardiologist?

A. Gavazzi, M. Ponzetta, C. Inserra, M. Giraldi, R. Sebastiani, C. Campana, A. Raisaro, M. Laudisa, E. Colombi, B. Dal Bello and E. Arbustini

Introduction

Cardiomyopathies are no longer considered as heart muscle diseases of unknown cause [1], but are defined as diseases of the myocardium associated with cardiac dysfunction, and classified by the dominant pathophysiology or, if possible, by etiological and pathogenetic factors [2].

During the last decade there has been a flurry of research attempting to identify factors which may contribute to the development of dilated cardiomyopathy (DCM) and a considerable amount of data has been produced regarding this issue.

Three basic mechanisms have been recognised: 1) genetic factors, 2) immunological factors, 3) viral infections. These causal mechanisms are not mutually exclusive, and several may combine to produce clinical disease in susceptible patients.

The consequences of this increasing understanding of etiopathogenesis are relevant and have major implications in the clinical and therapeutical approach to this heterogeneous group of diseases.

The purpose of this report is to review the most important experimental and clinical studies focused on development and progression of DCM, and to examine the implications that may derive in clinical practice.

Genetic Factors

Frequency of Familial DCM

The fact that DCM may be familial has been known for a long time, yet familial association was considered a rare event and the prevalence of a genetic trasmission was usually estimated to be less than 10% [3, 4].

However recent controlled studies, using a prospective method and a more careful evaluation of relatives, suggest that genetic factors are more frequently involved than previously suspected [5, 6]. Table 1 shows the frequency of familial DCM reported by different investigators [3-12].

In retrospective studies carried out during the 1980s, the frequency of familial DCM was estimated to be very low, from 2% to 9% [3, 4, 7-9];

Table 1. Frequency of familial dilated cardiomyopathy (DCM)

Author	DCM pts (n)	Familial DCM frequency	Methods
Fuster, 1981 [3]	104	2%	Retrospective history
Michels, 1985 [4]	169	6%	Retrospective questionnaires
Fragola, 1988 [7]	12	33%	Prospective evaluation of relatives
Griffin, 1988 [8]	32	10%	Study of children
Valantine, 1989 [9]	184	9%	Retrospective history
Keren, 1990 [10]	16	56%	Mildly DCM study
Mestroni, 1990 [11]	165	7%	Prospective study of suspect families
Michels, 1992 [5]	59	20%	Prospective evaluation of relatives
Zachara, 1993 [12]	105	13%	Retrospective study of suspect families
Keeling, 1995 [6]	40	25%	Prospective evaluation of relatives

conversely the prospective studies conducted during the last decade show that a familial form occurs in 20% to 33% of patients with DCM [5, 6, 10]. Some authors suggest that the real frequency is still understimated and may be even higher [13].

Familial Cardiomyopathy - The Pavia Experience

Between December 1994 and March 1997, 51 consecutive cases of DCM were diagnosed at our institution. The clinical suspicion of DCM was confirmed invasively in every patient by demonstrating: (1) absence of significant coronary artery disease (<50% luminal diameter reduction of a major coronary artery branch) by coronary angiography, (2) absence of specific heart muscle disease or active myocarditis by endomyocardial biopsy, and (3) reduced left ventricular ejection fraction (< 55%) by cineangiography.

All patients had a two- to three-generation pedigree constructed and were offered screening irrespective of family history or the presence of suspected familial disease.

Prospective screening of these 51 families resulted in 208 relatives, mean age 32 ± 17 years (range 4-73); 122 (58%) were first degree relatives, 59 (28%) second degree, 27 (14%) third degree.

Screening consisted of history, clinical examination with blood pressure measurement, 12-lead electrocardiogram, two dimensional Doppler echocardiography, signal averaged electrocardiogram (SAECG) and blood sampling for serum creatine-kinase (CK).

Echocardiograms were performed by three experienced echocardiographers; echocardiographic measurements of chamber size and wall thickness were obtained at the level of the papillary muscle from two dimensional M-mode-guided recordings in the parasternal long axis view. Left ventricular enlargement was defined as a left ventricular end-diastolic diameter index > 32 mm/m^2 [14] and a depressed left ventricular systolic function was defined either as fractional shortening < 25% or ejection fraction < 50%.

According to these definitions, the screened relatives were classified as having an echocardiogram compatible with DCM, left ventricular enlargement, depressed left ventricular systolic function or being normal. Familial disease was considered to be present when at least one relative was affected by DCM. Screening was extended to involve all living relatives when an affected relative was identified, or to involve the next generation when a minor echocardiographic abnormality was detected.

DCM was documented in 19 relatives (9%) coming from 12 families, who represented 23.5% of those screened. Of the remaining 189 relatives, 32 (15%) had left ventricular enlargement, 25 (12%) had presence of late ventricular potentials at SAECG (2/3 criteria), 11 (5.2%) had depressed fractional shortening, and 10 (4,6%) had an ejection fraction < 50%.

This preliminary survey confirms the results of the most recent studies, showing that a genetic transmission occurs in almost one fourth of patients with DCM.

The Mode of Transmission

In DCM different modes of inheritance are observed. Although autosomal dominant is the most frequent pattern of transmission [15], matrilineal [16], X-linked and autosomal recessive [11, 17] inherited forms have been reported. The hypothesis of a genetic heterogeneity in DCM, generated by clinical studies, has been confirmed by molecular genetic studies. The results of molecular genetic investigations are limited mainly by inadequate samples, because of the low penetrance of the disease, premature deaths, and lack of criteria for the preclinical diagnosis. The identification of disease genes is still in progress. Currently, known disease gene loci for different forms of DCM have been mapped on four different chromosomes: chromosome 1 contains the CDDC1 locus (1q1-p1) [18], and the familial DCM2 locus (1q31-q32) [19], chromosome 3 the CDDC2 locus (3p22-p25) [20], chromosome 9 the familial DCM1 locus (9q13-q22) [21], and chromosome X the dystrophin gene [22, 23].

Clinical Implications

The notion that DCM is a genetic disease in a significant proportion of patients, has relevant clinical implications. First of all, an accurate investigation of the family history is mandatory in every patient with DCM and a systematic screening of first degree relatives (parents, siblings and offspring) should be performed to identify affected individuals. Newly diagnosed DCM patients, even when asymptomatic, may benefit from early medical treatment, including drug therapy with ACE-inhibitors and probably, in selected cases, with beta-blockers, and of a regular follow-up, to monitor disease progression and treat complications appropriately.

A great problem arising from screening for familial DCM is represented by the criteria to identify early disease. Current diagnostic criteria have been developed for overt forms of DCM, while early clinical markers have not yet been classified; only prospective follow-up analyses will clarify the significance of mild left ventricular enlargement or dysfunction as preclinical signs of disease. In the near future we will have to define the likelihood of an affected individual of transmitting the disease to offspring and to develop practical guidelines of genetic counselling in DCM.

Subclinical skeletal muscle involvement in DCM patients should always be considered, and this possibility can be adressed by a careful evaluation of skeletal muscle and by a simple test such as serum CK determination. If serum CK is increased, dystrophinopathy or another muscle dystrophy should be suspected.

Once the gene or genes responsible for the disease are identified, "molecular diagnosis" of DCM will become possible. This will rely on new simple tests, which should allow the identification of carriers of the disease gene before the appearance of clinical manifestations. In these subjects an early diagnosis of DCM may permit the application of new treatments, genotype-based, which could modify the causative pathogenetic mechanisms.

Immunologic Factors

During the last decade the possible role of immunologic factors in the pathogenesis and progression of DCM has been extensively investigated.

An increased expression of the major histocompatibility complex (MHC) class II molecules, which regulate many immune responses, occurs in several autoimmune diseases. Caforio et al. identified HLA-DR positivity in endomyocardial bioptic tissue obtained from DCM patients [23]. HLA-DR expressing T lymphocytes are increased in affected DCM patients compared to controls [24]. In addition specific HLA-DR subtypes have been associated with the disease: a meta-analysis of five different studies published between 1987 and 1991 [25-28], including the investigation carried out in Pavia [29], clearly shows an increased expression of HLA-DR4 antigen in 361 DCM patients. However, to date no studies have documented a significant correlation between expression of a peculiar HLA-DR haplotype and clinical characteristics, such as age, gender, symptom duration or severity, or disease progression.

Circulating antibodies to the ADP-ATP carrier protein, the nucleotide transporting protein of the inner mithocondrial membrane, were found in a significant proportion of DCM patients [30, 31]. These antibodies can cause disturbance of cellular metabolism and myocardial dysfunction, but whether they are relevant to the pathogenesis of DCM, or merely represent a non-specific response to the cardiac disease process is unknown.

Modulation of beta-adrenergic receptors has been extensively studied, and anti-beta-adrenergic receptor antibodies have been demonstrated in 30% to 40% of DCM patients, compared with 15% of ischemic or valvular heart disease patients [32]. Although theoretically elimination of these antibodies should ameliorate the course of the disease, immunosuppression did not produce any improvement [33]. Organ-specific cardiac antibodies, which were specific for alpha-myosin chains have been recently detected by indirect immunofluorescence or enzyme-linked immunosorbent assay techniques. Caforio and colleagues documented a higher frequency of organ-specific antibodies at diagnosis in DCM patients than in patients with other cardiac diseases or in normal controls (30% versus 1% and 3.5%) [34]. Among DCM patients the prevalence of organ-specific cardiac antibodies is significantly higher in patients with shorter disease duration and less severe functional impairment; moreover these antibodies become undetectable as the disease progresses [35]. Interestingly, organ-specific cardiac antibodies were more frequent in familial than in nonfamilial DCM cases (24% versus 15%, $p = 0.03$) and were observed in 20% of asymptomatic DCM relatives [36]. However, whether these organ-specific cardiac antibodies have a direct pathogenetic role or are secondary to the disease state is still unknown.

Myocarditis

A number of experimental and clinical studies provides evidence of a link between myocarditis and the subsequent development of DCM [37-39]. The diagnosis of myocarditis is difficult: clinical criteria are notoriously unreliable and, although endomyocardial biopsy remains the only accurate diagnostic technique, histologic criteria used to differ among centers. In an overview of the series published between 1978 and 1986 among 270 out of 2350 patients presenting with heart failure of unknown cause or DCM, a bioptic diagnosis of myocarditis was established in 11% of cases, but with a very wide range (from 0% to 69%) [40]. In the attempt to standardize these different histologic criteria, in 1987 a panel of expert cardiac pathologists established the "Dallas" criteria [41]: myocarditis was defined as the presence of inflammatory infiltration of the myocardium, with necrosis and/or degeneration of adjacent myocytes. This definition applies only if adequate sampling (at least 4 fragments) is obtained and multiple levels are examined; furthermore drug toxicity and coronary artery disease must be excluded. However, even using the "Dallas" criteria, the prevalence of histologic evidence of myocarditis in DCM patients remains usually low (10%) [42]. For instance, in the ten-year overall experience with endomyocardial biopsy at our institution in Pavia, among 601 patients presenting with unexplained heart failure, an histologically proven myocarditis was demonstrated in 26 cases (4.3%) by "Dallas" criteria: a lymphocytic myocarditis was diagnosed in 21, a border-line myocarditis in 2, a giant cell myocarditis in 2, and a eosinophylic myocarditis in 1 [43]. The efficacy of immunosuppression in biopsy-proven myocarditis is controversial because most of the studies are small and uncontrolled. In a recent controlled trial in patients with biopsy-proven myocarditis according to the "Dallas" criteria, immunosuppressive therapy failed to reduce mortality and to improve ventricular function [42]. Recent investigations, which compared histological and immunohistochemical examinations of myocardial samples, demonstrated that the sensitivity of endomyocardial biopsy for the diagnosis of myocarditis was considerably greater when immunohistological procedures were added [44].

Therefore in 1995 a Consensus Report of the German Association for Internal Medicine proposed new rules to diagnose acute myocarditis in endomyocardial biopsy, which integrate the "Dallas" criteria with immunohistochemical criteria [45]. Immunohistochemistry provides additional information on the lymphocytic infiltrate characteristics, myocytolysis, increased expression of HLA class I and class II antigens, and of adhesion molecules, and increased binding of immunoglobulins IgG, IgA, and IgM. Lack of correlation between antibody status and biopsy features has recently been shown by Caforio et al. in patients with clinical myocarditis [46]. This bulk of evidence suggests that diagnosis of myocarditis should probably not rely on histology alone, as immune markers (autoantibodies or immunohistological features) may provide adjunct diagnostic tools to identify patients who may potentially benefit from immunomodulatory therapy.

Preliminary studies suggest that immunosuppressive treatment in the subset of DCM patients, who show active ongoing myocardial inflammation by immunohistological criteria, may result in clinical, hemodynamic, and immunohistological improvement in a substantial proportion of cases [47].

Clinical Implications

Although abnormalities in cellular and humoral immunity have been clearly demonstrated in DCM, their clinical and therapeutic implications remain uncertain. Organ-specific autoimmunity as early serological marker potentially allows the identification of family members at risk of developing the disease. In these cases the pre-clinical introduction of appropriate treatment, either with ACE-inhibitors or immunomodulatory agents, could be considered. A role of the cardiac-specific autoantibodies as non-invasive prognostic marker for patients in the early stages of disease, has been suggested but not yet firmly established.

In patients with overt DCM, therapy with various anti-inflammatory agents failed to produce beneficial effects on ventricular function, exercise tolerance or survival [48, 49].

Given these negative results, at present no specific immunosuppressive therapy appears to be justified for unselected DCM patients in clinical practice. Patient characterization and diagnosis of myocarditis are still difficult. The diagnosis of myocarditis should not be based solely on endomyocardial biopsy, but the evaluation should incorporate immunohistology and autoantibody testing. So far the scarce evidence of benefit of immunosuppressive therapy in myocarditis according to "Dallas" criteria prevents recommendation of such a treatment in clinical practice.

Viral Infections

Serological studies have long been used to examine viral involvement in DCM patients [50]. However, these data provided only circumstantial evidence, but not definite proof, of a viral etiology. Isolation of viruses from heart tissue is rare, and Coxackie viruses have been detected in few cases from the hearts of patients with neonatal acute fulminant myocarditis [51]. Most recently the presence of virus in heart tissue of patients with myocarditis and DCM has been demonstrated using molecular techniques. The enteroviruses contain a positive strand of RNA as genetic material; probes that are complementary to the viral genome can be used to detect viral RNA in endomyocardial biopsy tissue samples. The slot-blot probe hybridization was the first to detect enteroviral RNA in DCM patients [52], but has some cross-reactivity to uninfected cardiac tissue. Polymerase chain reaction (PCR), a rapid, sensitive and specific molecular technique, detected viral RNA in very small amounts of cardiac tissue. In-situ hybridization is technically more difficult, but offers the advantage of visualizing the specific cells infected in a field of non-infected cells and therefore is currently the method of choice. The results of several molecular studies are contradictory: enteroviral genomic sequences were detected in the heart tissue of 0% to 45% of patients studied, who had either DCM or acute myocarditis (Table 2) [53-63]. Average frequencies of viral genome detection, derived from published studies, are of 15% in DCM and of 25% in myocarditis.

These conflicting results are probably related to the different techniques and experimental procedures applied, and underscore the need for strict quality control in molecular diagnosis.

The presence of viral RNA in cardiac tissue does not imply pathogenicity

Table 2. Detection of enterovirus (EV) in myocardial tissue

Author		Source	Methodology	DCM EV-positive	Myocarditis EV-positive
Kandolf	1989 [52]	EMB Expl. heart	ISH	3/20 (15%) 4/19 (21%)	19/81 (23%)
Archard	1990 [53]	EMB Expl. heart	Slot blot H.	28/67 (42%) 6/19 (32%)	13/37 (35%)
Tracy	1990 [54]	EMB	ISH	1/9 (11%)	2/8
Jin	1990 [55]	EMB	RT-PCR	3/42 (7%)	2/6
Cochrane	1991 [56]	Expl. heart	Northern blot	0/19 (0%)	–
Weiss	1991 [57]	EMB Expl. heart	RT-PCR	0/11 (0%)	1/15 (7%)
Grasso	1992 [58]	Expl. heart	RT-PCR	0/21 (0%)	–
Keeling	1992 [59]	EMB	RT-PCR	6/50 (12%)	–
Satoh	1994 [60]	EMB	Nested-PCR	17/35 (17%)	-
Giacca	1994 [61]	EMB Expl. heart	Nested-PCR	4/ 53 (7.5%)	1/3
Figulla	1995 [62]	EMB	ISH	20/77 (26%)	-

EMB, endomyocardial biopsy; Expl. heart, explanted heart; ISH, in-situ hybridization; slot blot H, slot blot hybridization; RT, reverse transcription; PCR, polymerase chain reaction.

or active infection, and its clinical significance remains to be established. Bowles showed that enteroviral RNA persists in the heart of a substantial portion of patients with end-stage DCM, in absence of a continuing cell-mediated or humoral immune response [64]. Archard observed that enteroviral RNA-positive patients have a significantly poorer prognosis than enteroviral RNA-negative ones [65]. Why found that the presence of enteroviral RNA is an independent predictor of clinical outcome [66]. In contrast, Figulla recently reported that enterovirus-positive patients have better survival and hemodynamic course than enterovirus-negative patients [63]; a benign response was observed after interferon treatment in a subset of enterovirus-positive patients.

Clinical Implications

Although the presence of viral genome in myocardial tissue from DCM patients has been demonstrated by several authors using different molecular techniques, there is no definite evidence that this finding is relevant to pathogenesis or progression of the disease. Technical advances will result in more sensitive and reliable methods to approach this problem, particularly in assays for viral identification and quantitation of viral replication.

The diagnosis of a viral myocardial infection may have important therapeutic consequences, but to date no controlled studies on anti-viral therapy have been performed.

Conclusion

The rapid integration of molecular and cellular biology with cardiovascular medicine is particularly evident in the field of etiopathogenesis of cardiomyopathies.

Recent advances in etiopathogenesis of DCM should continue to result in improvement in diagnostic techniques, as well as in the generation of new therapeutic strategies and agents. To approach this goal a closer cooperation between basic scientists and clinical cardiologists is mandatory.

References

1. Report of the WHO/ISFC task force on the definition and classification of cardiomyopathies (1980) Br Heart J 44:672-673
2. Richardson P, McKenna WJ, Bristow M, Maisch B, Mautner B, O' Connell J, Olsen E, Thiene G, Goodwin J, Gyarfas I, Martin I, Nordet P (1996) Report of the 1995 World Organization/International Society and Federation of Cardiology Task Force on the definition and classification of cardiomyopathies. Circulation 93:841-842
3. Fuster V, Gersh BJ, Giuliani ER, Tajik AJ, Brandenburg RO, Frye RL (1981) The natural history of idiopathic dilated cardiomyopathy. Am J Cardiol 47:525-531
4. Michel VV, Driscoll DJ, Miller FA (1985) Familial aggregation of idiopathic dilated cardiomyopathy. Am J Cardiol 55:1232-1233
5. Michels VV, Moll PP, Miller FA, TajiK AJ, Chu JS, Briscoll DJ, Burnett JC, Rodeheffer RJ, Chesebro JH, Tazelaar HD (1992) The frequency of familial dilated cardiomyopathy in a series of patients with idiopathic dilated cardiomyopathy. N Engl J Med 326:77-82

6. Keeling PJ, Gang G, Smith G, Seo H, Bent SE, Murday V, Caforio ALP, McKenna WJ (1995) Familial dilated cardiomyopathy in the United Kingdom. Br Heart J 73:417-421

7. Fragola PV, Autore A, Picelli A, Sommariva L, Cannata D, Sangiorgi M (1988) Familial dilated cardiomyopathy. Am Heart J 115:912-914

8. Griffin ML, Hernandez A, Martin TC, Goldring D, Bolman RM, Spray TL, Strauss AW (1988) Dilated cardiomyopathy in infants and children. J Am Coll Cardiol 11:139-144

9. Valantine HA, Hunt SA, Fowler MB, Billingham ME, Schoeder JS (1989) Frequency of familial nature of dilated cardiomyopathy and usefulness of cardiac transplantation in this subset. Am J Cardiol 63:959-963

10. Keren A, Gottlieb S, Tzivoni D, Stern S, Yarom R, Billingham ME, Popp RL (1990) Mildly dilated congestive cardiomyopathy. Use of prospective diagnostic criteria and description of the clinical course without heart transplantation. Circulation 81:506-517

11. Mestroni L, Miani D, Di Lenarda A, Silvestri F, Bussani R, Filippi G (1990)Clinical and pathologic study of familial dilated cardiomyopathy. Am J Cardiol 65:1449-1453

12. Zachara E, Caforio ALP, Carboni GP, Pellegrini A, Pompili A, Del Porto G, Scarra A, Bosman C, Boldrini R, Prati Pl, McKenna WJ (1993) Familial aggregation of idiopathic dilated cardiomyopathy: clinical features and pedigree analysis in 14 families. Br Heart J 69:129-135

13. Mestroni L, Milasin J, Vatta M, Pinamonti B, Sinagra G, Rocco C, Matulic M, Falaschi A, Giacca M, Camerini F and the heart muscle disease study group (1996) Genetic factors in dilated cardiomyopathy. Arch Mal Coeur 89:15

14. Gavazzi A, De Maria R, Renosto G, Moro A, Borgia M, Caroli A, Castelli G, Ciaccheri M, Pavan D, De Vita C, Baroldi G, Camerini F (1993) The spectrum of left ventricular size in dilated cardiomyopathy: Clinical correlates and prognostic implications. Am Heart J 125:410-422

15. Mestroni L, Krajinovic M, Severini GM, Pinamonti B, Di Lenarda A, Giacca M, Falaschi A Camerini F (1994) Familial dilated cardiomyopathy. Br Heart J 72 [Suppl 6]:S35-S41

16. Zeviani M, Gellera C, Antozzi C, Rimoldi M, Morandi L, Villani F, Tiranti V, Di Donato S (1991) Maternally inherited myopathy and cardiomyopathy: association with mutation in mitochondrial DNA tRNA Leu (UUR). Lancet 338:143-147

17. Berko B, Swift M (1987) X-linked dilated cardiomyopathy. N Engl J Med 316:1186-1191

18. Kass S, MacRae C, Graber HL, Sparks EA, McNamara D, Boudoulas H, Basson CT, Baker PB 3rd, Cody RJ, Fishman MC (1994) A gene defect that causes conduction system disease and dilated cardiomyopathy maps to chromosome 1p1-1q1. Nature Genet 7:546-551

19. Durand JB, Bachinski LL, Bieling LC, Czernuszewicz GZ, Abche AB, Tao Yu Q, Tapscot T, Hill R, Ifegwu J, Marian AJ, Brugada R, Daiger S, Gregoritch JM, Anderson JL, Quinones M, Towbin JA, Roberts R (1995) Localization of a gene responsible for familial dilated cardiomyopathy to chromosome 1q32. Circulation 92:3387-3389

20. Olson TM, Keating MT (1996) Mapping a cardiomyopathy locus to chromosome 3p22-p25. J Clin Invest 97:528-532

21. Krajinovic M, Pinamonti B, Sinagra GF, Batta M, Severini GM, Milasin J, Falaschi A, Camerini F, Giacca M, Mestroni L and the heart muscle disease study group (1995) Linkage of familial dilated cardiomyopathy to chromosome 9. Am J Hum Gen 57:846-852

22. Muntoni F, Cau M, Ganau A, Congiu R, Arvedi G, Mateddu A, Marrosu MG, Cianchetti C, Realdi G, Cao A, Melis MA (1993) Deletion of the dystrophin muscle-promoter region associated wiyh X-linked dilated cardiomyopathy. N Engl J Med 329:921-925

23. Caforio ALP, Stewart JT, Bonifacio E, Burke M, Davies MJ, McKenna WJ, Bottazzo GF (1990) Inappropiate major histocompatibility complex expression on cardiac tissue in dilated cardiomyopathy. Relevance for autoimmunity? J Autoimmunity 3:187-200

24. Ronnblom LE, Forsberg H, Evrin PE (1991) Increase level of HDL-DR expressing T lynphocytes in peripheral blood from patients with idiopathic dilated cardiomyopathy. Cardiology 78:161-167

25. Carlquist JF, Menlove RL, Murray MB, O'Connell JB, Anderson JL (1991) HLA Class

II (DR and DQ) antigen associations in idiopathic dilated cardiomyopathy. Circulation 83:515-522

26. Zerbe TR, Kaufmann C, Colson Y, Duquesnoy R (1988) Associations of HLA-A,B, DR antigens with primary disease in cardiac allograft recipients. Am J Cardiol 61:1359-1361

27. Limas CJ, Limas C (1989) HLA antigens in idiopathic dilated cardiomyopathy. Br Heart J 62:379-383

28. Komajda M, Raffoux C, Salame E, Colombani J, Grosgogeat Y, Cabrol C, Dausset J (1987) HLA A-B and DR antigens in dilated cardiomyopathy. Arch Mal Coeur Vaiss 80:1233-1237

29. Arbustini E, Gavazzi A, Pozzi R, Grasso M, Pucci A, Campana C, Graziano G; Martinetti M, Cuccia M, Salvaneschi-L (1989) The morphologic spectrum of dilated cardiomyopathy and its relation to immune-response genes. Am J Cardiol 64:991

30. Schultheiss HP (1987) The mitochondrium as antigen in inflammatory heart disease. Eur Heart J 8:203-210

31. Michels VV, Poll PP, Rodeheffer RJ, Miller-FA Jr, Tajik-AJ, Burnett-JC Jr, Driscoll-DJ, Thibodeau-SN, Ansari-AA, Herskowitz-A (1994) Circulating heart autoantibodies in familial as compared with non familial idiopathic dilated cardiomyopathy. Mayo Clin Proc 69:24-27

32. Limas CJ, Goldemberg IF, Limas C (1989) Autoantibodies against beta-adrenoceptors function in human dilated cardiomyopathy. Circ Res 64:97-103

33. Sindhwani R, Yuen J (1994) Genetic basis of myocarditis: a paradigm based on myosin heavy chain polymorphisms. Heart Failure 2:12-25

34. Caforio ALP, Bonifacio E, Stewart JT, Neglia D, Parodi O, Bottazzo GF (1990) Novel organ-specific circulating cardiac antibodies in dilated cardiomyopathy. J Am Coll Cardiol 15:1527-1534

35. Caforio ALP, Goldman JH, Baig MK (1997) Cardiac autoantibodies in dilated cardiomyopathy become undetectable with disease progression. Heart 77:62

36. Caforio LP, Keeling PJ, Zachara E, Mestroni L, Camerini F, Mann JM, Bottazzo GF, Mc Kenna WJ (1994) Autoimmunity in dilated cardiomyopathy: evidence from family studies. Lancet 344:773-777

37. Matsumori A, Kawai C (1982) An animal model of congestive (dilated) cardiomyopathy: dilatation and hypertrophy of the heart in the chronic stage in DBA/2 mice with myocarditis caused by encephalomyocarditis virus. Circulation 66:355

38. O'Connell JB, Mason JW (1989) Diagnosing and treating active myocarditis. West J Med 150:431-435

39. Kasper EK, Agema WR, Hutchins GM, Deckers JW, Hare JM, Baughman KL (1994) The cause of dilated cardiomyopathy: a clinicapathologic review of 673 consecutive patients. J Am Coll Cardiol 23:586-590

40. O'Connell JB (1992) Endomyocardial biopsy in the diagnosis and treatment of myocarditis. In: Fowles RE (ed) Cardiac biopsy. Futura Publishing Inc, Mount Kisko NY, pp 165-179

41. Aretz HT, Billingham ME, Edwars WD, Factor-SM, Fallon-JT, Fenoglio-JJ Jr, Olsen-EG, Schoen-FJ (1987) Myocarditis: a histopathologic definition and classification. Am J Cardiovasc Pathol 1:3-14

42. Mason JW, O'Connel JB, Herskowitz A, Rose NR, McManus BM, Billingham ME, Moon TE and the myocarditis treatment trial investigators (1995) A clinical trial of immunosoppressive therapy for myocarditis. N Engl J Med 333:269-275

43. Arbustini E, Gavazzi A, Dal Bello B, Morbini P, Campana C, Diegoli M, Grasso M, Fasani R, Banchieri N, Porcu E, Pilotto A, Ponzetta M, Bellini O, Lucreziotti S, Viganò M (1997) Ten-year experience with endomyocardial biopsy in myocarditis presenting with congestive heart failure: frequency, pathologic characteristics, treatment and follow-up. G Ital Cardiol 27:209-223

44. Kuhl U, Noutsias M, Schultheiss HP (1995) Immunohistochemistry in dilated cardiomyopathy. Eur Heart J 16 [Suppl O]: 100-106

45. Strauer BE, Kandolf R, Mall G, Maisch B, Mertens T, Schwatzkopff B, Schultheiss HP (1996) Myocarditis - Cardiomyopathy. Consensus Report of the German Association for Internal Medicine. Acta Cardiologica 51 (4):347-371

46. Caforio ALP, Goldman JH, Haven AJ, Baig MK, Dalla Libera L, McKenna WJ, and the Myocarditis Treatment Trial Investigators (1997) Circulating cardiac-specific autoantibodies as markers of autoimmunity in clinical and biopsy-proven myocarditis. Eur Heart J 18:270-275
47. Kuhl U, Strauer BE, Schultheiss HP (1994) Methylprednisolone in chronic myocarditis. Br Heart J 72 [Suppl]: S30 - S34
48. Parrillo JE, Cunnion RE, Epstein SE, Parker MM, Suffredini AF, Brenner M, Schaer GL, Palmeri ST, O.Cannon R, Alling D, Wittes JT, Ferrans WJ, Rodriguez ER, Fauci AS (1989) A prospective, randomized, controlled trial of prednisone for dilated cardiomyopathy. N Engl J Med 321:1061-1069
49. Latham RD, Mulrow JP, Virmani R, Robinowitz M, Moody JM (1989) Recently diagnosed idiopathic dilated cardiomyopathy: incidence of myocarditis and efficacy of prednisone therapy. Am Heart J 117:876-882
50. Cambridge G, MacArthur CGC, Waterstone AP, GoodwinGF, Oakley CN (1979) Antibodies to Coxackie B viruses in congestive cardiomyopathy. Br Heart J 41:692-696
51. Woodroof JF (1980) Viral myocarditis: a review. Am J Pathol 101:427-479
52. Bowles N, Richardson P, Olsen E, Archard L (1986) Detection of Coxackie-B-virus-specific RNA sequences in myocardial biopsy samples from patients with dilated cardiomyopathy and myocarditis. Lancet 1:1120-1123
53. Kandolf R, Hofschneider PH (1989) Enterovirus-induced cardiomyopathy. In: Notkins AL, Oldstone MBA, (eds) Concepts in viral pathogenesis III. Springer-Verlag, New York pp 282-290
54. Archard LC, Bowles NE, Cunningam L, Freeke CA, Morgan Capner P, Olsen EGS, Banner NR, Rose ML, Yacoub MH, Meany BT, Richardson PJ, (1990) Enterovirus RNA sequences in hearts with dilated cardiomyopathy: a pathogenetic link between virus infection and dilated cardiomyopathy. In: Baroldi G, Camerini F, Goodwin JF, (eds) Advances in cardiomyopathy. Springer-Verlag, Berlin, pp 194-198
55. Tracy S, Wiegand V, McManus B, Gauntt C, Pallansch M, Beck M, Chapman N (1990) Molecular approaches to enteroviral diagnosis in idiopathic cardiomyopathy and myocarditis. J Am Coll Cardiol 15:1688-1694
56. Jin O, Sole MJ, Butany JW, Chia WK, McLaughlin PR, Liu P, Liew CC (1990) Detection of Enterovirus RNA in myocardial biopsies from patients with myocarditis and cardiomyopathy using gene amplification by polymerase chain reaction. Circulation 82:8-16
57. Cochrane HR, May FEB, Ashcroft T, Dark JH (1991) Enteroviruses and idiopathic dilated cardiomyopathy. J Pathol 163:129-131
58. Weiss LM, Liu XF, Chang KL, Billingham ME (1992) Detection of enteroviral RNA in idiopathic dilated cardiomyopathy and other human cardiac tissue. J Clin Invest 90:156-159
59. Grasso M, Arbustini E, Silini E, Diegoli M, Percivalle E, Ratti G, Bramerio M, Gavazzi A, Viganò M, Milanesi G (1992) Search for coxsackievirus B3 RNA in idiopathic dilated cardiomyopathy using gene amplification by polimerase chain reaction. Am J Cardiol 69:658-664
60. Keeling PJ, Jeffery S, Caforio ALP, Taylor R, Bottazzo GF, Davies MJ, McKenna WJ (1992) Similar prevalence of enteroviral genome in myocardium from patients with idiopathic dilated cardiomyopathy and controls by the polymerase chain reaction. Br Heart J 68:554-559
61. Satoh M, Tamura G, Segawa I, Hiramori K, Satodate R (1994) Enteroviral RNA in dilated cardiomyopathy. Eur Heart J 15:934-939
62. Giacca M, Severini GM, Mestroni L, Salvi A, Lardieri G, Falaschi A, Camerini F (1994) Low frequency of detection of enterovirus RNA in endomyocardial tissue of patients with idiopathic dilated cardiomyopathy by nested polymerase chain reaction. J Am Coll Cardiol 24:10-33
63. Figulla HR, Stille-Siegener M, Mall G, Heim A, Kreuzer H (1995) Myocardial enterovirus infection with left ventricular dysfuction: a benign disease compared with idiopathic dilated cardiomyopathy. J Am Coll Cardiol 25:1170-1175
64. Bowles NE, Rose ML , Taylor P, Banner NR, Morgan Capner P, Cunningham L, Archard LC, Yacoub MH (1989) Persistence of Enterovirus RNA in myocardium at

cardiac transplantation and lack of immune response. Circulation 80:1128-1136
65. Archard LC, Bowles NE, Cunningham L, Freeke CA, Olsen EG, Rose ML, Meany B, Why HJ, Richardson PJ (1991) Molecular probes for detection of persisting enterovirus infection of human heart and their prognostic value. Eur Heart J 12 [Suppl D):56-59
66. Why HG.F, Meany BT, Richardson PJ (1994) Clinical and prognostic significance of detection of enteroviral rna in the myocardium of patients with myocarditis or dilated cardiomyopathy. Circulation 89:2582-2589

The Italian Multicentric Study: Natural History of Dilated Cardiomyopathy

R. De Maria and M. Parolini on behalf of the Italian Study Group
on Cardiomyopathies (SPIC), Subproject on Dilated Cardiomyopathy

Dilated cardiomyopathy was defined as a heart muscle disease of unknown cause characterized by left ventricular or biventricular dilatation and impaired systolic function [1]. The natural history of the disease is difficult to ascertain, as asymptomatic ventricular dilatation and dysfunction may be present for long periods. Prognosis of the disease from the onset of symptoms was generally described as poor [2-3]. These retrospective studies usually analysed patients with advanced heart failure, who have been mostly evaluated in a period preceding the widespread use of echocardiography as a diagnostic tool, in tertiary referral centers. Whether earlier diagnosis and careful follow-up would substantially impact on the reportedly dire prognosis was at the moment unclear. These considerations prompted a cooperative effort involving 15 Italian centers in a multicenter Registry, which started in January 1986. The aim of this registry was the prospective study of the natural history of dilated cardiomyopathy, with particular attention to early manifestations of disease.

In the late eighties and early nineties, a number of retrospective reports challenged the unfavourable outcome to some extent [4-9], and related improved prognosis to selection of less severely diseased patients [4-7] and to evolving therapy in heart failure [8,9]. The present report describes the long term course of dilated cardiomyopathy of unknown origin in a large prospective series, selected on the basis of uniform diagnostic criteria, and puts into perspective the impact of early diagnosis, careful follow-up and changing medical treatment on prognosis.

The SPIC Registry. Enrollment and Study Methods

Patients referred to the participating centers because of heart failure and/or high grade ventricular arrhythmias and/or severe depression of ventricular function (echocardiographic left ventricular fractional shortening < 20%) of unknown etiology, or a combination of signs and symptoms including dyspnea, supraventricular or ventricular arrhythmias, ECG abnormalities and left ventricular dilation or dysfunction, underwent a complete screening. Non-invasive evaluation included physical examination, 12-lead electrocardiogram, M-mode and two-dimensional echocardiography, 24-hour dynamic electrocardiographic monitoring, exercise stress testing and biochemistry, including thyroid function tests. Patients with systemic hypertension, cor pulmonale, valvular heart disease, thyroid dysfunction or systemic diseases were excluded. Excessive alcohol consumption was recorded and analysed as a potential risk factor.

Patients with end-stage cardiomyopathy, who had been specifically referred for heart replacement and entered in the transplant waiting list, were not included in this series.

The clinical suspicion of dilated cardiomyopathy was confirmed invasively in every patient by demonstrating (1) reduced left ventricular ejection fraction (< 50%) at cineangiography, (2) absence of significant coronary artery disease (> 50% luminal diameter reduction of a major coronary artery branch) at coronary angiography, (3) absence of specific heart muscle disease or active myocarditis at endomyocardial biopsy. All patients underwent non-invasive and invasive evaluation within one month.

Functional status was classified according to New York Heart Association criteria.

Echocardiographic measurements were obtained according to previously published standards [10] and normalized for body surface area. M-mode images were recorded under two-dimensional guidance, selecting an orthogonal plane to the ultrasound beam. Left ventricular volumes were obtained from the apical four chamber view; left ventricular ejection fraction was calculated with the single-plane area-length method [11].

Left and right heart catheterization was performed with fluid filled catheters and low volume displacement transducer. Mean right atrial, right ventricular end-diastolic, pulmonary artery, capillary wedge, left ventricular end diastolic and aortic pressures were recorded. Patients with restrictive pattern of ventricular pressure recordings were excluded from the study. Cardiac output was measured with the thermodilution method; the mean of three measurements was given and corrected for body surface area to obtain cardiac index.

Left ventricular angiography was accomplished in the 30 degree right anterior oblique projection. Mean normal values for left ventricular ejection fraction in the participating hemodynamic laboratories were 72% ± 8%; thus 50% (below two standard deviations from the normal value) was chosen as upper limit of left ventricular ejection fraction, to indicate left ventricular dysfunction. Selective coronary angiography was performed according to Judkins' technique.

Right ventricular endomyocardial biopsy was accomplished through the right femoral vein with King's College bioptome or through the right internal jugular vein with Caves' bioptome; in a minority of patients left ventricular endomyocardial biopsy was performed. In each biopsy procedure at least four tissue specimens were obtained and processed for histological diagnosis; Dallas criteria [12] were used to rule out myocarditis.

Dynamic electrocardiogram was recorded for at least 24 hours. The total number of ventricular premature complexes in 24 hours, their mean hourly frequency and the total number of ventricular pairs (2 consecutive ventricular premature complexes) in 24 hours and their hourly frequency were calculated. The number of ventricular tachycardia episodes (≥3 consecutive ventricular premature complexes) per 24 hours, their hourly frequency and the number of beats per episode were also evaluated.

When clinically feasible, a symptom-limited exercise stress test was performed in the upright position at bicycle cycloergometer with 25 watt steps every 3 minutes or 10 watt steps every minute.

Medical treatment was administered according to the clinical judgement of the attending physician at each center, along common guidelines. These included limitation of dietary salt intake, restriction of physical activity, digoxin, diuretics (usually furosemide) to relieve congestive symptoms, and vasodilators, prevalently ACE-inhibitors, which were administered even in asymptomatic patients from 1992. Amiodarone was prescribed for complex ventricular arrhythmias or atrial fibrillation and flutter; other antiarrhythmic agents were used in a minority of cases, when amiodarone was contraindicated or not tolerated.

Clinical examination and noninvasive tests were repeated yearly during follow up. The study began after completion of the baseline evaluation and terminated at December 1996 or at the patient's death or transplantation. Circumstances of death were investigated by interviewing relatives or attending physicians. Classification of the type of death was based on evaluation of the state of circulation immediately before death [13]. Death was distinguished in (a) *sudden*, if it occurred instantaneously or within minutes or during sleep, in patients in NYHA class I to III, and was not preceded by deteriorating cardiac failure, or (b) *secondary to heart failure*, when resulting from ongoing deterioration of heart performance, (c) of *unknown cause* when the mechanism of death could not be ascertained with certainty, or (d) *noncardiac*, when a cardiac cause could be ruled out (e.g. suicide, accident, cancer).

Statistical analysis. Continuous data are expressed as mean values ± standard deviation. Product limit survival was calculated with Kaplan-Meier curves. Cox proportional hazards model was used to analyse the relationship between survival and prognostic indices. The Statistical Package for the Social Science Program (SPSS, SPSS Inc. Chicago, Ill.) and Biomedical Computer Program (BMPD Statistical Software Inc., Los Angeles CA) softwares were used. A p value < .05 was considered significant.

Results

Study Population

In December 1996, the total population enrolled in the Registry included 525 patients. A history of alcohol abuse was elicited in 84 cases (16%), who were excluded from the present analysis. The remaining 441 cases are the subject of this report. Patients ranged in age from 8 to 69 years (mean 44 ± 13). The mean interval from symptom onset or first evidence of a cardiac abnormality

Table 1. Patient characteristics

	% patients
Men	71
History of familial disease	15
Casual detection of dilated cardiomyopathy	20
Selection criteria	
Unexplained heart failure	52
Ventricular arrhythmias	6
Severe LV dysfunction	12
Combination of criteria	30
NYHA class III-IV	35
Atrial fibrillation	10
Left bundle branch block	32
Complex ventricular arrhythmias	68
Advanced AV block	3
Cardiothoracic ratio >0.50	67

Table 2. Laboratory findings

	Mean±SD
Left ventricular end-diastolic diameter (mm/m²)	39±6
Left ventricular end-systolic diameter (mm/m²)	33±6
Left atrial diameter (mm/m²)	23±5
Ventricular premature complexes/hour	111±214
Ventricular pairs/hour	2.16±7.8
Ventricular tachycardia episodes/hour	0.17±1.18
Pulmonary wedge pressure (mmHg)	14±9
Left ventricular end-diastolic pressure (mmHg)	16±10
Cardiac index (l/min/m²)	3.2±1.08
Left ventricular ejection fraction %	30±10
Exercise duration (seconds)	547±229

to enrolment into the Registry was 27 ± 42 months. The main clinical and laboratory characteristics of study patients are presented in Tables 1 and 2. The spectrum of left ventricular ejection fraction in the study series is depicted in Figure 1; although the majority of patients had severe left ventricular dysfunction, 17% of cases showed only mild contractile impairment.

Medical treatment included digitalis in 348 patients (79%), furosemide in 278 (63%), ACE-inhibitors in 366 (83%), beta-blockers in 172 (39%), amiodarone in 154 (35%), other antiarrhythmic agents in 49 (11%), and oral anticoagulants in 154 (35%).

Outcome

During a mean follow-up of 55±32 months (range 15 days - 134 months), 88 patients died of cardiac causes (20%) and 52 underwent heart transplantation (12%); 9 patients died of non-cardiac causes, while in 7 cases the mechanism of death could not be ascertained. Death was sudden in 52 patients (12%)

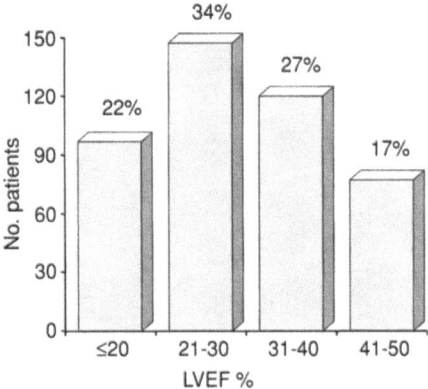

Fig. 1. Distribution of left ventricular ejection fraction (LVEF) in 441 patients with dilated cardiomyopathy of unknown origin

and due to heart failure in 35 (8%); one patient died of pulmonary embolism (confirmed at autopsy).

Product limit survival was calculated according to Kaplan and Meier. Survival (all cause mortality) and transplant-free survival curves are shown in Figure 2; 90%, 76% and 66% of patients were alive at two, five and eight years respectively. Transplant-free survival at the same intervals was 85%, 68% and 56% respectively.

Time to death or transplantation averaged 34 ± 26 months; the mean inter-

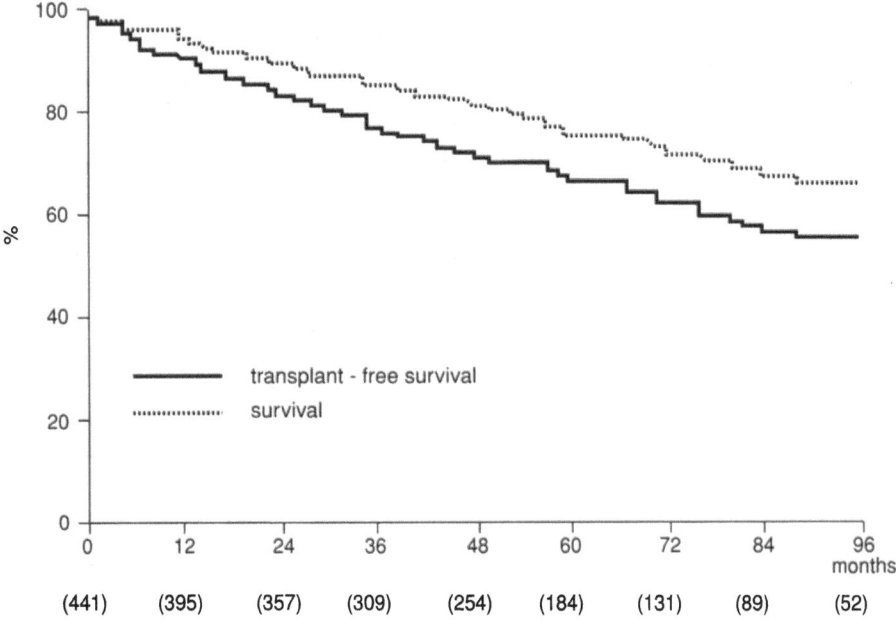

Fig. 2. Product-limit survival (dotted line) and transplant-free survival (continuous line) in the study series; in parentheses the number of patients alive at each time interval

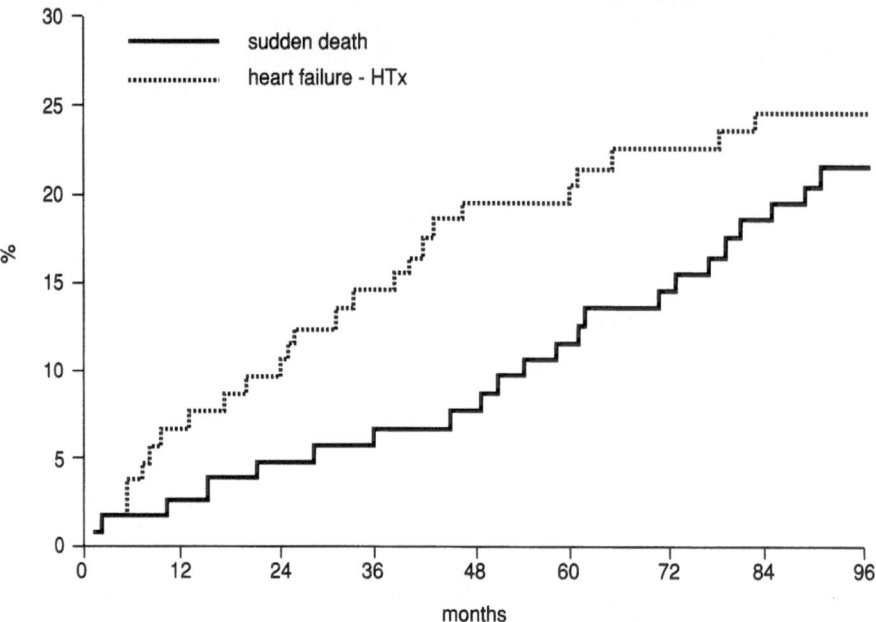

Fig 3. Cumulative mortality due to heart failure or heart transplantation (dotted line) or sudden death (continuous line) in the study series

val between entry into the study and outcome classification for non-transplanted survivors was 66 ± 29 months.

The time course of heart failure death or transplantation vs sudden death is shown in Figure 3. Cumulative mortality related to progressive heart failure, including death or heart transplantation, rose steeply during the first three to four years (mean time to death 28 ± 24 months, $p < .001$ vs sudden death) and tended to plateau thereafter, while sudden deaths show a smoother increase (mean time to death 44 ± 28 months) with a late peak after the first five years.

Functional Evaluation at Follow-up

The latest follow up data were available at a mean interval of 36±24 months

Table 3. Criteria for definition of functional outcome at follow-up

	improved	stable	deteriorated
NYHA class	decreased ≥ 1	unchanged	increased ≥ 1
LV end diastolic diameter	decreased > 10%	from −10% to +10%	increased > 10%
LV ejection fraction	increased > 5 pp	from −5 pp to +5 pp	decreased > 5 pp
Exercise duration	increased > 20%	from −20% to +20%	decreased > 20%

LV, left ventricular; pp, percent points.

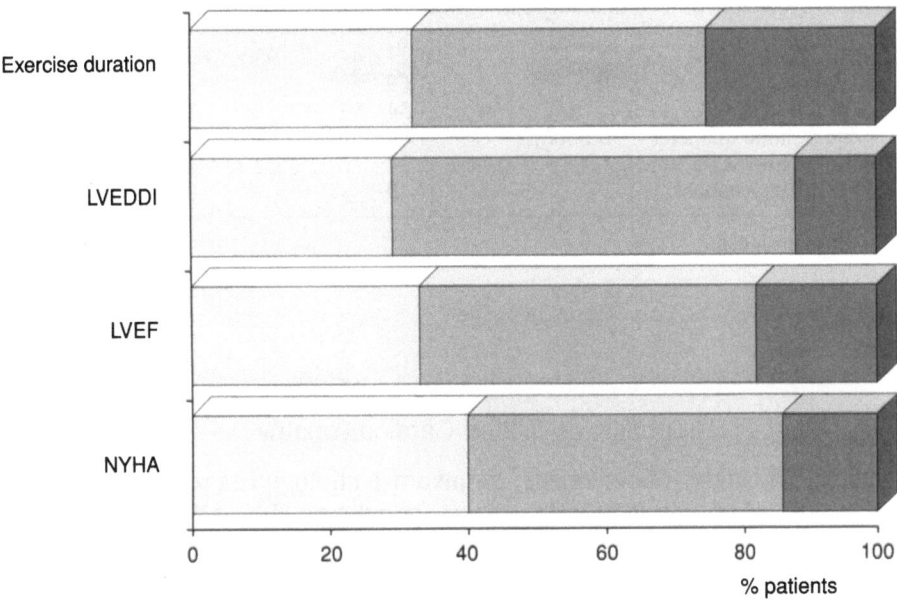

Fig. 4. Percent distribution of long term improvement (☐), stability (▨) or deterioration (■) in clinical and functional parameter in the study series (see text for details). LVEDDI, left ventricular end diastolic diameter index; LVEF, left ventricular ejection fraction; NYHA, New York Heart Association functional class

from baseline evaluation in 312 cases. Patients were classified as improved, stable or deteriorated according to the changes in functional parameters shown in Table 3.

Functional outcome at follow-up is summarized in Figure 4: the largest percent of improvement was observed in the symptomatic status (40% of cases had a decrese of at least one NYHA class), while about one third of cases showed an increase in LV ejection fraction and exercise duration at exercise stress testing, or a decrease in left ventricular dimensions. When a global score incorporating all of the above variables was calculated, 40 patients (14% of those with available data) had improved their functional status, ejection fraction and left ventricular dimensions at follow-up.

Predictors of Prognosis

Independent predictors of total mortality and heart transplantation by Cox multivariate analysis included advanced NYHA functional class, a longer symptomatic period, increased left ventricular end systolic dimensions and pulmonary wedge pressure (Table 4); beta-blocker treatment on the contrary was associated to a reduced mortality. When predictors of sudden death or progressive heart failure death or transplantation were separately analysed, the findings were similar: in particular no arrhythmic variable predicted sudden death.

Table 4. Predictors of total mortality and heart transplantation by Cox multivariate analysis

	Relative risk	95% Confidence intervals
Symptom duration > 6 months	1.69	1.18-2.40
NYHA class III-IV	1.54	1.08-2.20
LV end systolic diameter $\geq$ 30 mm/m^2	1.56	1.00-2.45
Wedge pressure $\geq$ 15 mmHg	2.28	1.59-3.28
Beta-blocker treatment	0.40	0.27-0.60

LV, left ventricular.

Discussion

The Changing Prognosis of Dilated Cardiomyopathy

Although dilated cardiomyopathy of unknown etiology is a relatively uncommon cause of heart failure in the general population [14], it is, particularly in the younger age group [15], a leading indication to heart transplantation, a solution limited by the scarcity of available donor hearts. Accordingly, changes in the dire prognosis of this disease would have a substantial impact in terms of human suffering and economic implications related to the use of sophisticated and costly medical procedures. Older series, which were often heterogeneous as to diagnostic criteria, and studied in the pre-echocardiography, pre-vasodilator era, included mostly severely symptomatic patients, and indicated two- and five-year survival rates around 60% and 40% respectively [2-4]. Subsequent, still mainly retrospective and heterogeneous reports, which included patients with less advanced disease [5,6], population based series [7] or referral series enrolled in the vasodilator era, demonstrated improved prognosis, with two- and five-year survival rates around 85% and 70% respectively on a total of 459 patients. Another study [9] examined changes in the prognosis of dilated cardiomyopathy over the last 20 years: survival increased significantly during time and outcome was related to the use of ACE-inhibitors and beta-blockers. Improved survival has also been demonstrated in three subsequent cohorts of patients with advanced heart failure [16] of various origin, following the implementation of optimal drug treatment.

The present prospective series included patients with moderately depressed left ventricular function, mild hemodynamic impairment and heart failure symptoms; moreover 83% of patients were on ACE-inhibitors. Not surprisingly in this series survival closely paralleled the one reported in the population-based study by Sugrue et al [7]: the combination of early diagnosis, careful follow-up and optimal medical management are probably responsible together for these findings. Despite these encouraging results, 8-year mortality is still a substantial 34%. Beta-blocker treatment, consistently with the findings of randomized clinical trials [17-19], seems to confer significant protection against mortality and transplantation.

Dilated cardiomyopathy of unknown cause is a leading cause of heart transplantation, a procedure which may substantially alter the natural history of this disease, as shown by a recent report [20]. In this study, 60 of 172 idiopathic dilated cardiomyopathy patients (35%) suffered progressive heart failure during follow-up; only 8% of them died, while the vast majority (77%) underwent heart transplantation. Therefore heart transplantation should probably be included in the analysis of outcome of this disease. The relative impact of the implementation of the National Heart Transplant Program in Italy on mortality from dilated cardiomyopathy may be estimated from the difference between the two curves reported in Fig. 2. If one considers transplantation as aborted death from progressive heart failure, a further ten percent should be added to the 8-year mortality burden posed by dilated cardiomyopathy, even in a population with mild to moderate disease.

Mechanisms of Death

In the present series, half of all deaths were sudden, representing one third of all negative outcomes, while progressive heart failure leading to death or transplantation comprised 56% of negative outcomes. Sudden death is common in dilated cardiomyopathy: in different series it has ranged from onethird to twothirds of deaths [21] and has shown a relative increase since many patients with progressive heart failure, particularly in the younger age group, undergo transplantation [17]. Sudden death represents a continuing threat, as its incidence tends to increase during later follow-up (Figure 3), and it typically affects patients in good clinical conditions: 73% of our patients who died suddenly were in NYHA class I or II at their last follow-up observation. In the present series the same variables predicted both sudden death and death from progressive heart failure, indicating that, even in patients with mild to moderate disease, whichever the mechanism of demise, the degree of functional impairment is the main determinant of outcome.

Follow-up data indicate that about one third of patients will show an improvement in symptoms, left ventricular dimensions or function. However approximately one in six patients will experience long-term improvement when all parameters are considered together, while the majority will remain stable during time.

In conclusion, although the natural history of dilated cardiomyopathy of unknown origin has changed over the last fifteen years and survival appears significantly prolonged, optimism as to the long-term outcome of this disease is not yet justified. However, the careful exploitation of optimal medical management holds promise for further improvement in prognosis.

Centres participating in the SPIC
(Studio Policentrico Italiano Cardiomiopatie)

Milano: Ospedale Niguarda Ca' Granda, Dipartimento di Cardiologia "A. De Gasperis" Claudio De Vita, Antonella Moreo, Maurizio Ferratini, Antonio Pezzano, Fabio Recalcati, Edgardo Bonacina; **Firenze**: Ospedale Careggi, Servizio di Cardiologia San Luca: Alberto Dolara, Mauro Ciaccheri, Gabriele Castelli, Vito Troiani, Franca Gori, Maurizio Nannini; **Milano**: Ospedale San Carlo, Divisione di Cardiologia: Franco Casazza, Angela Capozzi,

Roberto Mattioli; **Pisa:** Servizio di Cardiostimolazione, Istituto di Fisiologia Clinica del C.N.R.: Andrea Biagini, Oberdan Parodi, Marco Baratto, Danilo Neglia, Gualtiero Pelosi, Annalisa Tongiani, Fabio Vernazza; **Pavia:** I.R.C.C.S. Policlinico San Matteo, Divisione di Cardiologia: Antonello Gavazzi, Carlo Campana, Marina Ponzetta, Eloisa Arbustini, Carlo Montemartini; **Trieste:** Ospedale Maggiore, Divisione di Cardiologia: Fulvio Camerini, Andrea Di Lenarda, Gerardina Lardieri, Luisa Mestroni, Bruno Pinamonti, Andrea Perkan, Furio Silvestri, Gianfranco Sinagra, Massimo Zecchin, Dario Gregori, Elena Bernobich, Fulvia Longaro, Luca Salvatore; **Varese:** Ospedale di Circolo, Divisione di Cardiologia: Giovanni Binaghi, Sergio Repetto, Marcella Luvini; **Monza:** Ospedale San Gerardo, Divisione e Servizio di Cardiologia: Franco Valagussa, Alessandro Bozzano, Antonio Cadel, Bruno Pria; **Milano:** Istituto Villa Marelli, Servizio di Cardiologia: Aldo Sachero, Erminia Giagnoni, Luciano Beretta; **Napoli:** Ospedale Monaldi, Ia Divisione di Medicina: Massimo Cafiero, Massimo Borgia , Franco Costantino, Attilio De Santis, Raffaele D'Oriano; **Vicenza**: Ospedale Civile, Divisione di Cardiologia: Mario Vincenzi, Luigi La Vecchia; **Treviso**: Presidio Ospedaliero Multizonale, Divisione di Cardiologia: Paolo Stritoni, Giuliano Renosto, Agnese Moro; **Roma:** Ospedale San Camillo, Divisione di Cardiologia: Pierluigi Prati, Elisabetta Zachara; **Cagliari:** Ospedale Nuovo San Michele, Divisione di Cardiologia: Antonio Sanna, Maurizio Porcu, Stefano Salis, Francesco Uras.
Scientific Committee: Giorgio Baroldi, Istituto Fisiologia Clinica del CNR, Sezione di Milano; Fulvio Camerini, Ospedali Riuniti, Divisione di Cardiologia, Trieste; Claudio De Vita, Ospedale Niguarda Cà Granda, Dipartimento di Cardiologia "A. De Gasperis", Milano.
Scientific Secretariat: Renata De Maria, Istituto Fisiologia Clinica del CNR, Sezione di Milano; Antonello Gavazzi, Divisione di Cardiologia, I.R.C.C.S. Policlinico San Matteo, Pavia.
Statistical Analysis: Marina Parolini, Istituto Fisiologia Clinica del CNR, Sezione di Milano.

References

1. Report of the WHO/ISFC Task Force (1980) on the definition and classification of cardiomyopathies. Br Heart J 44:672-673
2. Fuster V, Gersh BJ, Giuliani ER, Tajik AJ, Branderburg RO, Frye RL (1981) The natural history of idiopathic dilated cardiomyopathy. Am J Cardiol 47:525-531
3. Gavazzi A, Lanzarini L, Cornalba C, Desperati M, Raisaro A, Angoli L, De Servi S, Specchia G (1984) Dilated (congestive) cardiomyopathy. Follow up study of 137 patients. G Ital Cardiol 11:492-498
4. Diaz RA, Obasohan A, Oakley CM (1987) Prediction of outcome in dilated cardiomyopathy. Br Heart J 58:393-399
5. Ikram H, Williamson HG, Won IG, Wells EJ (1987) The course of idiopathic dilated cardiomyopathy in New Zealand. Br Heart J 57:521-527
6. Komajda M, Jaist JP, Reeves F, Goldfarb B, Boubour JB, Juilleres Y, Lanfranchi I, Peycelon P, Geslin P, Carie D, Grosgogeat Y (1990) Factors predicting mortality in idiopathic dilated cardiomyopaty. Eur Heart J 11:824-831
7. Sugrue DD, Rodeheffer RJ, Codd MB, Ballard DJ, Fuster V, Gersh BR (1992) The clinical course of idiopathic dilated cardiomyopathy: a population-based study. Ann Intern Med 117:-23
8. Redfield MM, Gersh BJ, Bailey KR, Ballard DJ, Rodeheffer RJ (1993) Natural history of idiopathic dilated cardiomyopathy: effect of referral bias and secular trend. J Am Coll Cardiol 22:1921-1926
9. Di Lenarda A, Secoli G, Perkan A, Gregori D, Lardieri G, Pinamonti B, Sinagra G, Zecchin M, Camerini F (1994) Changing mortality in dilated cardiomyopathy. Br Heart J 72 [suppl]:S46-S51
10. Sahn DJ, De Maria AN, Kisslo J, Weyman A (1976) The committee on M-mode standardization of the American Society of Echocardiography: Recommendations regarding quantitation in M-mode echocardiography. Results of a survey of echocardiographic measurements. Circulation 58:1072-1083

11. Folland ED, Parisi AF, Moynihan PF, Jones DR, Feldman CL, Tow DE (1979) Assessment of left ventricular ejection fraction and volumes by real-time two-dimensional echocardiography. A comparison of cineangiographic and radionuclide techniques. Circulation 60:760-766
12. Aretz HT, Billingham ME, Edwards WD, Factor S, Fenoglio J, Olsen EG, Schoen F (1986) Myocarditis: a histopathologic definition and classification. Am J Cardiovasc Pathol 1:3-14
13. Hinkle L, Thaler J (1982) Clinical classification of cardiac deaths. Circulation 65:457-464
14. Codd MB, Sugrue DD, Gersh BJ, Melton LJ (1989) Epidemiology of idiopathic dilated and hypertrophic cardiomyopathy. Circulation 80:564-572
15. Hosenpud JD, Novick RJ, Breen TJ, Keck B, Daily P (1995) The registry of the Internaitonal Society for Heart and Lung Transplantation : twelfth official report - 1995. J Heart Lung Transplant 14:805-815
16. Stevenson WG, Stevenson LW, Middlekauf HR, Fonarow GC, Hamilton MA, Woo MA, Saxon LA, Natterson PD, SteimleA, Walden JA, Tillisch JH (1995) Improving survival for patients with advanced heart failure: a study of 737 consecutive patients. J Am Coll Cardiol 26:1417-1423
17. Waagstein F, Bristow MR, Swedberg K, Camerini F, Foxler MB, Silver MA, Gilbert EM, Johnson MR, Goss FG, Hjalmarson A (1993) Beneficial effects of metoprolol in idiopathic dilated cardiomyopathy. Lancet 342:1441-1446
18. CIBIS Investigators and Committees (1994) A randomized trial of beta-blockade in heart failure. The cardiac insufficiency bisoprolol study (CIBIS). Circulation 90:1765-1773
19. Packer M, Bristow MR, Cohn JN, Colucci WS, Fowler MB, Gilbert EM, Shusterman NH (1996) The effect of carvedilol on morbidity and mortality in patients with chronic heart failure. N Engl J Med 334:1349-1355
20. Goldman JH, Keeling PJ, Slade A, Elliot P, Caforio A, Poloniecki J, McKenna WJ (1995) The improved prognosis of idiopathic dilated cardiomyopathy in the era of modern therapeutics. J Am Coll Cardiol 25-I:386 (abs)
21. Dec GW, Fuster V (1994) Idiopathic dilated cardiomyopathy. N Engl J Med 331:1564-1575

Mildly Dilated Cardiomyopathy

M. Porcu, R. De Maria and A. Gavazzi, on behalf of the Italian Study Group
on Cardiomyopathies (SPIC), Subproject on Dilated Cardiomyopathy

Introduction

Dilated cardiomyopathy is considered a disease of uncertain and probably
heterogeneous origin, characterized by dilatation and impaired systolic function
of the left or both ventricles [1]. Although this definition underscores the typical pathological aspect of dilated cardiomyopathy, there is increasing evidence
that a larger spectrum of morphological conditions can be included in this unexplained heart muscle disease. In fact, patients with impairment of systolic function of unknown cause show a wide range of left ventricular dimensions, from
very enlarged to absolutely normal chambers [2]. In the past, different studies
attributed a prognostic significance to the degree of left ventricular dilatation,
that was considered as one of the factors predicting mortality in patients with
dilated cardiomyopathy [3-6]. However, other observations on small series have
recently shown that patients with an idiopathic reduction of contractility may
have an unfavorable outcome despite the absence of relevant left ventricular
enlargement [7,8]. Moreover, a preliminary analysis of 144 patients enrolled in
the SPIC (Italian Multicentric Study on Cardiomyopathies) Registry and
followed up for about three years did not confirm the role of ventricular dilatation as an independent negative prognostic factor [9].

The aim of this study was to define the clinical aspects and long-term prognosis of a large series of patients with idiopathic impairment of left ventricular systolic function and normal or mildly dilated left chamber (MDCM),
compared to patients with typically dilated cardiomyopathy (DCM).

Methods

The study population is a consecutive series of patients prospectively enrolled
in the Registry of the Italian Multicenter Cardiomyopathy Study. One of the aim
of this Registry was to define the clinical characteristics and the natural history
of patients with idiopathic systolic dysfunction, with particular emphasis on the
early phase of the disease. Enrollment criteria and protocol have been described
in detail elsewhere [9,2]. Briefly, patients with signs or symptoms of heart failure and/or high-grade ventricular arrhythmias and/or depression of left ventricular function (defined as an echocardiographic shortening fraction <20%) of

unknown cause underwent a complete clinical and laboratory evaluation to confirm the suspicion of dilated cardiomyopathy. Baseline noninvasive study included 12-lead electrocardiogram, chest X-ray, complete echocardiographic evaluation, 24-hour Holter monitoring and, when clinically feasible, symptom-limited exercise stress test. All echocardiographic measurements were obtained according to the American Society of Echocardiography criteria and normalized for body surface area [10]. Left and right heart catheterization, including coronary angiography, left ventriculography, and right ventricular endomyocardial biopsy was performed in all cases.

Patients were not enrolled in the Registry if they had angiographic left ventricular ejection fraction >0.50, coronary narrowing >50% in a major branch, hemodynamic signs of restrictive cardiomyopathy, histological evidence of specific heart disease or active myocarditis, according to Dallas criteria [11]. Systemic hypertension, cor pulmonale, primitive valvular heart disease, thyroid dysfunction, systemic disease were also considered as exclusion criteria. Patients on the waiting list for heart transplantation were also excluded. Patients with excessive alcohol consumption were included in the present analysis and daily alcohol intake was evaluated as a potential risk factor.

From January 1986 until December 1995, five hundred and twenty five patients fulfilled these diagnostic criteria and were prospectively followed up. Among this large group of patients, we evaluated for this study only subjects with a left ventricular ejection fraction ≤0.40. Following previously accepted criteria, we considered 32 mm/m^2 as the upper normalcy value for left ventricular end-diastolic diameter index [7,8]. Accordingly, all cases with an end-diastolic ventricular diameter not exceeding 15% of this value, i.e. 37 mm/m^2, were arbitrarily defined as MDCM. Patients with DCM, showing end-diastolic left ventricular diameter at enrollment ≥40 mm/m^2, were chosen as controls. Patients with left ventricular end-diastolic diameter >37 and <40 mm/m^2 were not considered in this analysis, to avoid inclusion of a possibly confusing intermediate population.

Medical treatment was adjusted independently by the cardiologists at each participating center, following guidelines which suggested the use of vasodilators (particularly ACE inhibitors) and, according to clinical status, digoxin, diuretics and beta-blockers. Routine yearly follow-up included a complete noninvasive re-evaluation. Right heart catheterization was repeated only according to clinical need.

Out-of-hospital causes of death were recorded contacting relatives or general pratictioners. Mode of death was defined according to the criteria indicated by Hinkle and Thaler [12]. Primary end-points were all-cause mortality and heart transplantation.

Statistical Analysis

The Statistical Package for the Social Science Program (SPSS, SPSS Inc. Chicago, Ill.) and Biomedical Computer Program (BMPD Statistical Software Inc., Los Angeles CA) software were used for statistical analysis.

Continuous data are expressed as mean values ± standard deviation. Comparisons between groups were performed with two-tailed unpaired Student's t test for continuous variables and with chi-square test with Yates' correction for discrete variables. Cumulative survival was calculated with Kaplan-Meier curves. A p value <0.05 was considered significant

Results

According to the above defined criteria, among the whole population of 415 patients with left ventricular ejection fraction ≤0.40 enrolled in the SPIC Registry, one hundred-seventy patients (41%) were included in the MDCM group, one hundred-eighty patients (43%) were considered as DCM controls and sixty-five patient with left ventricular end-diastolic diameter >37 and <40 mm/m² were excluded from the analysis. The baseline clinical characteristics of the patients with MDCM and DCM are shown in Table 1.

In the typically dilated group, a significantly larger number of patients had severe functional impairment (NYHA class III-IV), higher prevalence of left bundle branch block and lower mean left ventricular ejection fraction.

Despite smaller left atria, the prevalence of atrial fibrillation was signifi-

Table 1. Baseline clinical and laboratory findings in 180 patients with typically dilated (DCM) and 170 patients with mildly dilated (MDCM) cardiomyopathy

	MDCM (n=170)	p	DCM (n=180)
Age	45±11	ns	43±13
Male (%)	141 (83)	.001	121 (67)
NYHA class III-IV (%)	57 (33)	.02	84 (47)
Alcohol >100g/day (%)	30 (19)	ns	26 (15)
Digitalis	129 (76)	.01	157 (87)
ACE-inhibitors (%)	139 (82)	ns	159 (88)
Furosemide (%)	99 (58)	.003	133 (74)
Anticoagulants (%)	53 (31)	.002	85 (47)
Amiodarone%	64 (38)	ns	71 (39)
Beta-blockers%	67 (39)	ns	59 (33)
Heart rate (b/m)	86±16	ns	85±17
Left bundle branch block (%)	48 (28)	ns	80 (45)
Atrial fibrillation (%)	30 (18)	.0001	8 (4)
Left atrial diameter (m/m²)	22±4	.0001	26±5
Ventricular tachycardia episodes/hour	0.10±0.4	ns	0.21±1.5
Left ventricular ejection fraction (%)	29±7	.0001	24±8
Wedge pressure (mmHg)	15±9	ns	16±10
Mean aortic pressure (mmHg)	91±15	.0001	84±14
Cardiac index (l/m/m²/)	3.13±1.2	ns	2.97±0.9
Exercise duration (sec)	538±252	ns	512±234

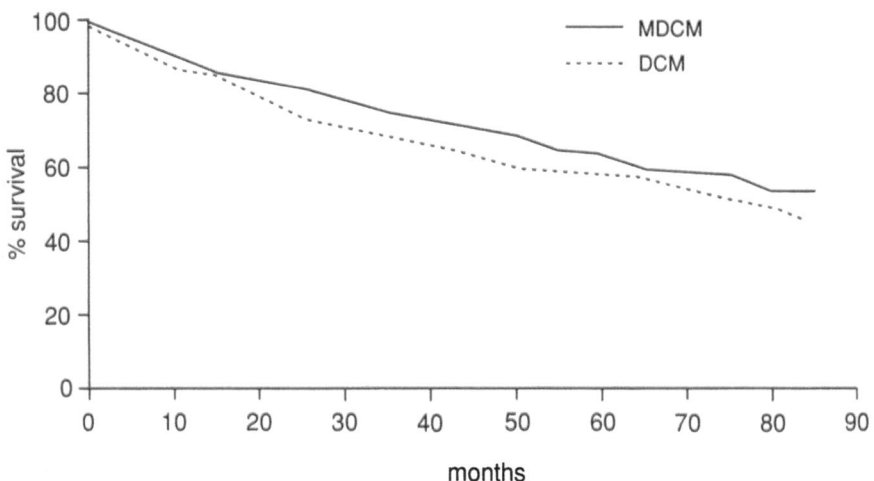

Fig. 1. Seven-year transplant-free survival in typically dilated (DCM) and mildly dilated (MDCM) patients

cantly higher in MDCM group than in DCM (18% vs 4 %, p=0.0001).This higher prevalence was not associated to a higher alcohol consumption or to hemodynamic factors, such as degree of mitral regurgitation or left ventricular end-diastolic filling pressure.

A similar number of patients were treated with ACE-inhibitors, beta-blockers and amiodarone, but more DCM patients received digoxin, furosemide and anticoagulants.

Seven-year transplant-free survival was not significantly different between the two groups, with an annual mortality rate of approximately 6% (Fig.1).

Sixty-eight patients (40%) in the MDCM group and eighty-seven (48%)

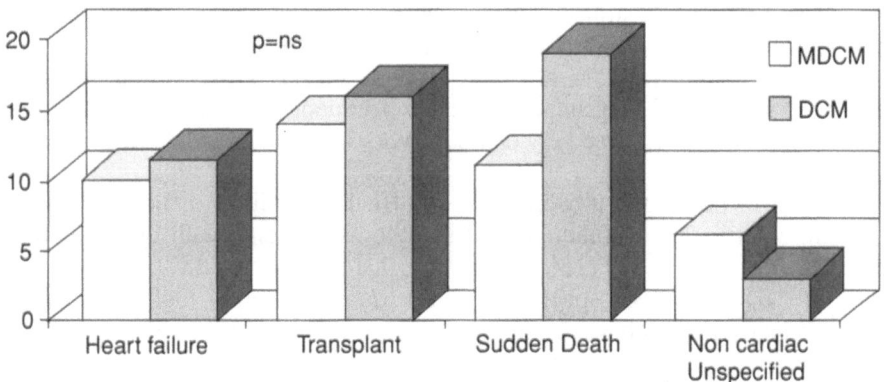

Fig. 2. The rate of negative outcomes in DCM and MCM patients at a mean follow-up of 53 ± 32 months

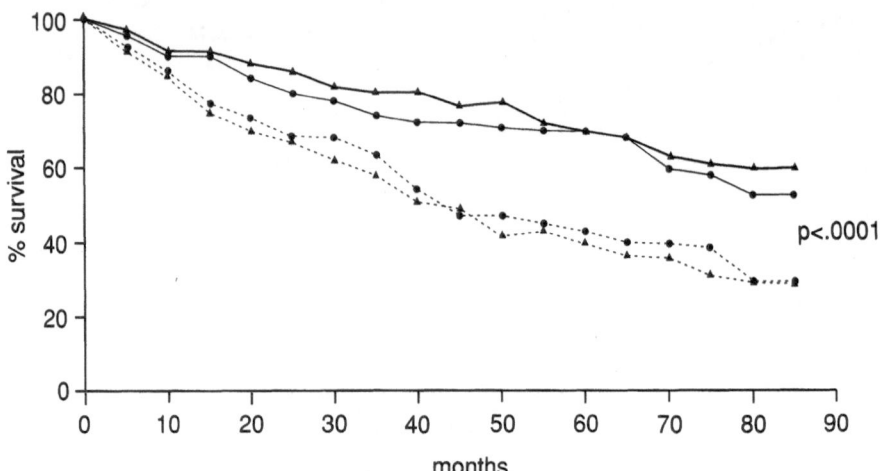

Fig. 3. Survival in MDCM (*triangles*) and DCM (*circles*) patients according to the severity of baseline ventricular dysfunction and symptoms. *Dotted lines*: ejection fraction < 0.30 and NYHA III-IV; *Continuous lines*: ejection fraction > 0.29 and NYHA I-II

in the DCM group died or were transplanted during follow-up. The rate of negative outcomes did not differ significantly between the two groups (Fig.2).

To better define the prognostic role of ventricular dilatation over time, we evaluated the outcome according to the evolution of left ventricular chamber size at a mean follow-up of about two years. This time interval from enrollment, at which survival rate in the entire population was almost 90%, was chosen to avoid a selection bias towards inclusion in the analysis of late survivors only.

In the MDCM group, 16 (13%) out of 120 patients who underwent the scheduled follow-up vs 11 (8%) out of 142 in DCM group showed a progressive enlargement of the left ventricle, defined as an increase greater than 10% from baseline end-diastolic diameter. Progressive dilatation over follow-up was significantly more frequent among MDCM patients with an unfavorable outcome than in survivors (26% vs 7%, p=0.001). This finding was not observed in the DCM group, where the frequency of further ventricular enlargement did not differ between survivors and dead/transplanted patients (5% vs 12%, p=ns).

Patients in both groups were then stratified according to the severity of baseline ventricular dysfunction and symptoms. Patients with ejection fraction less than 0.30 and NYHA class III-IV, that represented 38% of DCM and 25% of MDCM cases respectively, showed a significantly higher mortality, independently from left ventricular dimension at baseline (Fig.3). The excess of mortality in MDCM group was not associated to a significant progression to dilatation, which occurred in only 12% of cases during long-term follow-up.

Discussion

Left ventricular enlargement has classically been considered the chief morphological feature of dilated cardiomyopathy [13]. More recently, several studies have shown that idiopathic left ventricular systolic dysfunction can be dissociated from a significant degree of dilatation, even in the late course of the disease and in the absence of a restrictive hemodynamic profile [2,8,9]. Why left ventricular size can vary widely among patients with idiopathic impairment of contractility is unclear, even if there is some evidence that alterations in myocyte ultrastructure, as a higher degree of myofibrillar loss, could determine the extent of remodeling [7].

Moreover, the clinical aspects of the cardiomyopathies with reduced contractility and minimal dilatation have been insufficiently characterized and, for that reason, in the recent report of the WHO/ISFC Task Force these forms were defined as unclassified [1].

One of the main aims of the SPIC Registry was to evaluate the natural history of patients with idiopathic left ventricular systolic dysfunction, which was defined with very strict diagnostic criteria and detected as early as possible in the course of the disease. As left ventricular dilatation was not considered an inclusion criteria, this Registry allows epidemiological, clinical and prognostic information to be obtained on a very large population of patients with depressed contractility, independently of the presence of chamber enlargement. Impressively, patients with minimal or no dilatation represent a substantial amount of the whole population with idiopathic impairment of systolic function. In fact, in this prospective multicenter study, 41% of patients with an ejection fraction ≤0.40 had normal or slightly increased left ventricular end-diastolic dimension at enrollment. We reasoned that this finding might reflect the enrollment of patients in the early stage of the cardiomyopathic process. The baseline clinical and laboratory profile of DCM patients seemed in fact to characterize a group with more severe disease than MDCM: typically dilated patients were more symptomatic, as indicated by a more advanced NYHA functional class, had a higher prevalence of left bundle branch block and greater ejection fraction impairment, and were more frequently treated with digoxin, furosemide and anticoagulants. Although the mean time elapsed from diagnosis to enrollment was similar in the two groups, these clinical differences would suggest that DCM patients might have been evaluated initially in a later phase of the disease. Only atrial fibrillation, a rhythm disturbance possibly expression of long-standing disease, was significantly more frequent in MDCM (18% vs. 4%). This higher prevalence could not be explained on the basis of atrial enlargement, degree of mitral regurgitation, or a restrictive hemodynamic pattern. Although excess alcohol consumption has been related previously to atrial fibrillation [14,15], the daily alcohol intake of MDCM and DCM patients was similar; this is consistent with the data recently published by Prazak et al. who found no difference in the prevalence of atrial fibrillation in patients with alcoholic and non-alcoholic cardiomyopathy [16]. Other unexplained factors may predispose MDCM patients to the atrial arrhythmia. On the other hand, atrioventricular block and ventricular arrhythmias were equally distributed between MDCM and DCM. This finding confirms the absence of correlation between ventricular dilatation and severity of ventricular arrhythmias [17] previously observed by our group, and might justify the similar rate of sudden death observed in the present study in the long-term follow-up of dilated and non-dilated patients.

Long-term outcome data do not however confirm that preserved ventricular size is an indicator of an early cardiomyopathic process in all MDCM cases. In fact in this series, 7-year transplant-free survival for both MDCM and DCM groups was about 60%. The finding is consistent with the recent data reported by several authors [3,6] and indicates that in the last decade the prognosis of patients with idiopathic systolic dysfunction has considerably improved, if compared to older observations [4,18-20]. Ventricular dimensions do not then play a significant prognostic role during long-term follow-up: in fact, the survival curves of MDCM and DCM patients did not diverge over time and the annual rate of death/transplantation was about 6% in both groups. Furthermore, two years after enrollment in the Registry, the tendency to progressive ventricular enlargement was similar in the two groups: an increase in chamber size occurred in 13% of patients with baseline small ventricles and in 8% of typically dilated subjects. Within MDCM group, 10 patients evolved to a typically dilated form during follow-up; from this figure, an indirect estimate of the rate of progression to DCM would then be about 2.5% per year.

Within MDCM group, the negative prognostic value of progressive left ventricular dilatation, previously observed in 2 out of the 12 patients described by Keren et al. [8], was confirmed in our study. In fact, among the 120 patients with baseline small chambers who had a clinical and laboratory assessment after an average of two years, dilatation was significantly more frequent in patients with poor outcome as compared to survivors.

In patients with typically enlarged left ventricles, the prognostic value of severe symptoms and marked depression of ventricular function, either independently or in association, was already focused on by several authors [2,3, 11,21] and is confirmed by our findings. In the present series, even in MDCM patients, the combination of a LVEF <0.30 and NYHA functional class III-IV at baseline, which was observed in one fourth of mildly dilated patients, identified a subgroup with an unfavorable outcome: the 46% mortality/transplantation rate at 7-year follow-up is double when compared to MDCM patients with LVEF < 0.30 and NYHA class I-II. However, this negative prognosis seems not to be related to progressive dilatation over time, as 88% of MDCM patients with poor ventricular function and severe symptoms did not change left ventricular dimensions during their entire follow-up. Therefore an idiopathic cardiomyopathy with severe pump dysfunction, preserved ventricular size and a poor prognosis is not uncommon and deserves appropriate clinical attention from the very beginning of follow-up, despite a normal or mildly dilated left ventricle.

Conclusion

A substantial amount of patients with idiopathic systolic dysfunction can have normal or minimally enlarged left ventricles, when first observed. In the majority of cases, these patients maintain a stable morphological identity over time, with no tendency to overt dilatation. On the other hand, some typically dilated forms may represent the evolution of an initially mildly dilated cardiomyopathy, which was detected later in its clinical course. The objective difficulty to observe the true initial phase of the disease limits our possibility to clarify this doubt. More efforts must be addressed to understand the pathophysiological mechanisms which underlie such a different morphological ventricular response to the idiopathic impairment of contractility.

The lesson we can learn from the data of this large prospective Registry is that, from a clinical and prognostic standpoint, MDCM must not be considered an entity dissociated from the classical form of DCM.

Centres partecipantig to the SPIC
Studio Policentrico Italiano Cardiomiopatie

Milano: Ospedale Niguarda Ca' Granda, Dipartimento di Cardiologia "A. De Gasperis" Claudio De Vita, Antonella Moreo, Maurizio Ferratini, Antonio Pezzano, Fabio Recalcati, Edgardo Bonacina; **Firenze:** Ospedale Careggi, Servizio di Cardiologia San Luca : Alberto Dolara, Mauro Ciaccheri, Gabriele Castelli, Vito Troiani, Franca Gori, Maurizio Nannini; **Milano:** Ospedale San Carlo, Divisione di Cardiologia: Franco Casazza, Angela Capozzi, Roberto Mattioli; **Pisa:** Servizio di Cardiostimolazione, Istituto di Fisiologia Clinica del C.N.R.: Andrea Biagini, Oberdan Parodi, Marco Baratto, Danilo Neglia, Gualtiero Pelosi, Annalisa Tongiani, Fabio Vernazza; **Pavia:** I.R.C.C.S. Policlinico San Matteo, Divisione di Cardiologia: Antonello Gavazzi, Carlo Campana, Marina Ponzetta, Eloisa Arbustini, Carlo Montemartini; **Trieste:** Ospedale Maggiore, Divisione di Cardiologia: Fulvio Camerini, Andrea Di Lenarda, Gerardina Lardieri, Luisa Mestroni, Bruno Pinamonti, Andrea Perkan, Furio Silvestri, Gianfranco Sinagra, Massimo Zecchin, Dario Gregori, Elena Bernobich, Fulvia Longaro, Luca Salvatore; **Varese:** Ospedale di Circolo, Divisione di Cardiologia: Giovanni Binaghi, Sergio Repetto, Marcella Luvini; **Monza:** Ospedale San Gerardo, Divisione e Servizio di Cardiologia: Franco Valagussa, Alessandro Bozzano, Antonio Cadel, Bruno Pria; **Milano:** Istituto Villa Marelli, Servizio di Cardiologia: Aldo Sachero, Erminia Giagnoni, Luciano Beretta; **Napoli:** Ospedale Monaldi, Ia Divisione di Medicina: Massimo Cafiero, Massimo Borgia, Franco Costantino, Attilio De Santis, Raffaele D'Oriano; **Vicenza:** Ospedale Civile, Divisione di Cardiologia: Mario Vincenzi, Luigi La Vecchia; **Treviso:** Presidio Ospedaliero Multizonale, Divisione di Cardiologia: Paolo Stritoni, Giuliano Renosto, Agnese Moro; **Roma:** Ospedale San Camillo, Divisione di Cardiologia: Pierluigi Prati, Elisabetta Zachara; **Cagliari:** Ospedale San Michele, Divisione di Cardiologia: Antonio Sanna, Maurizio Porcu, Francesco Uras, Stefano Salis.
Scientific Committee: Giorgio Baroldi, Istituto Fisiologia Clinica del CNR, Sezione di Milano; Fulvio Camerini, Ospedali Riuniti, Divisione di Cardiologia, Trieste; Claudio De Vita, Ospedale Niguarda Cà Granda, Dipartimento di Cardiologia "A. De Gasperis", Milano.
Scientific Secretariat: Renata De Maria, Istituto Fisiologia Clinica del CNR, Sezione di Milano, Antonello Gavazzi Divisione di Cardiologia, Policlinico San Matteo, Pavia.
Statistical Analysis: Marina Parolini, Istituto Fisiologia Clinica del CNR, Sezione di Milano.

References

1. Report of the 1995 World Health Organization /International Society and Federation of Cardiology Task Force on the definition and classification of cardiomyopathies (1996) Circulation 93:841-842

2. Gavazzi A, De Maria R, Porcu, Beretta L, Casazza F, Castelli G, Luvini M, Parodi O, Recalcati F, Renosto G, Sinagra G, De Vita C, Camerini F, Baroldi G (1995) Cardiomiopatia dilatativa: una nuova storia naturale? L'esperienza dello Studio Italiano Policentrico Cardiomiopatie (SPIC). G Ital Cardiol 25:1109-1125
3. Komajda M, Jaist JP, Reeves F, Goldfarb B, Bouthour JB, Juillieres Y, Lanfranchi J, Peycelon P, Geslin PH, Carriett D, Grosgogeat Y (1990) Factors predicting mortality in idiopathic dilated cardiomyopaty. Eur Heart J 11:824-831
4. Diaz RA, Obasohan A, Oakley CM (1987) Prediction of outcome in dilated cardiomyopathy. Br Heart J 58:393-399
5. Gavazzi A, Lanzarini L, Cornalba C, Desperati M, Raisaro A, Angoli L, De Servi S, Specchia G (1984) Dilated (congestive) cardiomyopathy. Follow-up study of 137 patients. G Ital Cardiol 11: 492-498
6. Di Lenarda A, Secoli G, Perkan A, Gregori D, Lardieri G, Pinamonti B, Sinagra G, Zecchin M, Camerini F and the Heart Muscle Disease Study Group (1994) Changing mortality in dilated cardiomyopathy. Br Heart J 72 [Suppl]: S46-S51
7. Keren A, Billingham ME, Weintraub D, Stinson EB, Popp RL (1985) Mildly dilated congestive cardiomyopathy. Circulation 72:302-309
8. Keren A, Gottlieb S, Tzivoni D, Yarom R, Billingham ME, Popp RL (1990) Mildly dilated congestive cardiomyopathy. Use of prospective diagnostic criteria and description of the clinical course without heart transplantation. Circulation 81:506-517
9. Gavazzi A, De Maria R, Renosto G, Moro A, Borgia M, Caroli A, Castelli G, Ciaccheri M, Pavan D, De Vita C, Baroldi G, Camerini F (1993) on behalf of the SPIC Group: The spectrum of left ventricular size in dilated cardiomyopathy: clinical correlates and prognostic implications. Am Heart J 125:410-422
10. Sahn DJ, De Maria AN, Kisslo J, Weyman A, (1976) The committee on M-mode standardization of the American Society of Echocardiography: Recommendations regarding quantitation in M-mode echocardiography. Results of a survey of echocardiographic measurements. Circulation 58:1072-1083
11. Aretz HT, Billingham ME, Edwards WD, Factor SM, Fallon JT, Fenoglio JJ Jr, Olsen EGJ, Schoen FJ (1986) Myocarditis: a histopathologic definition and classification. Am J Cardiovasc Pathol 1:3-14
12. Hinkle L, Thaler J (1982) Clinical classification of cardiac deaths. Circulation 65: 457-464
13. Dec GW, Fuster V (1994) Idiopathic dilated cardiomyopathy. N Engl J Med 23:1564-1575
14. Regan TJ (1990) Alcohol and the cardiovascular system. JAMA 264:377-38
15. Urbano-Marquez A, Estruch R, Navarro-Lopez F, Grau JM, Mont L, Rubin E (1989) The effects of alcoholism on skeletal and cardiac muscle. N Engl J Med 320:409-415
16. Prazak P, Pfisterer M, Osswald S, Buser P, Burkart F (1996) Differences of disease progression in congestive heart failure due to alcoholic as compared to idiopathic dilated cardiomyopathy. Eur Heart J 17:251-257
17. De Maria R, Gavazzi A, Caroli A, Ometto R, Biagini A, Camerini F (1992) Ventricular arrhythmias in dilated cardiomyopathy as an independent prognostic hallmark. Am J Cardiol 69:1451-1457
18. Roberts WC, Siegel RJ, McManus BM (1987) Idiopathic dilated cardiomyopathy: analysis of 152 necropsy patients. Am J Cardiol 60:1340-1355
19. Fuster V, Gersh BJ Giuliani ER, Tajik AJ, Brandenburg RO, Frye RL (1981) The natural history of idiopathic dilated cardiomyopathy. Am J Cardiol 47:525-531
20. Ikram H, Williamson HG, Won IG, Wells EJ (1987) The course of idiopathic dilated cardiomyopathy in New Zealand. Br Heart J 57:521-517
21. Hofmann T, Meinertz T, Kasper W, Geibel A, Zehender M, Hohnloser S, Stienen U, Treese N, Just H (1988) Mode of death in idiopathic dilated cardiomyopathy: a multivariate analysis of prognostic determinants. Am Heart J 116:1455-146

DILATED CARDIOMYOPATHY
Treatment

Immunosuppressive Treatment for Inflammatory Dilated Cardiomyopathy (Myocarditis)

B. Maisch, G. Hufnagel, S. Pankuweit, M. Herzum, U. Schönian,
C. Bethge, I. Portig and A. Wilke

Introduction

Controversy still exists on whether immusuppressive treatment is beneficial in myocarditis. This contribution examines the immunologic rationale for immunosuppressive therapy in inflammatory dilated cardiomyopathy by revisiting currently available data in man and experimental animals.

Recently the WHO/ISFC task force has reclassified dilated cardiomyopathy [1]. Within this new definition dilated cardiomyopathies also include viral heart disease, autoreactive myocarditis and active or chronic inflammatory processes of the heart. The diagnostic matrix of Fig. 1 outlines this new concept with respect to inflammatory and dilated heart muscle diseases.

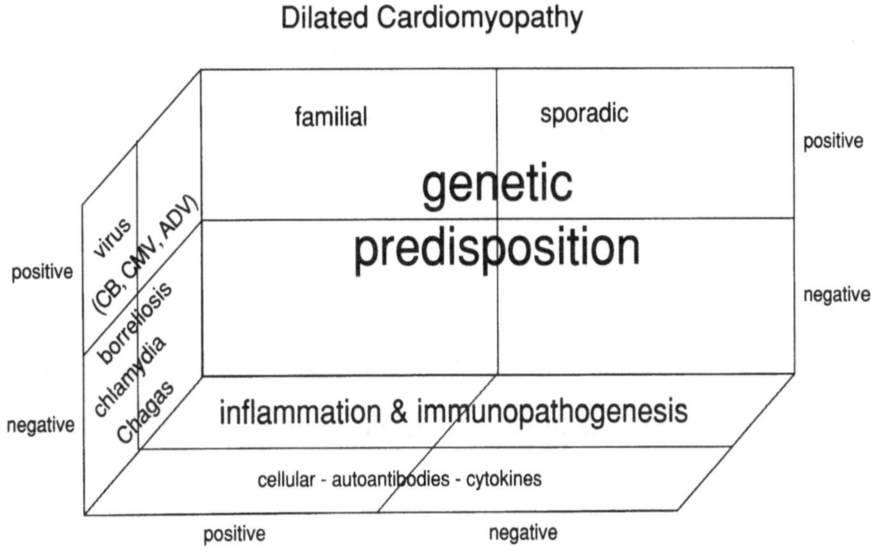

Fig. 1. Diagnostic matrix for primary and secondary heart muscle diseases. Myocarditis and inflammatory heart disease is but one facet of DCM

Clinical Diagnosis of Myocarditis

Historically the standards that have been used to diagnose inflammatory diseases of the myocardium and pericardium were cardiac symptoms, clinical observation and an allegedly typical electrocardiogram [2]. These criteria may be diagnostic in the course of a viral endemic also causing myocarditis, but are otherwise of low specificity for sporadic inflammatory heart muscle disease.

Recently other, more specific criteria have been proposed. Pericardial effusion and segmental wall motion abnormalities at time motion and two-dimensional echocardiography are specific noninvasive signs of a myocardial inflammatory process, particularly when coronary artery disease has been ruled out by coronary angiography [3].

Moreover in patients with pericardial effusion who undergo pericardiocentesis, pericardioscopically-guided epicardial biopsy may demonstrate a myocardial infiltrate with myocytolysis and edema [4]. There is some evidence that the sampling error by optically-guided epicardial biopsy is smaller than by the blinded endomyocardial biopsy [5].

Histopathological Diagnosis of Myocarditis

Controversy in the histopathological diagnosis of myocarditis has centered on the definition of inflammatory infiltrate and on whether light microscopy is the best diagnostic tool. The Dallas classification [6] has attempted to standardize diagnostic criteria, yet the diagnosis of inflammatory heart muscle disease retains a subjective component [7] and interobserver variability, even adopting Dallas criteria, remains high [8] due to various factors. Confusion may arise from misdiagnosed capillaries and myocyte interstial cells with conventional stainings. Endemic variability may also account for the differences in the frequency of myocarditis, which ranges from less than 1% to almost 100% in acutely dilated heart muscle disease.

The incidence of histologically ascertained active myocarditis barely reached 10% of patients screened because of suspected myocarditis in the American Myocarditis Trial [9,10]. Following the same histologic criteria of a lymphocytic infiltrate >5 cells per high power field, myocytolysis being not obligatory, only 1.6% of our patients [11,12], who underwent endomyocardial biopsy because of cardiac pain associated to segmental wall motion abnormalities or dilatation, received a diagnosis of histologic myocarditis or perimyocarditis (Table 1).

Conventional light microscopic evaluation of endomyocardial biopsies may then be a rather unsensitive tool to detect myocarditis. Using different histologic criteria of an inflammatory infiltrate [13,14], which had to include 14 or more cells/mm^2, and with the addition to conventional hematoxylin-eosin staining of monoclonal antibodies for leukocyte subsets on cryostat sections of myocardium, the European Study of Epidemiology and Treatment of Cardiac Inflammatory Disease (ESETCID) [14] reported focal

Table 1. Incidence (percent) diagnosis of heart muscle diseases in an endomyocardial biopsy series of 1250 patients and incidence of infiltrates (more than 5 lymphocytes per high power field) in these subgroups (from the Würzburg multicentre study; [11] and [12]

Clinical diagnosis	n° pts	incidence of diagnosis in total patient cohort	incidence of infiltrate in the subgroup analyzed
Myocarditis	20	1.6	100
Perimyocarditis	20	1.6	20
Status post myocarditis	22	1.76	0
Status post perimyocarditis	15	1.2	0
Postmyocarditic cardiomegaly	28	2.24	0
Dilated cardiomyopathy	50	4	0
Dilated cardiomyopathy with increased alcohol intake	20	1.6	10
Non-cardiac controls	17	0	0
Coronary artery disease	100	0	0

infiltrates in 24% out of 700 screened patients. Remarkably however only 27% of cases with focal infiltrates met the inclusion criterion of an ejection fraction below 45%.

From our registry of 4300 biopsied patients (Maisch, unpublished findings) the overall incidence of focal infiltrate > 14 cells/mm^2 is 1.25%, when the biopsy is assessed by light microscopy alone. With the addition of immunohistochemistry 19% of patients, who presented whith cardiac dilatation manifested within the last 6 months and the clinical suspicion of myocarditis, showed a focal or diffuse infiltrate, which met the Dallas definition of focal healing or borderline myocarditis. As myocytolysis was not compulsory, we have termed this infiltrate chronic myocarditis.

Therefore immunohistochemistry carried out on endomyocardial biopsies, with the use of monoclonal antibodies to leukocyte and lymphocite subsets, improves the sensitivity and specificity of the classic histological diagnosis [12, 15].

Further information on myocyte, non-myocyte [16, 17] and endothelial activation [18, 19] in inflamed tissue might come from the analysis of major histocompatibility complex (MHC) class I and II expression.

Assessment of Etiology of Myocarditis

Whereas serological evidence of infection with cardiotropic viruses does not prove that the infective agent itself is present in cardiac tissue, molecular biology and immunology techniques have enabled us to demonstrate the presence and persistence of enteroviral genome [20-24] or cytomegalovirus DNA in the myocardium [25] and particularly in the myocytes themselves [26, 27], in 20%-50% of patients with active myocarditis and dilated

Table 2. Demonstration of viral DNA and RNA by in situ hybridization, dot blot and PCR in myocardial tissue

Reference	Virus	Technique	% positive
Myocarditis			
Bowles et al 1986 [20]	enteroviruses	Northern blot	50
Jin et al 1990 [28]	enteroviruses	PCR	33
Kandolf et al 1985 [46]	enteroviruses	in situ hybridization	20-25
Sole (personal communication) Billingham group	enteroviruses	PCR	<10
Maisch & Wendl 1989 [25]	cytomegalovirus(in myoc)	in situ hybridization	20
Schönian et al 1991 [26]	cytomegalovirus	PCR/in situ hybridization	10
Giacca et al 1994 [30]	enterovirus	PCR	33
Schönian et al 1996	cytomegalovirus	PCR (2nd series 1992-96)	<6
Martin et al 1994 [31]	enteroviruses	PCR	23
	adenovirus	PCR	44
Dilated cardiomyopathy			
Jin et al 1990 [28]	enteroviruses	PCR	7
Kandolf et al 1985 [46]	enteroviruses	in situ hybridization	ca 20
Grasso et al 1992 [29]	enteroviruses	PCR	0
Schönian & Maisch 1993 [27]	cytomegalovirus	in situ hybridization	15
Giacca et al 1994 [30]	enteroviruses	PCR	7
Schönian et al 1997	cytomegalovirus	PCR (2nd series 1993-96)	5

cardiomyopathy (Table 2) although this prevalence may have been oversti-mated according to others [28-30]. Adenovirus was demonstrated by the polymerase chain reaction (PCR) even more frequently in children with myocarditis [31]. More than one viral genome may be found at the same time in the myocardium.

Whether the presence of viral genome bears pathogenetic impact remains, however, unsolved: viral persistence may only be a marker of former infec-tion or represent a defective mutant with an incomplete cycle of viral repli-cation. This has a direct clinical influence on therapeutic choices: antiviral therapy is useful only if an *active* virus is still present; conversely, immu-nosuppression may be hazardous if there is still a replicating virus in the myocardium. In experimental models of murine myocarditis or in isolated infected murine heart cells, virus has a direct lytic effect [32-34]. Whether after the first viral damage it is still the replicating virus rather than auto-reactive mechanisms that determine progression to deterioration and myocardial disease, preventing resolution of the infective process and the development of protective immunity is however uncertain.

Assessment of Immunopathogenesis of Myocarditis, a Prerequisite of Immunosuppressive Therapy

Immunohistochemical studies of a large number of endomyocardial biopsies [12] have demonstrated that, while immunoglobulin fixation of IgG isotype is present in various diseases, including myocarditis, dilated cardiomyopathy, and even in some patients with coronary artery disease and in few controls, IgM-binding and complement fixation indicate an ongoing autoreactive process.

In 1982 we first demonstrated in human myocarditis a cytolytic, complement-depending antibody that lysed isolated rat myocytes in vitro [35]. Further experiments demonstrated that, in coxsackie B myocarditis, this antibody and its cytolytic activity could be absorbed out with enteroviral proteins, thus clearly establishing that antigenic mimicry was one principle of autoimmune processes in the heart. Just recently we were able to define the proteins responsible for coxsackievirus-associated autoantibodies more clearly by Western Blot experiments [36]. Similar evidence could be compiled for influenza myocarditis [35].

Inflammatory heart muscle disease may elicit in man a polyclonal humoral immune response directed towards many cardiac structures: the adenine nucleotide translocator [37], the calcium channel [38], the beta-receptor [39, 40], myosin heavy chain, proteins from the extracellular matrix including laminin and collagen, the cardiac conduction system [41, 42] and the vascular endothelium have all been identified as targets of an antibody response. Moreover, immune complex depositions and increased class I, class II receptor expression [17], increased neopterin plasma levels [43] are evidence for an autoreactive or immunologic process. This evidence is important for the decision making in the therapy of myocarditis and/or dilated cardiomyopathy, since persistence of autoreactivity in the myocardium indicates an inflammatory process that may be treatable by immunosuppression.

Lessons for Treatment from Animal Models of Myocarditis

In experimental myocarditis most often models of murine coxsackie B3 (CVB3) myocarditis (Nancy strain) or derivatives, including different strains such as Balb/c mice, A/J mice, DBA 2 and NMRI mice, have been used [32, 44-47]. Another model uses the encephalomyocarditis (EMC) virus, which is not pathogenetic in humans [48-50]. In Balb/c mice inoculated with CVB3 virus [51, 52], cardiac inflammation was shown to be dependent upon functional T lymphocytes. Depletion studies and in vitro assays revealed at least two different effector T lymphocyte populations which mediates myocytolysis: a MHC class II restricted T cell that recognizes viral proteins expressed on infected cells, and a MHC class I restricted T cell, which reacts to a so far unknown structure on uninfected myocytes [53, 54]. Analysis of the T cell receptor $V\alpha$ genes using PCR products showed that infiltrating T cells express a restricted V gene repertoire, an indication that T lymphocytes recognize a specific antigen or antigens in the hearts of CVB3-infected mice [55]. Thus, attracted by the enhanced expression of intercellular adhesion molecule-1, which is stimulated by interferon and tumor necrosis factor (TNF-α) after virus inoculation, killer T cells infiltrate the myocardium, recognize specific antigens on cardiac cells and kill the cells by releasing the cytolytic factor perforin [56-58].

Although TNF-α has an antiviral effect in vitro, exogenous administration promotes viral spread in the myocardium, thus aggravating cardiac inflammation and necrosis in EMC-induced myocarditis; in contrast, antibodies to TNF-α given prior to virus inoculation, decrease disease severity [58].

Conflicting results have been published on the effects of exogenous interleukin-2 (IL2) in CVB3-induced murine myocarditis: early in the course of infection, both deterioration [59] and beneficial effects [60] were reported. When given late, starting from 7 days after viral inoculation, IL-2 increased the number of T-lymphocytes in the heart, exacerbating disease severity. Interleukins are also involved in the greater susceptibility to CVB3-virus of males and testosterone-treated female mice [61-63].

Several studies analysed the effects of immunosuppressive agents in various murine myocarditis models. In the EMC murine model [48, 49], steroids increased mortality, with respect to infected untreated control mice, when administered early, but had no effect when administered after 14 days, when substantial neutralizing antibodies to the virus could be measured. In the early phase of murine CVB3 myocarditis, steroids increased the severity of cardiac damage and lethality [64]. Prednisone given at the dose of 0.33 mg and 15 mg/Kg body weight did not reduce the amount of inflammation and necrosis in CVB3-infected Balb/c mice [34]. The immune response in Balb/c mice, in contrast to humans, is based principally on T-cells. In A/J mice, that have a balanced B- and T-cell immune response, a dose-dependent decrease in cardiac inflammation and necrosis, that ranged up to 90% in comparison to untreated mice, was observed. In DBA/2 mice with a predominantly humoral immune response, inflammatory lesions were reduced by 30% at day 7. In this group the amount of replicating virus did not increase, probably because prednisone does not greatly interfere with specific IgM production, or with natural killer activity. However corticosteroid treatment may prolong persistance of a replicating virus in the myocardium [65].

Cyclosporin A, a fungal metabolite with immunosuppressive properties, blocks IL-2 release from activated T-helper lymphocytes and the release of gamma-interferon by activated T-cells. The expression of the IL2-receptor and the responsiveness of activated T-cells to lymphokines are not altered, however. Cyclosporin may spare the activation of T suppressor cells in vitro and in vivo; in animal models, like azathioprine, it does not erase presensitization of lymphocytes [66]. In murine EMC virus myocarditis, early administration of cyclosporin 25 mg/kg/day increased mortality significantly, while later administration had no mortality effect with a tendency to deterioration. Balb/c, A/J and DBA/2 mice [32] treated early with cyclosporin A demonstrated increased necrosis, although leukocyte infiltrate was reduced to some extent; virus titres in the heart were not changed in any strain by the drug. This corresponds well with experimental data from O'Connell et al [67].

Evolution of Untreated Human Myocarditis: Spontaneous Improvement Also Plays a Role

Spontaneous improvement in clinically suspected viral myocarditis is remarkable [1,2]. Table 3 summarizes results obtained in biopsied and non-

Table 3. Spontaneous improvement in myocarditis (adapted from [71])

Reference	n° pts	improved	no change	deteriorated	follow-up
Helin 1986	12(CVB)	12	0	0	7 months
Bengtsson 1966	90	53	23	14	5 years
Gerzen 1972	18	8	5	5	12 months
Giesecke 1987	45	38	2	5(but alive)	3 months
Sainani 1975	19(CVB)	13	6	0	3 months
Edwards 1982	5	3	1	1	6-12 months
Fenoglio 87	18	7	8	3	12 months
Dec 1985	18	6	10	2	6-12 months
Anderson 1987	10	3	5	2	6-12 months
Maisch 1991	85	53	18	14(10 dead)	4,5 years
Maisch 1994	21	3	12	6	6 months
Mason 1995[a]	47	25	14	8	6-12 months
Total	388	224(58%)	104(22%)	60(15%)	3-60 months

[a] according to an oral presentation at the 3rd International Symposium on the Diagnosis and Treatment in Inflammatory and Dilated Heart Muscle Diseases, Berlin 1994.
CVB, coxsackie B virus.

biopsied patients treated with standard therapy and restricted physical activity alone: 58% of patients showed spontaneous improvement. In biopsied series, spontaneous improvement ranged from 14% in our own controlled study to 53% in the Myocarditis Treatment Trial; when improved and unchanged patients are considered togheter, patients who did not deteriorate ranged from 72% in ours to 83% in the Myocarditis Treatment Trial cohort [10].

Immunomodulating and Immunosuppressive Drugs in the Treatment of Inflammatory Cardiomyopathy in Man

With the above data in mind, we will revisit the principles of immunosuppression with respect to clinical studies (Fig. 2).

Recent reports suggest that in vivo corticosteroids reverse episodes of rejection after heart transplantation by indirectly blockade of the IL-1 dependent production of IL-2 from activated T cells, since they prevent IL-1 release from monocytes and monocyte chemotaxis [66]. In suspected viral myocarditis, small non-randomized trials or case-reports have demonstrated that application of corticosteroids may be useful. Benefit was shown in eight patients with influenza myocarditis (Table 4), in whom spontaneous improvement was not investigated. In human enteroviral myocarditis treated with immunosuppressives, lethal cases have been described (Table 5), but no control groups are available. Among the few cases from our older series, who had been treated with prednisone and azathioprine, and in whom PCR in the endomyocardial biopsy was retrospectively carried out,

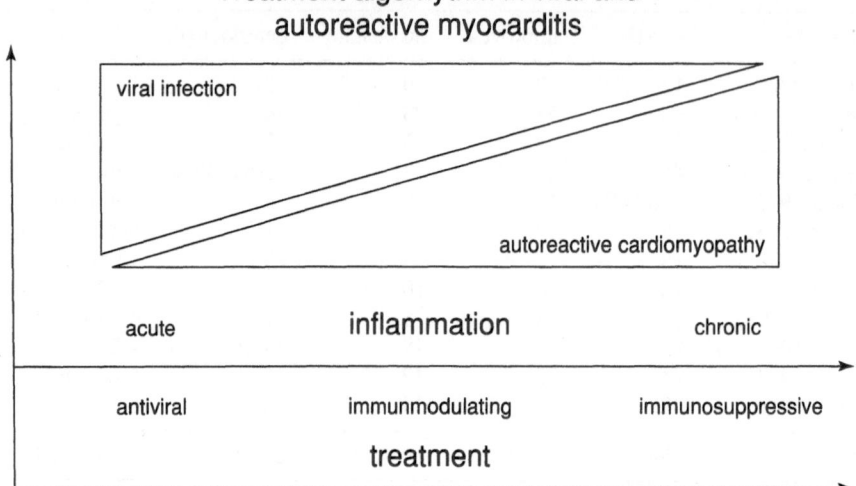

Fig. 2. Proposed scheme for the different indications of treatment in myocarditis. In the initial viral phase antiviral treatment may be beneficial, whereas immunosuppressive therapy is contraindicated. In the intermediate phase we advocate (hyper)immunoglobulin treatment, in the virus-negative late phase with autoreactive mechanisms predominating (chronic myocarditis) immunosuppressive treatment may still maintain its still unproven role

Table 4. Immunosuppressive treatment in Influenza myocarditis (from [71])

Reference	Age	Sex	Virus subtypes	Treatment	Outcome
Ainger 1965	3	m	A2	Prednisolone	improved
(n = 8)	0.5	m	A2	Prednisolone	improved
	1.5	m	A	Prednisolone	improved
	3.5	m	A	Prednisolone	improved
	4	f	B	Prednisone	improved
	2	f	B	Prednisolone	improved
	2,5	f	B	M-Prednisolone	improved

Table 5. Immunosuppressive treatment in enterovirus-positive myocarditis. Overview of published data (from [71])

Reference	Age	Sex	Virus	Treatment	Outcome
Sanyai 1965	13	f	CVB4	Prednisone	died
Glacjchen 1953	24	f	CVB1	Prednisone	deteriorated
Sutinen 1971	15	f	CVB3	Prednisone	died
Maisch 1995	21,32,44,45	f,f,m,m	CVB3(2); CBV4(2)	Prednisone + Azathioprin	3 improved, 1 unchanged

CVB, coxsackie B virus.

deterioration was not observed in those patients with a more chronic infiltrate. In an uncontrolled study, Mason et al. [68] reported the decrease of the inflammatory infiltrate by a regimen of prednisone and azathioprine. In another uncontrolled study Schultheiss et al. [11] and Kuhl and Schultheiss [69] demonstrated hemodynamic and clinical benefit with immunosuppression in patients with dilated heart muscle disease and an infiltrate who had not responded to conventional treatment.

In our own controlled study of patients with autoreactive myocarditis [70], where cases with cytomegalovirus-DNA or enteroviral-RNA persistence at PCR, or changes in the microneutralisation titres of enteroviruses were excluded, we could demonstrate in 15 patients on azathioprine plus prednisone therapy, a clear reduction of IgG and complement binding in the biopsy (95% in conventional vs 26% in immunosuppressive treatment group, $p < 0.05$) and an improvement of the hemodynamic status (15% vs 57%, $p < 0.05$). Lymphocyte infiltrates were reduced in both groups in the second biopsy, but more so in the active treatment group. Table 6 shows all trials with immunosuppressive treatment, with or without controls: improvement was shown in 61% of patients, no change or deterioration in 39%.

The Myocarditis Treatment Trial [10] and the ongoing ESETCID trial [71] are the only double blind randomized trials on immunosuppressive therapy, for acute and chronic or subacute myocarditis respectively, which

Table 6. Meta-analysis of immunosuppressive treatment in myocarditis: azathioprin (A) and prednisone (P) or cyclosporin A (CyA) (adapted from [71])

Reference	n	treatment	improved(%)	unchanged/ deteriorated %	controls
Mason 1980	8	P+(A+P)	4(50%)	4(50%)	no
Sekiguchi 1980	3	P	2(67%)	1(33%)	no
Edwards 1982	5	P	3(60%)	2(40%)	yes
Fenoglio 1983	18	P, A+P	7(39%)	11(61%)	yes
Hess 1983	6	A+P+ATG	6(100%)	0(0%)	no
Zee-Cheng 1984	8	A+P+(ATG)	5(62,5%)	3(37.5%)	no
Daly 1984	1	P(A+P)	0(0%)	1(100%)	no
Vignola 1984	6	A+P	5(83%)	1(17%)	no
Fenely 1984	2	A+P	2(100%)	0(0%)	no
Dec 1985	9	A+P	4(44%)	5(56%)	yes
Mortensen 1985	12	A+P, Cy A	8(67%)	4(33%)	no
Hosenpud 1985	6	A+P	0(0%)	6(100%)	no
Camerini 1991	28	A+P	8(29%)	20(71%)(dead:11(39%)	no
Hobbs 1989	34	A+P,P, Cy A	25(74%)	9(26%)	no
Chan 1990	13	A+P	6(46%)	7(54%)	no
Jones 1991	9	P,A+P,var	4(44%)	5(56%)	no
Ruzyllo 1980	20	A+P	10(50%)	10(50%)	no
Schultheiß 92,93	41	P	32(78%)	9(12%)	no
Maisch 1993	21	A+P	10(47%)	11(53%)	yes
Total	250	A+P,P,Cy A	141(61%)	97(39%)	

Table 7. Placebo-controlled and double blind randomized trials with immunosuppressives in myocarditis: A meta-analysis (modified from [71])

a) Controlled trials

Reference	treatment	Pts Tx/Co	Tx impr	Tx unch/det	co impr	co unch/det
Edwards 1982	P	5/5	3(60%)	2(40%)	3(60%)	2(40%)
Fenoglio 1983	P,A+P	18/4	7(39%)	11(61%)	2(50%)	2(50%)
Dec 1985	A+P	9/18	4(44%)	5(56%)	6(33%)	12(67%)
Anderson 1987	A+P	7/10	2(29%)	4/1(57%/14%)	3(30%)	5/2(50%/20%)
Marboe 1987	A+P;P	16/18	9(56%)	7(44)	7(39%)	8/3(44%/17%)
Maisch 1993/94	A+P	21/21	10(47%)	65(29%/24%)	3(14%)*	12/6(57%/29%)
All controlled Trials	**P,A+P**	**76/76**	**35(46%)**	**41(64%)**	**24(32%)**	**47(78%)**

b) Double-blind-randomized trials

Mason 1995	P+Cy A	64/47	49(76%)	15(24%)	25(53%)	14/8(30%/17%)

c) Metanalysis of all controlled and randomized trials

	P+A/CyA	140/123	84(60%)	56(40%)	49(40%)	69(56%)

Tx, treatment; co, control; impr, improved; det, deteriorated

have been carried out. Controlled, randomized trials show results similar to those of non randomized studies (Table 7).

In the Myocarditis Treatment Trial, immunosuppressive treatment consisted of a combination of cyclosporine A and prednisone, after the azathioprin arm was dropped very early. In the ongoing ESETCID trial, treatment follows 3 arms, under the rationale of a supposedly initial viral infection. In the early phase of virus infection or persistence of viral genome in the heart, as assessed by PCR or in situ hybridization, no immunosuppressives are given. In enteroviral myocarditis, interferon-alpha is part of the treatment protocol. In cytomegalovirus myocarditis, hyperimmunoglobulin treatment is initiated only in virus-negative chronic myocarditis, where the combination of azathioprin and prednisone is started and continued for 6 months.

The Double Blind Randomized Myocarditis Treatment Trial

It is the merit of the Myocarditis Treatment Trial [10] to have analysed the effect of treatment in patients with active myocarditis diagnosed according to Dallas criteria. Only 9.6% of the patients screened under the clinical suspicion of myocarditis met the Dallas criteria for diagnosis. Neither hemodynamic nor prognostic benefit were observed after a 6-month immunosuppressive treatment in 111 patients randomized either to cyclosporine A and prednisone or to placebo. However spontaneous improvement was also very impressive in about one third of patients. These findings were extensively debated [71-76] and many reasons have been proposed for the failure of this trial to demonstrate benefit of immunosuppression.

The *entrance criteria* of myocarditis relied on light microscopy. Today even M. Billingham from the Dallas panel of pathologists concedes that "these criteria have been misrepresented as a classification that is used as a sine qua non of the histological diagnosis of acute myocarditis" [77]. The requirement of necrosis, a finding indispensable for active myocarditis and almost impossible to diagnose in a tiny biopsy, might have excluded patients with chronic forms and autoreactive features, who might have profited most from immunosuppression. Advances in immunohistochemistry, including identification of lymphocyte subpopulations, expression of MHC class antigens, adhesion molecules and immunoglobulin binding to biopsy, have increased specificity and sensitivity. Light microscopy is no longer the only standard.

Other diagnostic tools were inadequate as well. Presence or persistence of viral genome in endomyocardial biopsy samples, which would today exclude patients from immunosuppression based on the experimental results in CVB3 infected animals, were not determined. Relevant immunohistological investigation were missing: only a nonspecific "immunostatus" was carried out. The lack of immunohistochemical assessment in the former therapeutical myocarditis trials leaves us with speculations on the interpretation of the effects of treatment. Was the "reactive group" in the treatment trial by Parrillo et al. [78] truly myocarditis if only two out of their 102 patients demonstrated infiltrating lymphocytes by electron microscopy as previously pointed out [79], or might it be a chronic inflammatory process as subsequenly postulated by the authors when discussing the findings of the Myocarditis Treatment Trial [73]? The conclusion that "a prominent immunologic response may be a benefit rather than a principal cause of the disease" remains questionable.

Trial duration might have been too short: a positive trend with immunosuppression was reported at six month, when treatment was discontinued.

In addition, not all immunosuppressives are alike. Cyclosporin A, that has made rejection after heart transplantation manageable, may be suitable to treat autoreactive forms of myocarditis when a defective T cell suppressor function is present, a finding postulated in human myocarditis by Eckstein et al. [80], but not confirmed by others. In man, our own limited experience of two cases with autoreactive myocarditis treated with corticosteroids and cyclosporin A, gave beneficial results on central hemodynamics and lymphocyte clearance in the follow-up biopsy. From controlled trials, azathioprin and prednisone were suggested to be more beneficial, since myocarditis is not only cellularly-driven, as rejection, but also humorally-mediated. These considerations remain unrefuted by Mason et al [76] in their reply; it was also acknowledged that giant-cell myocarditis is a contraindication to immunosuppression.

The negative results observed in the Myocarditis Treatment Trial might actually depend on the target population chosen [74], i.e. patients with active myocarditis, whereas the most effect by immunosuppressive therapy could be expected in patients with chronic myocarditis, a diagnosis that did not even exist for the interpretation of histological slides in that study. The Myocarditis Treatment Trial also showed, however, that steroid treatment is not detrimental to patients with active myocarditis, and better selection criteria are needed to distinguish patients that might benefit from immunosuppressive treatment from those that may not.

Implications for Immunosuppressive Treatment of Myocarditis in Man

From both human and animal studies it can be speculated that steroids cause little or no harm and that there may even be some benefit with prednisone therapy in selected subgroups of patients; but clearly this speculation is not substantiated by studies and more data are needed.

Some studies hint that benefit in man appears to be restricted to autoreactive chronic forms of myocarditis, when viral persistence is excluded. Without prescreening of patients for viral presence or persistence, or for immunohistochemical signs of autoreactivity, immunosuppressive treatment is not indicated. It is still experimental in man and should, when given, be restricted to autoreactive forms of myocarditis in the context of a randomized clinical trial, preselecting patients with autoreactive forms.

From a practical point of view, apart from clinical trials, it is still too early to advocate the general application of immunosuppressive therapy in myocarditis.

A detailed analysis of other immunosuppressive and immunoregulatory treatment has been presented elsewhere [81].

References

1. WHO/ISFC task force (Richardson P, McKenna W, Bristow M, Maisch B, Mautner B, O`Connel J, Olsen E, Thien G, Goodwin J, Gyarfas I, Martin I, Nordet P) (1996) Report of the 1995 World Health Organization/Inernational Society andFederation of Cardiology Task Force on the Definition and Classification of Cardiomyopathies. Circulation 93:841-842
2. Levine HD (1979) Virus myocarditis: a critique of the literature from clinical, electrocardiographic and pathological stand-points. Am J Med Sci 277:132-143
3. Maisch B, Salzer E, Ertl G, Kochsiek K (1987) Pericardial thickness and pericardial effusion as echocardiographic markers of acute or past pericardial, perimyocardial and myocardial disease. Eur Heart J 8[Suppl J]:109-114
4. Maisch B, Drude L (1991) Pericardioscopy-a new diagnostic tool in inflammatory disease of the pericardium. Eur Heart J 12[Suppl D]:2-6
5. Maisch B, Drude L (1992) Epi- and pericardial biopsy by pericardioscopy. Circulation 82 [Suppl 3]:417 (A1658)
6. Aretz HT, Billingham ME, Edwards WD et al (1986) Myocarditis- a histopathologic definition and classification. Am J Cardiovasc Pathol 1:3-14
7. Doerr W (1956) Morphologie der Myokarditis. Verh Dtsch Ges Inn Med 77:301-335
8. Shanes JG, Gahli J, Billingham ME et al (1987) Interobserver variability in the pathological interpretation of endomyocardial biopsy results. Circulation 75: 401-405

9. Hahn EA, Hartz VL, Moon TE, O'Connel JB, Herskowitz A, McManus BM, Mason JW for the Myocarditis Treatment Trial Investigators (1995) The Myocarditis Treatment Trial: design, methods and patient enrolment Eur Heart j 76 (Suppl):162-167
10. Mason JW, O'Connel JB, Herskowitz A et al (1995) A clinical trial of immunosuppressive therapy for myocarditis. N Engl J Med 333:0269-275
11. Maisch B (1986) Immunologic regulator and effector function in perimyocarditis, postmyocarditic heart muscle disease and dilated cardiomyopathy. Basic Res Cardiol 81[Suppl 1]:217-242
12. Maisch B, Bauer E, Hufnagel G, Pfeifer U, Rohkamm R (1988) The use of endomyocardial biopsy in heart failure. Eur Heart J 9[Suppl H]:59-71
13. Kühl U, Schultheiss H-P (1995) Treatment of chronic myocarditis with corticosteroids. Eur Heart J 16[Suppl O]:168-172
14. Maisch B, Hufnagel G, Schönian U, Hengstenberg C for the ESETCID Investigators (1995) The European Study of Epidemiology and Treatment of Cardiac Inflammatory Disease (ESETCID). Eur Heart J 16 [Suppl O]:173-175
15. Kühl U, Daun B, Seeberg B, Schultheiss H-P, Strauer BE (1992) Dilated Cardiomyopathy - a chronic myocarditis? Immunohistological characterization of lymphocytic infiltrates. Herz 17:97-106
16. Hershkowitz A, Baughman KL, Rose NR et al (1988) Introduction of major histocompatibility (MHC) antigens on myocardial cells in patients with active myocarditis and idiopathic cardiomyopathy. In : Schultheiß HP, ed. New Concepts in Viral Heart Disease. Springer Verlag, Berlin, Heidelberg, New York; pp 93-104
17. Hufnagel G, Maisch B (1991) Expression of MHC class I and II antigens and the IL-2 receptor in rejection, myocarditis and dilated cardiomyopathy. Eur Heart J 12 [Suppl D]:137-140
18. Hengstenberg C, Rose ML, Olsen EGJ, Maisch B (1991) Immune response to the endothelium in myocarditis, dilated cardiomyopathy and rejection after heart transplantation. Eur Heart J 12 [Suppl D]:144-146
19. Maisch B, Weyerer O, Hufnagel G, Hengstenberg C, Schönian U, Haverich A, Kochsiek K (1989) The vascular endothelium as target of humoral autoreactivity in myocarditis and rejection. Z Kardiol 78 [Suppl 6]:95-99
20. Bowles NE, Richardson PJ, Olsen EGJ, Archard LC (1986) Detection of coxsackie-B-virus-specific RNA sequences in myocardial biopsy samples from patients with myocarditis and dilated cardiomyopathy. Lancet I:1120-1123
21. Kandolf R, Hofschneider PH (1984) Effect of interferon on the replication of coxsackie B3 virus in cultured human foetal heart cells. In: Bolte HD (ed) Viral heart disease. Springer, Berlin-Heidelberg-New York pp 57-63
22. Kandolf R, Ameis D, Kirchner P, Canu A, Hofschneider PH (1987) In situ detection of enteroviral genomes in myocardial cells by nucleic acid hybridization: an approach to the diagnosis of viral heart disease. Proc Natl Acad Sci USA 84: 6272-6276
23. Tracy S (1984) A comparison of genomic homologies among the coxsackievirus B group: use of fragments of the cloned coxsackievirus B3 genome as probes. J Gen Virol 65:2167-2172
24. Tracy S, Hufnagel G, Chapman N (1992) Interesting problems in enteroviral inflammatory heart disease. Herz 17:79-84
25. Maisch B, Wendl J (1989) Cytomegalovirus DNA in endomycardial biopsies of patients with (peri)myocarditis. Eur Heart J 9[Suppl]:1000 (abstr)
26. Schönian U, Crombach M, Maisch B (1991) Does CMV infection play a role in myocarditis? New aspects from in-situ hybridization. Eur Heart J 12[Suppl D]: 65-99
27. Schönian U, Crombach M, Maisch B (1993) Assessment of cytomegalovirus DNA and protein expression in patients with myocarditis. Clin Immunol Immunopathol 68:229-233
28. Jin O, Sole MJ, Butany JW, Chia WK, McLaughlin PR, Liu P, Liew CC (1990) Detection of Enterovirus RNA in myocardial biopsies from patients with myocarditis and cardiomyopathy using gene amplification by polymerase chain reaction. Circulation 82:8-16
29. Grasso M, Arbustini E, Silini E, Diegoli M, Percivalle E, Ratti G, Bramerio M, Gavazzi A, Viganò M, Milanesi G (1992) Search for coxsackievirus B3 RNA in idiopathic

dilated cardiomyopathy using gene amplification by polimerase chain reaction. Am J Cardiol 69:658-664

30. Giacca M, Severini GM, Mestroni L, Salvi A, Lardieri G, Falaschi A, Camerini F (1994) Low frequency of detection of enterovirus RNA in endomyocardial tissue of patients with idiopathic dilated cardiomyopathy by nested polymerase chain reaction. J Am Coll Cardiol 24:10-33

31. Martin AB, Webber S, Fricker FJ, Jaffe R, Demmler G, Kearney D, Zhang Y-H, Bodurtha J, Gelb B, Ni J, Bricker T, Towbin JA (1994) Acute Myocarditis - Rapid dignosis by PCR in children. Circulation 90:330-339

32. Herzum M, Huber SA, Weller R, Grebe R, Maisch B (1991) Treatment of experimental murine coxsackie B3 myocarditis. Eur Heart J 12 [Suppl D]:200-201

33. Herzum M, Maisch B (1988) Humoral and cellular immune response in human myocarditis and dilated cardiomyopathy. Pathol Immunopathol Res 7:240-250

34. Herzum M, Ruppert V, Küytz B, Jomaa H, Nakamura I, Maisch B (1994) Coxsackievirus B 3 infection leads to cell death of cardiac myocytes. J Mol Cell Cardiol 26:907-913

35. Maisch B, Trostel-Soeder R, Stechemesser E, Berg PA, Kochsiek K (1982) Diagnostic relevance of humoral and cell-mediated immune reactions in patients with acute viral myocarditis. Clin Exp Immunol 48:533-545

36. Maisch B, Bauer E, Cirsi M, Pankuweit S, Schönian U, Kochsiek K (1993) Cytolytic cross-reactive antibodies directed against the cardiac membrane and viral protein in coxsackie virus B3 and B4 myocarditis-characterization and pathogenetic relevance. Circulation 87[Suppl IV]: IV-49 - IV-65

37. Schultheiss H-P (1989) The significance of autoantibodies against the ADP/ATP carrier for the pathogenesis of myocarditis and dilated cardiomyopathy-clinical and experimental data. Springer Semin Immunopathol 11:15-30

38. Kühl U, Melzner B, Schäfer B, Schultheiss HP, Strauer BE (1991) The Ca-channel as cardiac autoantigen. Eur Heart J 12(Suppl D) 99-104

39. Limas CJ, Limas C (1991) Beta-adrenoceptor antibodies and genetics in dilated cardiomyopathy-an overview and review. Eur Heart J 12[Suppl D]: 175-177

40. Wallukat G, Morwinski M, Kowal K, Förster A, Boewer V, Wollenberg A (1992) Autoantibodies against the ß-adrenergic receptor in human myocarditis and dilated cardiomyopathy: ß-adrenergic agonism without desensitization. Eur Heart J 17[Suppl D]:178-181

41. Maisch B, Lotze U, Schneider J, Kochsiek K (1986) Antibodies to human sinus node in sick sinus syndrome. PACE 9:1101-1112

42. Lotze U, Maisch B (1989) Humoral immune response to cardiac conducting tissue. Springer Semin Immunopathol 11:409-422

43. Samsonov M, Nassonov E, Kostin S, Samk A, Alexandrova L, Masenko V, Naumov V, Mareev V, Shevlyagin S, Zhadanov V (1991) Serum neopterin-possible immunological marker of myocardial inflammation in patients with dilated heart muscle disease. Eur Heart J 12 (Suppl D):151-153

44. Lyden DC, Feran M, Olszewski J, Job LP, Huber SA (1987) Coxsackievirus B-3 induced myocarditis: Effect of sex steroids on viremia and infectivity of cardiocytes. Am J Path 126:432-438

45. Weller A, Huber S, Herzum M (1982) Genetics in viral heart disease. J Mol Genetics 27:332-338

46. Kandolf R, Hofschneider PH (1985) Molecular cloning of the genome of a cardiotropic coxsackie B3 virus: full-length reverse-transcribed recombinant cDNA generates infectious virus in mammalian cells. Proc Natl Acad Sci USA 82: 4818-4822

47. Mall G, Klingel K, Albrecht M, Seemann M, Rieger P, Kandolf R (1991) Natural history of coxsackievirus B3-induced myocarditis in ACCA/Sn mice: viral persistence demonstrated by quantitative in situ hybridization histochemistry. Eur Heart J 12[Suppl D]:121-123

48. Matsumori A, Kawai C (1989) Immunomodulating therapy in experimental myocarditis. Springer Semin Immunopathol 11:77-88

49. Matsumori A, Yamada T, Kawai C (1991) Immunomodulating therapy in viral myocarditis: Effects of tumour necrosis factor, interleukin 2 and anti-interleukin-2 receptor antibody in an animal model. Eur Heart J 12 [Suppl D]:203-205

50. Matsumori A (1992) Lessons from animal experiments in myocarditis. Herz 17:107-111
51. Woodruff JF, Woodruff JJ (1974) Involvement of T lymphocytes in the pathogenesis of coxsackievirus B3 heart disease. J Immunol 113:1726-1734
52. Huber SA, Job LP (1983) Cellular immune mechanisms in coxsackievirus group B, type 3 induced myocarditis in Balb/c mice. In: Spitzer JohnJ (ed): Myocardial Injury. Plenum Publishing Corporation, New York, pp 491-508
53. Huber SA, Lodge PA (1984) Coxsackie B-3 myocarditis in Balb/c mice: evidence for autoimmunity to myocyte antigens. Am J Pathol 116:21-29
54. Guthrie M, Lodge PA, Huber SA (1984) Cardiac injury in myocarditis induced by coxsackievirus group B, type 3 in Balb/c mice is mediated by Lyt2+ cytolytic lymphocytes. Cell Immunol 88:558-567
55. Seko Y, Yagita H, Okumura K, Yazaki Y (1994) T-cell receptor Vb gene expression in infiltrating cells in murine hearts with acute myocarditis caused by coxsackievirus B3. Circulation 89:2170-2175
56. Seko Y, Matsuda H, Kato K, Hashimoto Y, Yagita H, Okumura K, Yazaki Y (1993) Expression of intercellular adhesion molecule-1 in murine hearts with acute myocarditis caused by coxsackievirus B3. J Clin Invest 91:1327-1336
57. Seko Y, Shinkai Y, Kawasaki A, Yagita H, Okumura K, Yazaki Y (1993) Evidence of perforin-mediated cardiac myocyte injury in acute murine myocarditis caused by coxsackievirus B3. J Pathol 170:53-58
58. Yamada T, Matsumori A, Sasayama S (1994) Therapeutic effect of anti-tumor necrosis factor-α antibody on the murine model of viral myocarditis induced by encephalomyocarditis virus. Circulation 89:846-851
59. Huber SA, Polgar J, Schultheiss P, Schwimmbeck P (1994) Augmentation of pathogenesis of coxsackievirus B3 infections in mice by exogenous administration of interleukin-1 and interleukin-2. J Virol 68:195-206
60. Kishimoto C, Kuroki Y, Hiraoka Y, Ochiai H, Kurokawa M, Sasayama S (1994) Cytokine and murine coxsackievirus B3 myocarditis. Interleukin-2 suppressed myocarditis in the acute stage but enhanced the condition in the subsequent stage. Circulation 89:2836-2842
61. Lyden DC, Huber SA (1984) Aggravation of coxsackie virus B-3 induced myocarditis and increase in cellular immunity of myocyte antigens in pregnant Balb/c mice and animals treated with progesterone. Cell Immunol 87:462-472
62. Lyden D, Olszewski J, Huber SA (1987) Influence of sex hormones on coxsackie virus group B, type 3 induced myocarditis in Balb/c mice. Eur Heart J 8 [Suppl. J]:389-391
63. Huber SA, Pfaeffle B (199a) Differential Th1 and Th2 cell response in male and female BALB/c mice infected with coxsackievirus group B type 3. J Virol 68:5126-5132
64. Kilbourne ED, Wilson CB, Perrier D (1956) The induction of gross myocardial lesions by a coxsackie(pleurodynia) virus and cortisone. J Clin Invest 35:362-367
65. Tomioka N, Kishimoto C, Matsumori A, Kawai C (1986) Effects of prednisolone on acute viral myocarditis in mice. J Am Coll Cardiol 7:868-872
66. Strom TB (1984) Immunosuppressive agents in renal transplantation. Kidney Int 26:353-362
67. O'Connell JB, Reap Ea, Robinson JA (1986) The effect of cyclosporine on acute murine coxsackie B3 myocarditis. Circulation 73:353-355
68. Mason JW, Billingham ME, Ricci DR (1980) Treatment of acute inflammatory myocarditis asssisted by endomyocardial biopsy. Amer J Cardiol 45:1037-1044
69. Schultheiß HP, Kühl U, Janda I, Schanwell M, Strauer BE (1992) Immunosuppressive therapy in myocarditis. Herz 17:112-121
70. Maisch B, Schönian U, Hengstenberg C., Herzum M, Hufnagel G, Bethge C, Bittinger A, Neumann K (1994) Immunosuppressive treatment in autoreactive myocarditis-results from a controlled trial. Postgrad Med J 70 (Suppl. 1):S29-S34
71. Maisch B, Herzum M, Hufnagel, G, Bethge C, Schönian U (1995) Immunosuppressive treatment for myocarditis and dilated cardiomyopathy. Eur Heart J 16 [Suppl O]:153-161

72. McKenna WJ, Davies MJ (1995) Immunosuppression for myocarditis N Engl J Med 333; 312-313
73. Cunnion RE, Parrillo JE (1995) Immunosuppressive therapy for myocarditis. N Engl J Med 333:1713
74. Maisch B, Camerini F, Schultheiss H-P (1995) Immunosuppressive therapy for myocarditis. N Engl J Med 333:1713
75. Cooper LT, Shabetai R (1995) Immunosuppressive therapy for myocarditis. N Engl J Med 333:1713-1714
76. Mason JW, O'Connel JB, McManus BM (1995) Immunosuppressive therapy for myocarditis (authors reply). N Engl J Med 333:1714
77. Billingham M (1993) Histology of myocarditis. In: Banatrala JE (Ed) Viral Infections of the heart. Arnold Publ, p 47
78. Parillo JE, Cunnion RE, Epstein SE, Parker MM, Suffredini AF, Brenno M, Schaer GL, Palmeri ST, Cannon RO, Ailing D, Wittes JT, Ferrans VJ, Rodriguez ER, Fauci AS (1989) A prospective randomized, controlled trial of prednisone for dilated cardiomyopathy. N Engl J Med 321:1061-1068
79. Maisch B (1990) Myocarditis. Current opinion in Cardiology 5:320-327
80. Eckstein R, Mempel W, Bolte HD (1982) Reduced suppressor cell activity in congestive cardiomyopathy and in myocarditis. Circulation 65:1224-1229
81. Maisch B, Herzum M, Hufnagel G, Schönian U (1996) Immunosuppressive and immunomodulatory treatment for myocarditis. Current Opinion in Cardiology 11:310-324

Prevention of Sudden Death in Patients with Dilated Cardiomyopathy

M. Borggrefe, M. Block and G. Breithardt

Introduction

The prognosis of patients with congestive heart failure is poor. Depending on the severity of the disease, the annual mortality rate ranges between 10% and 50% [1-4]. The mode of death is circulatory failure or sudden cardiac death which accounts for approximately 50% of deaths [1,3-5]. There is a high prevalence of sudden death in patients with mild symptoms (50% sudden death rate) and in those with severe symptoms awaiting cardiac transplantation (25% sudden death rate). The proportion of sudden death however varies in different studies between 4% and 90%. This discrepancy may partly be explained by varying definitions, different patient populations and inclusion of non-classifiable deaths in the sudden death category. Non-ischemic (idiopathic) dilated cardiomyopathy (DCM) is the most common etiology. However, in some reports, no attempts have been made to differentiate non-ischemic from ischemic left ventricular dysfunction because in these studies only noninvasive diagnostic procedures were performed. This represents a major shortcoming of some large prospective studies in patients with heart failure as two completely different subgroups (ischemic vs. non-ischemic left ventricular dysfunction) are included. There are many clinical and hemodynamic parameters that might predict a poor prognosis due to impending circulatory failure. The identification of the patient at risk of sudden death however is difficult mainly because of different possible mechanisms and changes induced by the impaired left ventricular function.

Mechanisms of Sudden Death in DCM

Although no sufficient data are available concerning the mechanisms of sudden death in patients with DCM, it has been assumed that ventricular tachycardia degenerating into ventricular fibrillation or primary ventricular fibrillation are the most common modes of death. In addition, asystole has been documented as the primary electrical event in some patients with DCM. Recently, Luu et al. [5] reviewed the causes of cardiac arrest from electrocardiographic monitoring and from clinical and autopsy data in patients hospitalized for cardiac transplantation evaluation and management of heart failure. There were 21 cardiac arrests which occurred in 13 patients with a prior myocardial infarction and in another 7 patients with non-ischemic cardiomyopathy. The rhythm at the time of cardiac arrest was bradycardia or electromechanical dissociation in 13 patients (62%). In only 8 of 21 arrests (38%), ventricular tachycardia or ventricular fibrillation were recorded. Therefore, the predominant mechanism of cardiac arrest in patients with advanced heart failure may be a bradycardic arrest in a substantial number of patients. This is in contrast to out-of-hospital patients with coronary artery disease where the initial rhythm in out-of-hospital cardiac arrest patients has been shown to be ventricular tachycardia degenerating to ventricular fibrillation in approximately 40%-80% of arrests.

The extent to which antiarrhythmic drugs facilitate the development of bradyarrhythmias or electromechanical dissociation is unknown. As evident from post mortem examinations, sudden death may also be due to an embolic cerebral event or even pulmonary embolism, especially in patients with severe biventricular forms of heart failure. Therefore, taking these observations into account, sudden death in DCM is multifactorial, making risk stratification and management of patients extremely difficult.

Risk Stratification in DCM

Mortality in DCM is closely related to impaired left ventricular function as indexed by high ventricular filling pressures, high end-diastolic and end-systolic volumes and low ventricular ejection fraction [1,2]. Many studies suggest that left ventricular ejection fraction is the most potent predictor of death. However, although ejection fraction is a predictor of total deaths, it may not be the best predictor of arrhythmic death in DCM, where half of the deaths are sudden. Moreover, some reports suggest that sudden death is present in a higher proportion of functional class I and II patients compared to functional class Ill or IV patients in whom death due to progressive heart failure may be the usual cause of mortality [2].

The role of asymptomatic arrhythmias as detected during Holter monitoring for predicting sudden death is controversial. Atrial fibrillation is frequently encountered in patients with advanced heart failure (9%-35%) [3,4]. In the Veterans Administration Cooperative Trial [3], atrial fibrillation detected during Holter monitoring was not related to mortality. However, Middlekauff et al. [4], who recently examined the relationship of atrial fibrillation to prognosis in 390 patients with advanced heart failure, found that the presence of atrial fibrillation was associated with an increase in total mortality and in the rate of sudden death. ln most studies, nonsustained ventricular tachycardia during Holter monitoring has not been found to independently worsen prognosis [6,7]. Meinertz et al. [8] and von Olshausen et al. [9] studied the incidence and prognostic significance of ventricular arrhythmias in patients with idiopathic DCM. Both studies found that patients with poor left ventricular function and frequent nonsustained ventricular tachycardia had a high risk of dying. Although these studies support the prognostic significance of asymptomatic, complex ventricular arrhythmias, other investigators have not found a similar relationship. The sensitivity of Holter monitoring in detecting frequent ventricular ectopy or nonsustained ventricular tachycardia appears to be high, but the predictive value with regard to sudden death seems to be low.

The presence of ventricular late potentials on the signal-averaged ECG was associated with a poor prognosis in patients with ischemic heart disease. Several studies that have evaluated the use of signal-averaged electrocardiography in the assessment of individuals with diverse underlying clinical diagnosis have included small numbers of patients with non-ischemic DCM. Several small-scale studies have suggested the utility of the signal-averaged ECG in the prediction of malignant ventricular tachyarrhythmias in patients with DCM. In patients with coronary artery disease an abnormal signal-averaged ECG has successfully identified patients with a high propensity for sustained VT or even sudden cardiac death. The data has not been as conclusive in patients with DCM.

Mancini et al. [10] reported on 114 consecutive patients referred for evaluation for heart transplantation with non-ischemic DCM. In this report the utility of signal-averaged electrocardiography and the impact of bundle branch block QRS morphology on the development of malignant arrhythmic events and all-cause mortality were appraised. The best predictor of an adverse outcome defined as death, transplantation or occurrence of sustained VT was a higher New York Heart Association classification. On the other hand, the only other predictor of an adverse outcome was the presence of an abnormal signal-averaged ECG. Despite these promising results the clinical application of signal-averaged electrocardiography in patients with DCM has the same limitations as those inherent with its use in patients after myocardial infarction. The negative and positive predictive value for predicting sudden death or sustained VT were 100% and 45%, respectively. Thus, if interventions are considered in high risk patients, an excessive number of patients without risk may unnecessarily be treated. On the other hand, as it is true for post myocardial infarction patients, a negative signal-averaged ECG carries a good prognosis. Therefore, at the present time the value of this noninvasive technique for risk stratification of patients with DCM is unknown as no prospective, large scale studies in mildly symptomatic patients are available.

Various studies [11,12] have investigated the prognostic value of programmed ventricular stimulation in asymptomatic patients with DCM. Sustained ventricular tachycardia or fibrillation were inducible in up to 40% of patients. These studies demonstrate that programmed ventricular stimulation in patients with DCM has limited ability to identify those patients at risk of sudden death as

1. the yield of inducible monomorphic VT is low;

2. aggressive stimulation techniques lead to polymorphic VT or VF which may be unspecific.

In summary, available data suggest that risk stratification of patients with DCM is extremely problematic. Poor left ventricular function seems to be the most potent predictor for total cardiac mortality. The prediction of sudden death in patients with DCM is poor.

Antiarrhythmic Drug Therapy versus ICD Implantation in Asymptomatic Patients with DCM and Nonsustained Ventricular Tachycardia

Presently, studies with either class I antiarrhythmic drugs or amiodarone have failed to demonstrate a reduction in total mortality or sudden death in patients with DCM and nonsustained ventricular tachycardia. Furthermore, the risks of antiarrhythmic therapy are increased in patients with reduced left ventricular function: proarrhythmic effects occur more likely in these patients and exacerbation of heart failure may be observed in 4%-25% of cases especially with the use of class I drugs. As the role of asymptomatic, complex ventricular arrhythmias for determining prognosis in DCM is not known and the therapeutic end-point is not clear, it is likely prudent to avoid antiarrhythmic drug therapy in this group of patients. Whether non-pharmacological interventions, such as the implantation of an implantable cardioverter defibrillator (ICD) in asymptomatic patients with DCM may be beneficial, has to be proven by properly designed, prospective studies such as the Cardiomyopathy Trial (CAT) which has recently been started in Germany. This prospective randomized multicenter study was initiated by Karl-Heinz Kuck, Hamburg, and was first called the German Dilated Cardiomyopathy Study (GDCMS). The primary objective of CAT is to assess the impact of prophylactic ICD in patients with advanced DCM and no symptomatic ventricular arrhythmias. The inclusion criteria of CAT are as follows: DCM with left ventricular ejection fraction < 30% at angiography, NYHA class II or III, age between 18 and 70 years and absence of symptomatic ventricular arrhythmias. DCM had to be diagnosed within 9 months prior to inclusion. Up to June 1993, approximately 50 patients were randomized. Hopefully this Cardiomyopathy Trial will provide some evidence on whether implantation of an ICD in patients with heart failure is beneficial. Several retrospective studies have questionned the usefulness of ICD in patients with depressed left ventricular ejection fraction. It has been argued that the long-term benefits of ICD therapy can not be reasonably measured without taking into consideration intraoperative and perioperative mortality and morbidity. Kim et al. [13] suggested that ICD outcomes should be assessed in terms of total arrhythmic deaths, including not only sudden death during follow-up, but also perioperative surgical mortality and non-sudden death occurring as a consequence of an ICD-treated ventricular tachyarrhythmia. These Authors observed a poor outcome in ICD patients with reduced ejection fraction (<30%) compared with patients with better ejection fraction during a follow-up period of 31 ± 27 months. Although this study included only a small sample size, the potential benefit of an ICD in patients with low ejection fraction appeared questionable.

Until the results of large prospective studies in this group of patients are known, therapy of arrhythmias in DCM should be directed towards eliminating arrhythmogenic factors, i.e. hypokalemia, hypomagnesemia, activation of the sympathetic nervous system and the renin-angiotensin-aldosterone system, and the proarrhythmic effects of inotropic agents. Measures would therefore include the use of potassium-sparing diuretics, potassium and magnesium supplementation, careful use and titration of beta-blockers, angiotensin converting enzyme-inhibitors, digitalis and inotropic agents. Possibly, depending on the duration of runs of nonsustained ventricular tachycardia, programmed ventricular stimulation may be indicated in a subgroup of patients with DCM and electropharmacologic-guided therapy may be useful in some of them. However, no prospective studies are available to support this approach.

Management of Patients with Sustained Ventricular Tachycardia and/or Ventricular Fibrillation in DCM

Patients with sustained ventricular tachycardia or out-of-hospital ventricular fibrillation and DCM are at high risk of recurrent, life-threatening tachyarrhythmias and sudden cardiac death [14-17]. Several large studies have validated the use of electropharmacological testing in patients with sustained ventricular tachyarrhythmias. The usefulness of serial electropharmacological testing has been shown predominantly for patients with coronary heart disease and ventricular tachycardia. The value of a baseline electrophysiologic study and electropharmacological testing in patients with DCM is still controversial [14-19]. Several studies have addressed this issue. A total of 268 patients with DCM and ventricular tachyarrhythmias have been studied [14-19]. Sixty-three percent of patients had inducible ventricular tachycardia or fibrillation at baseline. Sustained ventricular tachycardia was more frequently induced in DCM patients with clinically documented sustained ventricular tachycardia than in those with clinical ventricular fibrillation [18]. Serial drug testing has been shown to be effective in preventing arrhythmia recurrence in those patients in whom ventricular tachycardia or fibrillation was reproducibly induced at baseline and rendered non-inducible, or more difficult to induce, following oral drug administration [18,19]. However, a favorable drug response was only obtained in 26%-53% of patients. Therefore, as one third of patients with DCM has no inducible ventricular tachycardia or fibrillation at baseline, or the reproducibility of ventricular tachycardia induction is poor, serial drug testing is not applicable in many patients. Several studies have shown a high recurrence rate of ventricular tachycardia or fibrillation or even sudden death in those patients not inducible at baseline [18,19]. Taking these findings into account, serial drug testing in patients with DCM is applicable only for those in whom ventricular tachycardia or fibrillation can reproducibly be induced at baseline off antiarrhythmic drugs, which may be true only for about 50%-60% of patients with DCM and a history of sustained ventricular tachycardia or fibrillation. However, a favorable drug response (i.e. suppression of inducibility of ventricular tachycardia) can only be obtained in a minority of patients (about 30%) [18]. Therefore, implantation of an ICD should be considered early in the management of patients with DCM and life-threatening ventricular tachyarrhythmias [20]. Based on the available information - prospective, randomized trials comparing serial drug testing and ICD implantation are presently lacking - the following approach is suggested in patients with DCM and sustained ventricular tachycardia or fibrillation, who are not primary candidates for heart transplantation: if sustained ventricular tachycardia or fibrillation cannot be induced or the reproducibility of induction during baseline electrophysiologic evaluation is lacking, implantation of an ICD should be performed. If sustained ventricular tachycardia or fibrillation is reproducibly inducible, the patients may undergo serial drug testing. About 30%-50% of patients may be controlled by antiarrhythmic drugs. If no drug is found to be effective, ICD implantation should be offered to those patients whose prognosis with regard to their left ventricular dysfunction is better than one year.

A retrospective analysis of our own series comprising 164 patients with DCM undergoing programmed electrical stimulation has shown that with the availability of the ICD (1984 first German implant), the prognosis of patients with DCM seems to be considerably improved with regard to freedom of sudden death. Between 1979 and 1987, 84 patients underwent therapy because of documented or suspected ventricular tachycardia or fibrillation (ICD implantation rate 5%). This group of patients was compared to a cohort studied between 1988 to 1991 (80 patients, ICD implantation rate 39%). Eleven percent of patients died suddenly in the early period (1979 to 1987) compared to 2.5% in the latter phase (1988 to 1991). Although the follow-up periods in both patient cohorts are not comparable, most arrhythmic events occurred during the first year following the initial electrophysiologic evaluation. Taking this limitation into account, the results of this non-randomized, retrospective study show a significant prognostic improvement with the availability of an ICD in this patient cohort.

Recently, Fazio et al. [20] analyzed the long-term outcome of 40 patients with DCM and ventricular tachycardia or fibrillation undergoing implantation of an ICD. The actuarial mortality at 1 and 4 years was 0% and 14% for sudden death. Compared with projected mortality rates, these results confirm a significant improvement in prognosis of patients with DCM and life-threatening ventricular tachyarrhythmias and are consistent with results from other groups in patients with ischemic heart disease undergoing implantation of an ICD. Recently, Grimm et al. [21] reported on 49 consecutive patients with idiopathic DCM. The mean ejection fraction was $27 \pm 11\%$. The patients were followed for 28 ± 28 months after ICD implantation. Eight-two percent of patients presented with cardiac arrest, 12% with syncope and 6% with sustained ventricular tachycardia. During 25 ± 25 months follow-up with active ICD 59% of patients received one or more spontaneous ICD shocks and 51% of patients received appropriate shocks. During follow-up two patients died suddenly with active ICD, while other two patients died suddenly with inactive ICD (in one patient the device was inactivated according to patient wish and another patient refused generator replacement after battery depletion). In this analysis the authors recognize a sudden death rate of 25% at five years if intention to treat analysis is performed. The total death rate in patients with and without spontaneous shocks implies that ICD therapy improves survival in shocked patients to a level comparable to patients without recurrent ventricular tachycardia or ventricular fibrillation. Trappe et al. [22] observed a correlation of total mortality to the underlying cardiac disease. The five year survival rate of 36 patients with DCM was 28% versus 54% of 203 patients with coronary artery disease. This difference was due to a higher non-sudden cardiac death rate in patients with DCM.

Although controlled, randomized trials in patients with DCM and ventricular tachycardia or fibrillation undergoing implantation of an ICD are not available at the present time, a remarkable rate of freedom from recurrent cardiac arrest has been observed as compared to the results that were reported prior to the use of ICDs. Therefore, especially with the use of subcutaneous implantation techniques of ICDs, patients with DCM and life-threatening tachyarrhythmias, not controlled by antiarrhythmic drugs or in the absence of inducibility at baseline or the lack of reproducibility of induction of ventricular tachycardia or fibrillation, should undergo implantation of a device. Presently, in patients with DCM and documented ventricular tachycardia or fibrillation data comparing serial drug testing to ICD implantation are lacking.

References

1. Massie B, Ports T, Chatterjee K (1981) Long-term vasodilator therapy for heart failure: Clinical response and its relationship to hemodynamic measurements. Circulation 63:269-278
2. Wilson JR, Schwartz JS, St. John Sutton M, Ferraro N (1983) Prognosis in severe heart failure: relation to hemodynamic measurements and ventricular ectopic activity. J Am Coll Card 2:403-409
3. Carson P (1991) Atrial fibrillation/flutter does not decrease survival in congestive heart failure J Am Coll Cardiol 17:90A (abstr)
4. Middlekauff HR, Stevenson WG, Stevenson LW (1991) Prognostic significance of atrial fibrillation in advanced heart failure. Circulation 84:40-48
5. Luu M, Stevenson WG, Stevenson LW, Baron K, Walden J (1989) Diverse mechanisms of unexpected cardiac arrest in advanced heart failure. Circulation 80:1675-1680
6. Franciosa JA, Wilen M, Ziesche S, Cohn JN (1983) Survival in men with severe chronic left ventricular failure due to either coronary heart disease or idiopathic dilated cardiomyopathy. Am J Cardiol 51:831-836
7. Huang SK, Messer JV, Denes P (1983) Significance of ventricular tachycardia in idiopathic dilated cardiomyopathy: Observation in 35 patients. Am J Cardiol 51:507-512
8. Meinertz T, Hofmann T, Kasper W (1984) Significance of ventricular arrhythmias in idiopathic dilated cardiomyopathy. Am J Cardiol 53:902-907
9. Von Olshausen K, Schafer A, Mehmel HC, Schwartz F, Senges J, Kuebler W (1984) Ventricular arrhythmia in idiopathic dilated cardiomyopathy. Br Heart J 51:195-201
10. Mancini DM, Wong KL, Simson MB (1993) Prognostic value of an abnormal signal-averaged electrocardiogram in patients with nonischemic congestive cardiomyopathy. Circulation 87:1083-1092
11. Stevenson WG, Stevenson LW, Weiss J, Tillisch JH (1988) Inducible ventricular arrhythmias and sudden death during vasodilator therapy of severe heart failure. Am Heart J 116:1447-1454
12. Meinertz T, Treese N, Kasper W, Geibel A, Hofinann T, Zehender M, Bohn D, Pop T, Just H (1985) Determinants of prognosis in idiopathic dilated cardiomyopathy as determined by programmed electrical stimulation. Am J Cardiol 56:337-341
13. Kim SG, Fisher JD, Furman S, Gross J, Zilo P, Roth JA, Ferrick KJ, Brodman R (1991) Benefits of implantable defibrillators are overestimated by sudden death rates and better represented by total arrhythmic death rate. J Am Coll Cardiol 17:1587-1592

14. Poll DS, Marchlinski FE, Buxton AE, Doherty JU, Waxman HL, Josephson ME (1984) Sustained ventricular tachycardia in patients with idiopathic dilated cardiomyopathy: Electrophysiologic testing and lack of response to antiarrhythmic drug therapy. Circulation 70:451-456
15. Brembilla-Perrot B, Donetti J, Terrier de la Chaise A, Sadoui N, Aliot E, Juilliere Y (1991) Diagnostic value of ventricular stimulation in patients with idiopathic dilated cardiomyopathy. Am Heart J 121:1124-1131
16. Constantin L, Martins JB, Kienzle MG, Brownstein SL, McCue ML, Hopson RC (1989) Induced sustained ventricular tachycardia in nonischemic dilated cardiomyopathy: Dependence on clinical presentation and response to antiarrhythmic agents. PACE 12:776-783
17. Milner PG, Dimarco IP, Lerman BB (1988) Electrophysiological evaluation of sustained ventricular tachyarrhythmias in idiopathic dilated cardiomyopathy. PACE 11:562-568
18. Liem LB, Swerdlow CD (1988) Value of electropharmacologic testing in idiopathic dilated cardiomyopathy and sustained ventricular tachyarrhythmias. Am J Cardiol 62:611-616
19. Rae AP, Spielman SR, Kutalek SP, Kay HR, Horowitz LN (1987) Electrophysiologic assessment of antiarrhythmic drug efficacy for ventricular tachyarrhythmias associated with dilated cardiomyopathy. Am J Cardiol 59:291-295
20. Fazio G, Veltri EP, Tomaselli G, Lewis R, Griffith LSC, Guarnieri T (1991) Long-term follow-up of patients with nonischemic dilated cardiomyopathy and ventricular tachyarrhythmias treated with implantable cardioverter defibrillators PACE 14:1905-1910
21. Grimm W, Hoffinann J, Marchlinski F (1993) Shock occurrence and survival in patients with idiopathic dilated cardiomyopathy and implantable cardioverter-defibrillaton. Eur Heart J 14(A):411
22. Trappe HJ, Fieguth HG, Klein H (1993) Role of the underlying etiology in patients with an implantable cardioverter-defibrillator. Med Klin 88:362-370

Medical Treatment of Heart Failure: Problems in Dilated Cardiomyopathy

J.N. Cohn

The management of dilated cardiomyopathy involves two distinct goals [1]. One is to relieve symptoms and improve the quality of life of patients who suffer congestive heart failure as a consequence of a dilated, remodeled ventricle. The second, equally important, goal is to delay the progressive remodeling process which appears to eventuate in premature death. It is this latter goal that has been the subject of most recent large-scale trials on the management of heart failure.

Ventricular Remodeling

A dilated ventricle implies that the ventricular muscle has hypertophied and remodeled. This process involves enlargement of the myocytes, usually with synthesis of sarcomeres, both in series and in parallel to make the cell both longer and thicker, and activation of the interstitium with increased collagen synthesis often accompanied by alterations in collagen degradation. Although the contractile dysfunction that characterizes cardiomyopathy may have been initiated by a decrease in excitation-contraction coupling, the contractile dysfunction exhibited by the dilated heart may at least in part represent an obligatory reduction in shortening mandated by the dilated chamber. The dilated chamber may eject a normal stroke volume with very little myocyte shortening; indeed, normal cell shortening in the presence of a dilated chamber would eject an exceedingly large and inappropriate stroke volume. This construct makes it possible to consider the structural remodeling of the left ventricle as the primary chronic defect in the cardiomyopathic disease state. Consequently, therapeutic efforts to alter that remodeling process become of critical importance in the management of this syndrome.

The etiology of dilated cardiomyopathy is varied and importantly dependent on the definition of terminology. The most common cause of a dilated heart and symptoms of congestive heart failure in Western societies is coronary disease. Although this initially may be manifested by regional ischemia and infarction leading to a regional wall motion abnormality, the remodeling process initiated by this ischemic event may eventually result in global chamber enlargement and global reduction of wall motion. Therefore the dilated cardiomyopathy observed in this setting might appear similar to that in patients who sustained a more diffuse myocardial insult. Nonetheless, coronary artery disease is often excluded in patients classified as having dilated cardiomyopathy and the residual population includes a wide range of known and unknown etiologies, many of which end up being classified as idiopathic. Regardless of the etiology, however, the remodeling appears to be a stereotypical myocardial response to injury.

The stimuli contributing to this ventricular remodeling process are not fully understood. Neurohormonal mechanisms are considered to play an important role and a wide range of hormonal factors are activated in the syndrome of dilated cardiomyopathy. The sympathetic nervous system usually is activated and plasma norepinephrine levels are high [2]. The renin angiotensin system exhibits stimulation in a considerable fraction of such patients and the plasma renin activity is increased, often to extraordinarily high levels [2]. Plasma endothelin levels also are increased [3] as are circulating levels of arginine vasopressin [4]. Activation of atrial natriuretic peptide (ANP) is a classical feature of dilated cardiomyopathy and its elevation has even been proposed as a clinical screening test to identify subclinical cases of cardiomyopathy [5, 6]. A number of peptides in this family have been identified and all appear to be increased, although ANP has its primary origin in the atrium and brain natriuretic peptide appears to be primarily of ventricular origin [7, 8]. All these agents not only exert natriuretic effects on the kidney, but also are dilator peptides that tend to counteract the vasoconstrictor effect of the other activated neurohormonal systems. Despite what appears to be compensatory activation of these atrial peptides, patients with heart failure continue to manifest vasoconstriction and sodium retention, thus suggesting that the striking elevation of peptide levels is not sufficient to overcome the vasoconstrictor stimuli in this syndrome.

Efforts to slow or halt the progressive remodeling process in the left ventricle, and thus to improve the prognosis of dilated cardiomyopathy, have involved the use of angiotensin converting enzyme (ACE) inhibitors [9, 10], the combination of isosorbide dinitrate and hydralazine [10], and more recently the beta-blockers including the newer generation beta-blockers, such as carvedilol [11]. All of these drugs appear to interfere with one or more of the mechanisms stimulating remodeling or to activate systems that inhibit remodeling. Thus the ACE-inhibitors are assumed to be acting via the renin-angiotensin-aldosterone system, the beta-blockers through the sympathetic nervous system, and isosorbide dinitrate by generating nitric oxide that stimulates cyclic GMP that is known to be growth inhibiting. These pharmacologic agents are effective in both animal models and in man in slowing the natural history of the progressive left ventricular remodeling process and reducing mortality [12-14]. It is now clear that one or more of these drugs should form part of the therapeutic armamentarium in every patient with dilated cardiomyopathy and symptoms of heart failure. ACE-inhibitors have been approved by the Food and Drug Administration for therapy of the dilated ventricle even in the absence of symptoms, based upon the observation in the SOLVD prevention trial that enalapril reduced the rate of development of overt heart failure in this population [15]. Whether beta-blockers and nitrates would share that favorable effect would need to be addressed in a large-scale trial.

A wide range of ACE-inhibitors is currently on the market and there is reason to suspect that all of these agents would share a favorable effect on left ventricular remodeling. The problem is that not all of these drugs have been subjected to controlled trials and therefore we must remain uncertain as to the appropriate dose to gain the desired effect in this patient population. Even where dosing data do exist, however, such as with enalapril and chronic heart failure, adequate data on dose response are not available to make an informed judgment regarding the optimal dose of the drug that must be employed. Although 10 mg twice daily enalapril has been effective in most clinical trials at producing a modest and highly significant reduction in mortality, some investigators feel that doses far higher than are generally used would produce an even more favorable long-term response. This issue also needs further investigation.

Beta-blockers have been utilized to treat dilated cardiomyopathy since the early observations of Waagstein in Sweden [16]. Only in recent years have large enough scale trials been undertaken to study the effect of these agents on remodeling and mortality. It is now apparent that careful initiation of low doses of either metoprolol or carvedilol in patients with dilated cardiomyopathy and congestive heart failure is adequately tolerated to allow most patients to be titrated to full doses of the drugs. A striking increase in left ventricular ejection fraction appears over the ensuing months [17] and at least one study has demonstrated a reduction in cumulative mortality [11]. Indeed the magnitude of the increase in ejection fraction observed in these trials suggests that the beta-blockers are having a profound effect on the structural remodeling process, leading to a reduction of ventricular volume and an improvement in prognosis. The mechanism by which this beta-blocker action takes place is unknown, and preliminary data suggesting that carvedilol may exert a more favorable effect than metoprolol raise the possibility that other pharmacologic actions of carvedilol, including its alpha-blocking vasodilator effect and its antioxidant effect, may be contributing to the overall salutary response.

Use of the nitric oxide generating nitrates is aimed at augmenting myocardial nitric oxide concentration in an effort to prevent further myocardial structural remodeling. The hydralazine which was studied in V-HeFT [10] as a component of this vasodilator regimen now appears to exert its primary chronic action on inhibiting nitrate tolerance that otherwise might occur during sustained administration of isosorbide dinitrate [18]. This action of hydralazine to reduce nitrate tolerance appears to be related to its antioxidant properties, that limit the production of superoxide radicals that cause degradation of the nitric oxide at the vascular smooth muscle site of action [19].

Symptom Relief

The agenda to relieve symptoms and improve quality of life in the patient with congestive heart failure usually represents the goal most apparent to the patient. Since fluid retention is a hallmark of the clinical syndrome, diuretic therapy is usually mandatory. When loop diuretics are required to optimize intravascular volume, the dosing of these agents must be carefully titrated to avoid either under-treatment or over-treatment that can have unwanted consequences. In practice it is most useful to utilize the central venous pressure and daily morning weight as guides to the optimal dosage of diuretics. Optimal weight is defined as that weight at which jugular venous pressure is normal and the hepatojugular reflux test is negative. Loop diuretic doses to maintain that body weight, augmented if necessary with a second diuretic such as metolazone, can successfully avoid inappropriate sodium retention and the need for recurrent hospitalizations.

Digitalis therapy is often utilized in patients with dilated cardiomyopathy, because of the demonstrated ability of this drug to produce modest improvement in symptoms [20]. Although this drug apparently does not produce any net benefit on long-term survival [21], the favorable effect on symptoms justifies its use as long as the dose is kept low enough to avoid toxicity. Digoxin is the preferable agent to use for this syndrome and should be titrated on the basis of an algorithm as utilized in the large scale DIG trial [21].

Vasodilator drugs also are effective in relieving symptoms and improving quality of life in heart failure. Both ACE-inhibitors and hydralazine isosorbide dinitrate have been demonstrated to be effective in this regard, but the benefit on symptoms is more modest than the benefit on hemodynamics and on the left ventricular remodeling progression.

The use of parenteral inotropic agents to produce short-term hemodynamic benefit and occasionally long-term symptomatic benefit has gained widespread use in patients with severe heart failure. Relatively poorly controlled data suggest that some patients exhibit marked benefit with outpatient administration of agents such as dobutamine or milrinone on an intermittent basis. Controlled trials suggest that these drugs may actually increase the risk of premature death [22], but many patients who have markedly impaired lifestyles are willing to exchange symptomatic improvement for an increased risk of mortality [23]. The use of these agents must be carefully considered and the pros and cons discussed with the patient prior to initiating such experimental therapy.

Dilated Cardiomyopathy versus Ischemic Heart Disease

Recent trials have generated considerable interest in the possibility that patients with coronary artery disease respond differently to therapeutic interventions than patients with nonischemic dilated cardiomyopathy. Review of a number of large-scale trials appears to suggest that therapeutic interventions with ACE-inhibitors and vasodilators in general produce a more favorable impact in patients with dilated cardiomyopathy, but this appears to be at most a quantitative rather than a qualitative difference in response. It is intuitive that the presence of coronary disease would introduce another mechanism for deterioration and for premature mortality, whereas the dilated cardiomyopathy state is a purer heart failure condition in which ischemic episodes should not contribute to morbidity. Therefore an agent which would favorably affect the function of the left ventricle or inhibit the remodeling process might be anticipated to have a more favorable effect in this population than in those who also have generalized atherosclerosis and are at risk for other ischemic events.

When one explores the overall therapeutic response in subgroups of patients from most of the trials, there appears to be no fundamental difference between the efficacy in coronary disease and dilated cardiomyopathy. Several recent trials have suggested significant quantitative differences in responsiveness that need to be confirmed in subsequent studies. The CIBIS trial demonstrated what appeared to be a favorable effect of the beta-blocker bisoprolol in patients with dilated cardiomyopathy, but not in those with coronary disease [24]. The PRAISE trial reported a favorable effect on mortality of amlodipine in patients with dilated cardiomyopathy, but not in those with coronary disease [25]. Similarly, amiodarone, the type III antiarrhythmic drug, exerted a favorable effect on mortality in a South American trial composed predominantly of patients with cardiomyopathy [26] and not in an American trial composed largely of patients with coronary disease [27]. Whether these studies have identified a previously unrecognized fundamental difference in these syndromes or rather have only identified the well described trend for a better response to drugs in dilated cardiomyopathy remains to be established.

Although the treatment of dilated cardiomyopathy now has advanced to the point where therapeutic interventions can be employed with insight into the desired mechanism of action and the desired end-point, the efficacy of therapy in slowing progression of this syndrome and reducing mortality remains inadequate. Newer knowledge about cellular mechanisms contributing to the remodeling process and neurohormonal stimuli that may be critical to the progression of this process may help to identify in the future more targeted therapies that can exhibit even greater efficacy.

References

1. Cohn JN (1996) Drug therapy: the management of chronic heart failure. N Engl J Med 335:490-498
2. Levine TB, Francis GS, Goldsmith SR, Simon A, Cohn JN (1982) Activity of the sympathetic nervous system and renin-angiotensin system assessed by plasma hormone levels and their relationship to hemodynamic abnormalities in congestive heart failure. Am J Cardiol 49:1659-1666
3. Cody RJ, Haas GJ, Binkley PF, Capers Q, Kelley R (1992) Plasma endothelin correlates with the extent of pulmonary hypertension in patients with chronic congestive heart failure. Circulation 85:504-509
4. Goldsmith SR, Francis GS, Cowley AW, Levine TB, Cohn JN (1983) Increased plasma arginine vasopressin in patients with congestive heart failure. J Am Coll Cardiol 1:1385-1390
5. Burnett JC Jr, Kao PC, Hu DC et al. (1986) Atrial natriuretic peptide elevation in congestive heart failure in the human. Science 231:1145-1147
6. Lerman A, Gibbons RJ, Rodeheffer RJ, Bailey KR, McKinley LJ, Heublein DM, Burnett JC Jr (1993) Circulating N-terminal atrial natriuretic peptide as a marker for symptomless left-ventricular dysfunction. Lancet 341:1105-1109
7. Sumida H, Yasue H, Yoshimura M, Okumura K, Ogawa H, Kugiyama K, Matsuyama K, Kikuta K, Morita E, Nakao K (1995) Comparison of secretion pattern between A-type and B-type natriuretic peptides in patients with old myocardial infarction. J Am Coll Cardiol 25:1105-1110

8. Hosoda K, Nakao K, Mukoyama M, Saito Y, Jougasaki M, Shirakami G, Suga S, Ogawa Y, Yasue H, Imura H (1991) Expression of brain natriuretic peptide gene in human heart: production in the ventricle. Hypertension 17:1152-1155
9. The SOLVD Investigators (1991) Effect of enalapril on survival in patients with reduced left ventricular ejection fraction and congestive heart failure. N Engl J Med 325:293-302
10. Cohn JN, Archibald DG, Ziesche S, Franciosa JA, Harston WE, Tristani FE, Dunkman WB, Jacobs W, Francis GS, Flohr KH, Goldman S, Cobb FR, Shah PM, Saunders R, Fletcher RD, Loeb HS, Hughes VC, Baker B (1986) Effect of vasodilator therapy on mortality in chronic congestive hearth failure. Results of a Veterans Administration Cooperative Study (V-HeFT). N Engl J Med 314:1547-1552
11. Packer M, Bristow MR, Cohn JN, Colucci WS, Fowler MB, Gilbert EM, Shusterman NH, for the US Carvedilol Heart Failure Study Group (1996) The effect of carvedilol on morbidity and mortality in patients with chronic heart failure. N Engl J Med 334:1349-1355
12. McDonald KM, Carlyle PF, Matthews J, Hauer K, Elbers T, Hunter D, Cohn JN (1990) Early ventricular remodeling after myocardial damage and its attenuation by converting enzyme inhibition. Trans Assoc Amer Physicians 103:229-235
13. McDonald KM, Francis GS, Matthews J, Hunter D, Cohn JN (1993) Long-term oral nitrate therapy prevents chronic ventricular remodeling in the dog. J Am Coll Cardiol 21:514-522
14. McDonald KM, Rector T, Carlyle PF, Francis GS, Cohn JN (1994) Angiotensin-converting enzyme inhibition and beta-adrenoceptor blockade regress established ventricular remodeling in a canine model of discrete myocardial damage. J Am Coll Cardiol 24:1762-1768
15. The SOLVD Investigators (1992) Effect of enalapril on mortality and the development of heart failure in asymptomatic patients with reduced left ventricular ejection fractions. N Engl J Med 327:685-691
16. Waagstein F, Hjalmarson A, Varnauskas E, Wallentin I (1975) Effect of chronic beta-adrenergic receptor blockade in congestive cardiomyopathy. Br Heart J 137:1022-1036
17. Bristow MR, Gilbert EM, Abraham WT, Adams KF, Fowler MB, Hershberger RE et al. for the MOCHA Investigators (1996) Carvedilol produces dose-related improvements in left ventricular function and survival in subjects with chronic heart failure. Circulation 94:2807-2816
18. Gogia H, Mehra A, Parikh S, Raman M, Uppal JA, Johnson JV, Elkayam U (1995) Prevention of tolerance to hemodynamic effects of nitrates with concomitant use of hydralazine in patients with chronic heart failure. J Am Coll Cardiol 26:1575-1580
19. Muenzel T, Kurz S, Rajagopalan S, Martin T, Berrington WR, Thompson JA, Fruman BA, Harrison DG (1996) Hydralazine prevents nitroglycerin tolerance by inhibiting activation of a membrane-bound NADH oxidase. J Clin Invest 98:1465-1470
20. Packer M, Gheorghiade M, Young JB, Constantini PJ, Adams KF, Cody RJ, Smith LK, Van Voorhees L, Gourey LA, Jolly MK for the RADIANCE Study (1993) Withdrawal of digoxin from patients with chronic heart failure treated with angiotensin-converting enzyme inhibitors. N Engl J Med 329:1-7
21. The Digitalis Investigation Group (1997) The effect of digoxin on mortality and morbidity in patients with heart failure. N Engl J Med 336:525-533
22. Packer M, Carver JR, Rodeheffer RJ, Ivanhoe RJ, Di Bianco R, Zeldis SM, et al for the PROMISE Study Research Group (1991) Effect of oral milrinone on mortality in severe chronic heart failure. N Engl J Med 325:1468-1475
23. Rector TS, Tschumperlin LK, Kubo SH, Bank AJ, Francis GS, McDonald KM, Keeler CA, Silver MA (1995) Use of the Living with Heart Failure Questionnaire to ascertain patients' perspectives on improvement in quality of life versus risk of drug-induced death. J Cardiol Failure 1:201-206
24. CIBIS Investigators and Committees (1994) A Randomized Trial of Beta-Blockade in Heart Failure. The Cardiac Insufficiency Bisoprolol Study (CIBIS). Circulation 90:1765-1773
25. Packer M, O'Connor CM, Ghali JK, Pressler ML, Carson PE, Belkin RN, Miller AB, Neuberg GW, Frid D, Wertheimer JH, Cropp AB, DeMets DL for the Prospective

Randomized Amlodipine Survival Evaluation Study Group (1996) The effect of amlodipine on morbidity and mortality in severe chronic heart failure. N Engl J Med 335:1107-1114

26. Doval HC, Nul DR, Grancelli H, Perrone SV, Bortman GR, Curiel R for Grupo de Estudio de la Sobrevida en la Insufficiencia Cardiaca en Argentina (GESICA) (1994) Randomised trial of low-dose amiodarone in severe congestive heart failure. Lancet 344:493-498

27. Singh SN, Fletcher RD, Gross Fisher SG, et al. (1995) Amiodarone in patients with congestive heart failure and asymptomatic ventricular arrhythmia. N Engl J Med 333:77-82

Treatment of Dilated Cardiomyopathies with β-adrenergic Blocking Agents

M.R. Bristow

Introduction

Anti-adrenergic therapy with β-adrenergic blocking agents has proved to be effective in the medical treatment of various dilated cardiomyopathies, including idiopathic, valvular and ischemic subtypes. This report will summarize the effects of β-blocker treatment on the dilated cardiomyopathy phenotype, as well as on clinical parameters.

Rationale for the Use of β-Blocking Agents in Chronic Heart Failure

The rationale for the use of β-blocking agents is simply that the chronically elevated cardiac adrenergic drive that characterizes chronic heart failure produces harmful biologic effects, which can be prevented by competitive antagonists of norepinephrine. Figure 1 summarizes some of these effects,

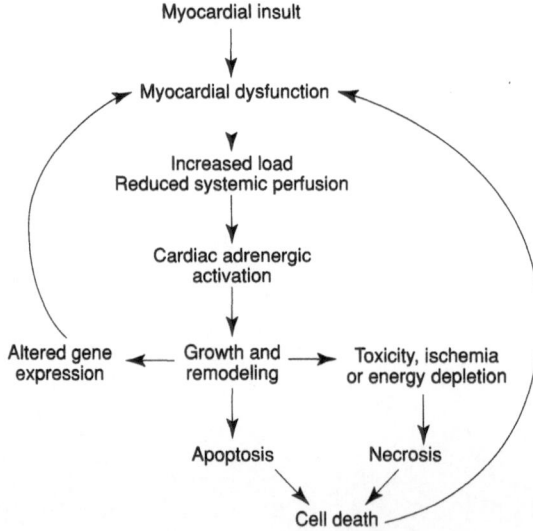

Fig. 1. Central role of cardiac adrenergic activation in producing adverse biologic effects which lead to progressive myocardial dysfunction, resulting in increased adrenergic activation

including exacerbation of ischemia [1], direct cardiotoxicity [2], induction of apoptosis [3-5], promotion of hypertrophy [6-8], and changes in myocardial gene expression that reduce contractile function [9,10].

Effects of β-Blocker Treatment on Ventricular Function

The most striking and consistent effect of β-blocking agents on the dilated cardiomyopathy phenotype is improvement in intrinsic systolic function [11]. Although the initial effect of β-blocking agents in chronic heart failure is to depress ventricular function by withdrawing the heart from ß-adrenergic support, after 2-3 months of treatment systolic function begins to improve [11]. An improvement in left ventricular (LV) function by β-blocking agents in chronic heart failure was first observed over 20 years ago in uncontrolled trials [12] and in 1990 in a placebo-controlled trial [13]. In that trial the ß-blocker/vasodilator bucindolol was shown to be superior to placebo in improving LV ejection fraction and other indices of LV performance [13]. Since then, more than 2000 patients with chronic heart failure from systolic dysfunction have been treated with β-blocking agents in placebo-controlled trials in which LV function has been measured. Without exception, in every study carried out for more than one month, LV ejection fraction (LVEF) increased with β-blocker therapy when compared to LVEF in the placebo group [11]. Most importantly, three human [14-16] and two animal studies [17,18] using several different β-blocking agents have shown that the

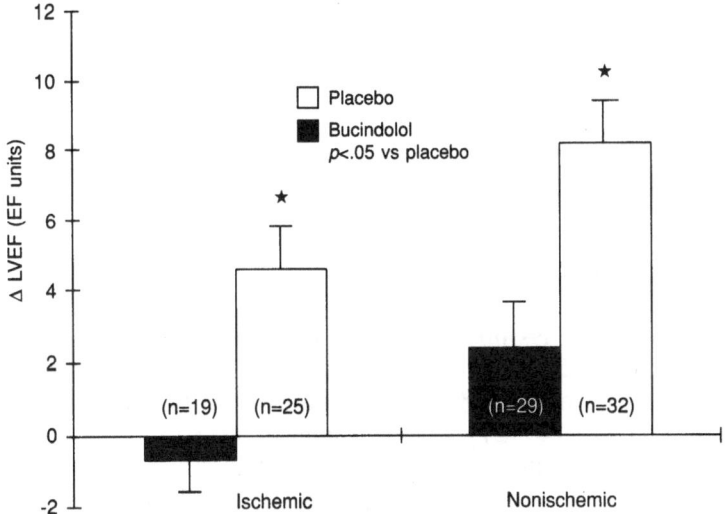

Fig. 2. Effects of 3 months treatment with bucindolol (200 mg/d) or placebo on left ventricular ejection fraction (LVEF) (3 month value minus baseline value) in ischemic vs non-ischemic cardiomyopathy

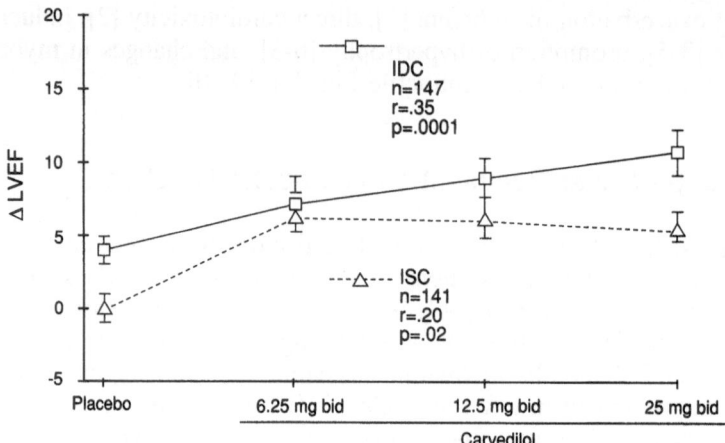

Fig. 3. Changes in left ventricular ejection fraction (ΔLVEF) according to ischemic/nonischemic etiology of dilated cardiomyopathy. Data from the MOCHA trial. Data are expressed as mean ± SEM

improvement in ventricular function is due to increased intrinsic systolic function, apparently due to enhanced cardiac myocyte contractility [18].

Several studies [19, 20] have suggested that β-blocking agents produce a quantitatively greater degree of improvement in LV function in idiopathic dilated (or "nonischemic dilated") cardiomyopathy compared to ischemic cardiomyopathy. Woodley et al [19] were the first to report this phenomenon, using bucindolol. However, a later and larger trial with bucindolol did not confirm this finding [21]. When the entire bucindolol Phase II trial data base is examined, a trend towards a greater degree of improvement in LV function is noted in idiopathic dilated vs. ischemic cardiomyopathy (Fig. 2), but some of the difference is in the greater placebo effect in the former subgroup. In the MOCHA trial [20] and the other U.S. carvedilol studies [22], a strong trend towards a greater quantitative effect in nonischemic vs. ischemic cardiomyopathy was noted (Fig. 3).

Effects of β–blocking Agents on Remodeling and Ventricular Geometry

In subjects with LV dysfunction β-adrenergic blocking agents prevent LV dilatation and remodeling [21, 23-25]. Interestingly, as subjects are treated over longer periods of time, β-blocking agents exert favorable effects on LV mass and geometry [26, 27]. Over a three-month period metoprolol treatment was associated with a reduction in LV volumes and improved LV function, but LV mass did not change [26]. However, by 18 months of treatment LV mass had regressed, and LV shape had became more elliptical [26]. This was the first demonstration that reversal of remodeling is possible in chronic heart failure. Similar results have recently been observed with the 3rd-generation ß-blocker carvedilol [27]. When compared to placebo, LV mass was significantly reduced after 4 months of treatment and the sphericity index was significantly increased (became more elongate) after 12 months of carvedilol therapy [27].

The relationship between the improvement in intrinsic myocardial function and reversal of remodeling associated with β-blocker treatment of chronic heart failure is interesting, as it appears that the improvement in function precedes the anti-remodeling effect [11]. In other words, it is possible that intrinsic myocyte dysfunction precedes remodeling, which apparently occurs in an attempt to stabilize cardiac output by increasing stroke volume. It is as if, when intrinsic myocardial function is improved, a larger end diastolic volume is no longer needed to maintain stroke volume, and remodeling then adaptively reverses. These events clearly need more vigorous investigation in the failing heart, particularly the relationships of reversal by antiadrenergic therapy. For the present, the data support only a relationship between myocyte dysfunction and remodeling, such that the presence of one will promote the other. The relationship between β-blocker improvement in LV function and reversal of remodeling is shown in Figure 4.

Clinical Effects of β-Blocking Agents on Subjects with Chronic Heart Failure from Dilated Cardiomyopathies.

It might be expected that the above salutary effects on myocardial function and geometry, which amount to an improvement in the biologic properties of the failing heart, would be accompanied by a substantial favorable effect on the natural history of heart failure [11]. As discussed below, this has proven to be the case for several clinical endpoints, including heart failure symptoms and hospitalizations. What has not been conclusively demonstrated is a favorable effect on mortality. Studies with the 2nd-generation compounds metoprolol and bisoprolol support such a favorable effect, since in clinical trials these compounds have been associated with reductions in mortality (by 20%,

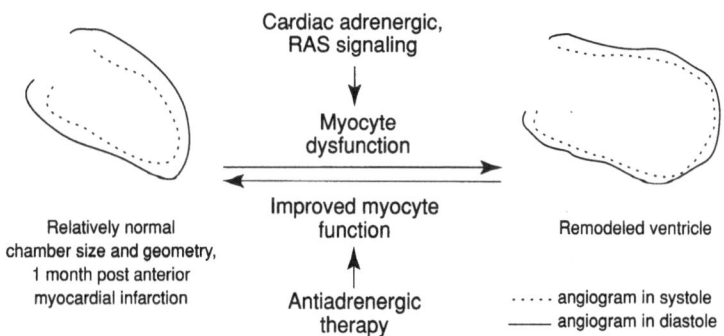

Fig. 4. Relationship between changes in myocyte and chamber remodeling, and effects of the adrenergic and renin angiotensin (RAS) systems on chamber remodeling

bisoprolol [28], or mortality and morbidity (by 35%, metoprolol [29]). However, because these trials were powered on unrealistic effect sizes, in neither case was the result statistically significant comparing the β-blocker arm to the placebo group. Nevertheless, the results are encouraging and follow-up, properly powered trials are underway with both agents.

The first individual clinical trial to demonstrate a reduction in mortality by a β-blocking agent was the "MOCHA" Trial [20]. Although this trial was not designed as a survival trial, it nevertheless demonstrated a marked reduction

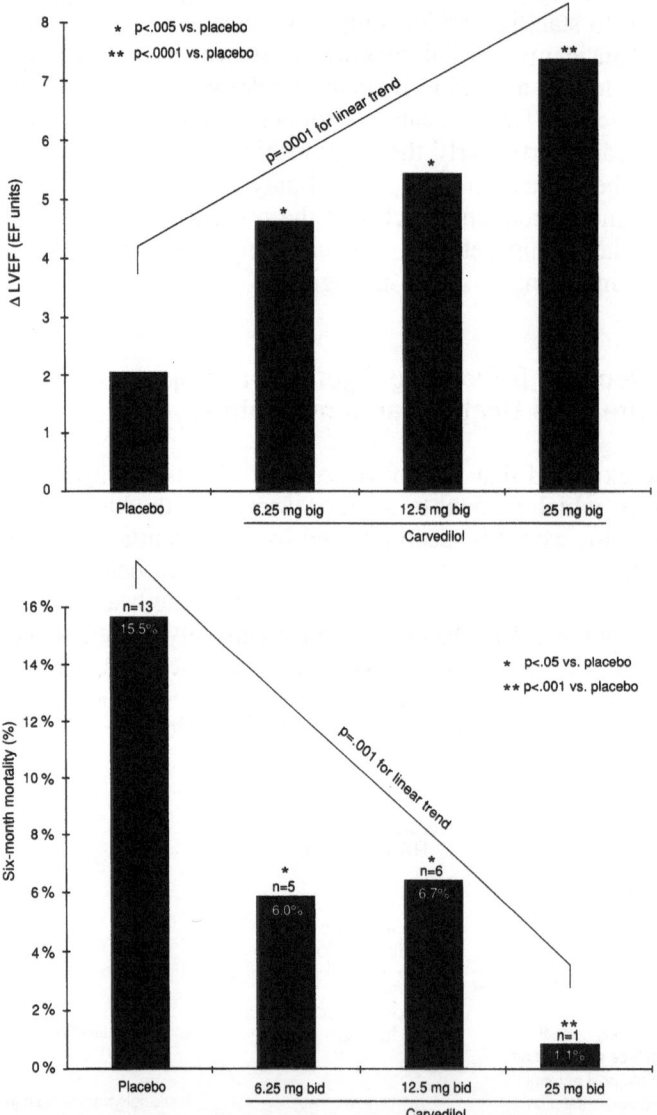

Fig. 5 - Carvedilol treatment was associated with a dose-related increase in LV ejection fraction (ΔLVEF) (*upper panel*) and also with a dose-related, near mirror-image reduction in mortality (*lower panel*)

in mortality (by 73%) over 6 months of follow-up in subjects with symptomatic heart failure from ischemic or nonischemic cardiomyopathy treated with the 3rd-generation β-blocker carvedilol [20]. Moreover, as shown in Figure 5 the reduction in mortality was dose-related, and agreed with a dose-related 'mirror image" improvement in LV function in patients treated with carvedilol. Importantly, sudden death was lowered in carvedilol treated subjects, something that has not been accomplished previously in placebo-controlled chronic heart failure trials. These data agree with results in the three other U.S. carvedilol trials, which were collectively analyzed with the MOCHA results for purposes of effects on mortality [30]. The data are also consistent with the hypothesis that 3rd-generation compounds, or carvedilol *per se,* produce more beneficial effects on the natural history of heart failure than do 2nd-generation compounds, an issue which is now being directly tested in the ongoing "COMET" trial of carvedilol vs metoprolol.

Despite these encouraging results, it should be noted that there has yet to be completed a properly powered, placebo-controlled long-term survival trial that demonstrates a reduction in mortality with a β-blocking agent. However, three such trials are underway (with metoprolol, bisoprolol and bucindolol), and the hope is that these trials will definitively demonstate the mortality-reducing benefit of β-blocking agents in chronic heart failure.

It is clear that β-blocker therapy can reduce symptoms and lower heart failure morbidity. The first placebo-controlled trial that demonstrated an improvement in symptoms was reported by Engelmeir et al, in idiopathic dilated cardiomyopathy using metoprolol [31]. Since that report multiple small and medium-sized trials have noted an improvement in heart failure symptoms, with metoprolol [29], bucindolol [21, 32] or carvedilol [33-36] as the active treatment. Both metoprolol [29] and carvedilol [20, 35, 36] have reduced hospitalizations in medium-sized clinical trials, and this effect was instrumental in the FDA approval of carvedilol. The reduction in hospitalizations obviously translates into a major reduction in the cost of caring for chronic heart failure patients, as this is the biggest single economic factor associated with this disorder [37]. Additionally, in idiopathic dilated cardiomyopathy, metoprolol has been shown to markedly lower the transplantation requirement. For this reason, all eligible idiopathic dilated cardiomyopathy subjects should receive a trial of β-blockade before being listed for transplant.

The effects of β-blocking agents on exercise tolerance have been mixed. In one small [31] and one medium-sized [29] trial metoprolol has improved maximal exercise time, but it has failed to do so in another small trial where the dose was slightly higher [38]. The 3rd-generation, nonselective β-blocker/vasodilator agents bucindolol and carvedilol have in general not improved maximal exercise time [20, 21, 35] but in smaller trials have tended to improve submaximal exercise time [33-35]. The reason β-blocking agents do not improve maximal exercise tolerance is almost certainly their inhibition of maximal heart rate [21] upon which the heart failure patient is dependent to increase cardiac output [39]. This failure to improve maximal exercise tolerance is not a drawback to the use of β-blocking agents in chronic heart failure, since patients feel better and tend to have improved submaximal exercise time, which correlates better with tasks of daily living.

Summary

β-blocking agents are a promising "new" treatment for dilated cardiomyopathies. Because their short-term use produces myocardial depression this treatment was originally thought by many to be counter-intuitive, and it has taken 25 years for this therapy to reach regulatory agency and physician approval. As further data is gathered, and better tolerated or more efficacious agents are developed, β-blocker therapy will likely become a cornerstone in the treatment of dilated cardiomyopathies.

Acknowledgement. This work was supported by NIH R01 HL48013.

References

1. Epstein SE, Braunwald E (1968) Inhibition of the adrenergic nervous system in the treatment of angina pectoris. Med Clin North Am 52:1031-1039
2. Mann DL, Kent RL, Parsons B, Cooper IV G (1992) Adrenergic effects on the biology of the adult mammalian cardiocyte. Circulation 85:790-804
3. Matsui T, Hajjar RJ, Kang JX, Rosenzweig A (1997) Norepinephrine directly induces apoptosis in neonatal rat myocytes. J Am Coll Cardiol 29 [Suppl 2]:230A
4. Communal C, Singh K, Pimental DR, Colucci WS (1997) The β-adrenergic pathway mediates norepinephrine-stimulated apoptosis in vitro in adult rat cardiac myocytes. Circulation 96 [Suppl I]:117
5. Geng YJ, Ishikawa Y, Vatner DE, Wagner TE, Bishop SP, Vatner SF, Homcy CJ (1996) Overexpression of Gsα accelerates programmed death (apoptosis) of myocardiocytes in transgenic mice. Circulation [Suppl 1] 94:1640
6. Bishopric NH, Sato B, Webster KA (1992) β-adrenergic regulation of a myocardial actin gene via a cyclic AMP-independent pathway. J Biol Chem 267:20932-20936
7. Kariya K, Karns LR, Simpson PC (1991) Expression of a constitutively activated mutant of the β-isozyme of protein kinase C in cardiac myocytes stimulates the promoter of the β-myosin heavy chain isogene. J Biol Chem 266: 10023-10026
8. Iwaki K, Sukhatme VP, Shubeita HE, Chien KR (1990) α- and β-adrenergic stimulation induces distinct patterns of immediate early gene expression in neonatal rat myocardial cells. J Biol Chem 265:13809-13817
9. Lowes BD, Minobe WA, Abraham WT, Rizeq MN, Bohlmeyer TJ, Quaife RA, Roden RL, Dutcher DL, Robertson AD, Voelkel NF, Badesch DB, Groves BM, Gilbert EM, Bristow MR (1997) Changes in gene expression in the intact human heart: down-regulation of α-myosin heavy chain in hypertrophied, failing ventricular myocardium. J Clin Invest 100:2315-2324
10. Bristow MR, Gilbert EM, Lowes BD, Minobe W, Shakar S, Quaife RA, Abraham WT (1997) Changes in myocardial gene expression associated with β-blocker-related improvement in ventricular systolic function. Circulation 96 [Suppl I]:92
11. Eichhorn EJ, Bristow MR (1996) Medical therapy can improve the biologic properties of the chronically failing heart: A new era in the treatment of heart failure. Circulation 94:2285-2296
12. Waagstein F, Hjalmarson A, Varnauskas E, Wallentin I (1975) Effect of chronic beta-adrenergic receptor blockade in congestive cardiomyopathy. Br Heart J 37:1022-1036
13. Gilbert EM, Anderson JL, Deitchman D, Yanowitz FG, O'Connell JB, Renlund DG, Bartholomew M, Mealey PC, Larrabee P, and Bristow MR (1990) Chronic β-blocker-vasodilator therapy improves cardiac function in idiopathic dilated cardiomyopathy: A double-blind, randomized study of bucindolol versus placebo. Am J Med 88:223-229

14. Eichhorn EJ, Bedotto JB, Malloy CR, Hatfield B, Deitchman D, Brown M, Willard JE, Grayburn PA (1990) Effect of beta-adrenergic blockade on myocardial function and energetics in congestive heart failure: improvements in hemodynamic, contractile, and diastolic performance with bucindolol. Circulation 82:473-483

15. Wisenbaugh T, Katz I, Davis J, Essop R, Skoularigis J, Middlemost S, Rothlisberger C, Skudicky D, Sareli P (1993) Long-term (3 month) effects of a new beta-blocker (nebivolol) on cardiac performance in dilated cardiomyopathy. J Am Coll Calrdiol 21:1094-1100

16. Eichhorn EJ, Heesch CM, Barnett JH, Alvarez LG, Fass SM, Grayburn PA, Hatfield BA, Marcoux LG, Malloy CR (1994) Effect of metoprolol on myocardial function and energetics in patients with non-ischemic dilated cardiomyopathy: A randomized, double-blind, placebo-controlled study. J Am Coll Cardiol 24:1310-1320

17. Glass MG, Fueihan F, Liao R, Lincolf AM, Chapados R, Hamlin R, Apstein CS, Allen PD, Ingwall JS, Hajjar R, Cory CR, O'Brien PJ, Gwathmey JK (1993) Differences in cardioprotective efficacy of adrenergic receptor antagonists in an animal model of dilated cardiomyopathy: Effects on gross morphology, global cardiac function, and twitch force. Circ Res 73:1077-1089

18. Tsutsui H, Spinale FG, Nagatsu M, Sehmid PG, Ishihara K, DeFreyte G, Cooper G, Carabello BA (1994), Effects of chronic β-adrenergic blockade on the left ventricular and cardiocyte abnormalities of chronic canine mitral regurgitation. J Clin Invest 93:2639-2648

19. Woodley SL, Gilbert EM, Anderson JL, O'Connell JB, Deitchman D, Yanowitz FG, Mealey PC, Volkman K, Renlund DG, Menlove R, Bristow MR (1991) β-blockade with bucindolol in heart failure caused by ischemic versus idiopathic dilated cardiomyopathy. Circulation 84:2426-2441

20. Bristow MR, Gilbert EM, Abraham WT, Adams KF, Fowler MB, Hershberger R, Kubo SH, Narahara KA, Ingersoll H, Krueger S, Young S, Shusterman N (1996) Carvedilol produces dose-related improvements in left ventricular function and survival in subjects with chronic heart failure Circulation 94:2807-2816

21. Bristow MR, O'Connell JB, Gilbert EM, French WJ, Leatherman G, Kantrowitz NE, Orie J, Smucker M, Marshall G, Kelly P, Deitchman D, Anderson JL, for the Bucindolol Investigators (1994) Dose-response of chronic β-blocker treatment in heart failure from either idiopathic dilated or ischemic cardiomyopathy. Circulation 89:1632-1642

22. Bristow MR (1996) Effect of carvedilol on survival and hospitalization in patients with ischemic or non-ischemic cardiomyopathy. Circulation 94 [Suppl] I-338

23. Quaife RA, Gilbert EM, Christian PE, Datz FL, Mealey PC, Volkman K. Olsen SL, Bristow MR (1996), Effects of carvedilol on systolic and diastolic left ventricular performance in idiopathic dilated cardiomyopathy or ischemic cardiomyopathy. Am J Cardiol 78:779-784

24. Australia-New Zealand Heart Failure Research Collaborative Group (1995) Effects of carvedilol, a vasodilator-β-blocker, in patients with congestive heart failure due to ischemic heart disease. Circulation 92:212-218

25. Australia-New Zealand Heart Failure Research Collaborative Group (1997) Randomized, placebo-controlled trial of carvedilol in patients with congestive heart failure due to ischaemic heart disease. Lancet 349:375-380

26. Hall SA, Cigarroa CG, Marcoux L, Risser RC, Grayburn PA, Eichhorn EJ (1995) Time course of improvement in left ventricular function, mass, and geometry in patients with congestive heart failure treated with β-adrenergic blockade. J Am Coll Cardiol 25:1154-1161

27. Lowes BD, Gill EA, Rodriguez-Larrain J, Abraham WT, Bristow MR, Gilbert EM (1996), Carvedilol is associated with a reversal of remodeling in chronic heart failure. Circulation 94:I-407

28. CIBIS Investigator and Committees (1994) A randomized trial of beta-blockade in heart failure: The Cardiac Insufficiency Bisoprolol Study (CIBIS). Circulation 90:1765-1773

29. Waagstein F, Bristow MR, Swedberg K, Camerini F, Fowler MB, Johnson M, Silver MA, Gilbert EM, Hjalmarson A (1993) Beneficial effects of metoprolol in idiopathic dilated cardiomyopathy. Lancet 342:1441-1446

30. Packer M, Bristow MR, Cohn JN, Colucci WS, Fowler MB, Gilbert EM, Shusterman NH, for the US Carvedilol Heart Failure Study Group (1996) The effect of carvedilol on morbidity and mortality in patients with chronic heart failure. N Engl J Med 334:1349-1355
31. Engelmeier RS, O'Connell JB, Walsh R, Rad N, Scanlon PJ, Gunnar RM (1985) Improvement in symptoms and exercise tolerance by metoprolol in patients with dilated cardiomyopathy: A double-blind, randomized, placebo-controlled trial. Circulation 72:536-546
32. Pollock SG, Lystash J, Tedesco C, Craddock G, Smucker ML (1990) Usefulness of bucindolol in congestive heart failure. Am J Cardiol 66:603-607
33. Metra M, Nardi M, Giubbini R, Dei Cas L (1994) Effects of short- and long-term carvedilol administration on rest and exercise hemodynamic variables, exercise capacity and clinical conditions in patients with idiopathic dilated cardiomyopathy. J Am Coll Cardiol 24:1678-1687
34. Olsen SL, Gilbert EM, Renlund DG, Mealey PC, Taylor DO, Yanowitz FD, Bristow M (1995) Carvedilol improves left ventricular function and symptoms in heart failure: A double-blind randomized study. J Am Coll Cardiol 25:1225-1231
35. Krum H, Sackner-Bernstein JD, Goldsmith RL, Kukin ML, Schwartz B, Penn J, Medina N, Yushak M, Horn E, Katz SD, Levin HR, Neuberg GW, DeLong G, Packer M (1995) Double-blind, placebo-controlled study of the long-term efficacy of carvedilol in patients with severe chronic heart failure. Circulation 92:1499-1506
35. Packer M, Colucci WS, Sackner-Bernstein JD, Liang CS, Goldscher DA, Freeman I, Kukin ML, Kinhal V, Udelson JE, Klapholz M, Gottlieb SS, Pearle D, Cody RJ, Gregory JJ, Kantrowitz NE, LeJemtel TH, Young ST, Lukas MA, Shusterman NH, for the PRECISE Study Group (1996) Double-blind, placebo-controlled study of the effects of carvedilol in patients with moderate to severe heart failure: The PRECISE Trial. Circulation 94:2793-2799
36. Colucci WS, Packer M, Bristow MR, Gilbert EM, Cohn JN, Fowler MB, Krueger S, Hershberger RE, Uretsky BF, Bowers JA, Sackner-Bernstein JD, Younj ST. Holcslaw TL, Lukas MA, for the US Carvedilol Heart Failure Study Group (1996) Carvedilol inhibits clinical progression in patients with mild symptoms of heart failure. Circulation 94:2800-2806
37. O'Connell JB, Bristow MR (1994) Economic impact of heart failure in the United States: Time for a different approach. J Heart Lung Transplant 13:S107-S112
38. Gilbert EM, Abraham WT, Olsen S, Hattler B, White M, Mealy P, Larrabee P, Bristow MR (1996) Comparative hemodynamic, LV functional, and antiadrenergic effects of chronic treatment with metoprolol vs. carvedilol in the failing heart. Circulation 94:2817-2825
39. Weber KT, Janicki JS (1985) Cardiopulmonary exercise testing for evaluation of chronic cardiac failure. Am J Cardiol 55:22A-31A

The Role of β-Blockers in the Management of Heart Failure: Results of Controlled Trials

R. Dougthy and N. Sharpe

Introduction

Congestive heart failure is a common clinical syndrome, the incidence of which apperars to be increasing. Over recent years there have been considerable advances in the understanding of both the pathophysiology and management of heart failure. However, despite these advances, morbidity and mortality remain high and heart failure is still a major public health problem. In New Zealand there are about 8000 admissions of about 5000 patients each year with heart failure, or the equivalent of 330 hospital beds being occcupied all year, every year by patients with heart failure [1]. Management of heart failure accounts for about 1.5% to 2% of total health budgets in Western countries [1,2].

There are now numerous data from the clinical trials regarding the effects of various therapeutic agents for the treatment of patients with heart failure. Angiotensin converting enzyme (ACE) inhibitors have an established role in the treatment of heart failure and asymptomatic left ventricular dysfunction. They are the only class of drugs which have been shown to improve all aspects of heart failure, including symptoms, exercise tolerance, and left ventricular function as well as reducing hospital readmissions and improving survival [3,4]. Diuretics remain the main agents used to relieve the symptoms of congestion although there are no data regarding the long-term effect of these agents on survival. Clinical research studies have also identified agents which, despite appearing favourable in short term clinical and hemodynamic studies may increase mortality with long term use [5]. Such agents do not have a role in the treatment of most patients with heart failure. The dissociation between short term clinical benefits and long term outcome has served to highlight the importance of reliable mortality data for the approval and widespread use of newer agents in the treatment of patients with heart failure. New agents are required that may be complementary to the ACE-inhibitors and which can further reduce the burden of this disease on both the patients and the health service. The β-adrenergic antagonists (β-blockers) are one group of drugs that may provide further benefit.

Rationale for the Use of B-Blockers in Heart Failure

The rationale for the use of β-blockers in the treatment of heart failure is now well established [6]. Several neurohormonal systems are activated in heart failure, including the renin-angiotensin-aldosterone and sympathetic nervous systems. In acute heart failure these systems provide support for the heart and circulation and activation may be considered compensatory. However in chronic heart failure, activation of these systems continues, contributing to the vasoconstriction, volume expansion and progressive left ventricular dysfunction which is characteristic of chronic heart failure. This "neurohormonal hypothesis" of heart failure progression [7] is central to the rationale for the use of β-blockers in treatment.

Blockade of the activated renin-angiotensin system with the ACE-inhibitors now has an established place in the treatment of heart failure [3,4]. However the sympathetic nervous system is activated earlier and to a greater degree than the renin-angiotensin system. Prolonged and excessive activation of the sympathetic nervous system, especially central cardiac sympathetic activity, has many potential adverse effects, including direct toxic effects on the myocardium [8] decreased coronary blood flow [9] and tissue anoxia from vasoconstriction [10] which may be linked to the genesis of ventricular arrhythmias in heart failure [9]. Consequently, the excessive sympathetic activity in heart failure appears as important as that of the renin-angiotensin-aldosterone system and contributes to the progression of the disease process and associated poor prognosis. Blockade of the sympathetic nervous system may provide clinical benefits which are complementary to the effects of ACE-inhibitors.

Clinical Trials of β-Blockers in Patients with Heart Failure

Traditionally the use of β-blockers in heart failure has been considered contra-indicated because of their negative inotropic effects. The first reports of the application of β-blockers in patients with heart failure were from a Swedish group in the mid-1970s [11,12]. These reports described patients with severe idiopathic dilated cardiomyopathy who had a favourable clinical response to metoprolol. Subsequent reports from the same group suggested that survival was improved in this situation [13], although comparison was with historical controls. Since then there have been 24 randomised, controlled trials of the effects of β-blockade in patients with heart failure (Table 1).

These trials have involved 3141 patients, approximately half of whom had ischemic heart disease as the underlying cause of heart failure with most of the remainder having idiopathic dilated cardiomyopathy.

Effects of β-Blockade on Symptoms

The results from the trials of the effects of β-blockade on symptoms in heart failure have been conflicting. Several trials have reported lessening of symp-

Table 1. Randomised trials of beta-blocker therapy in patients with congestive heart failure

Trial	N	Beta-Blocker	FU	Primary study end-points
Ikram[a] [14]	17	Acebutolol	1	LV function, exercise
Currie[a] [15]	10	Metoprolol	1	LV function, symptoms, exercise
Anderson [16]	50	Metoprolol	19	Mortality
Engelmeier [17]	25	Metoprolol	12	LV function, exercise
Sano [18]	22	Metoprolol	12	LV function
Leung[a] [19]	12	Labetalol	2	LV function, symptoms, exercise
Pollock [20]	20	Bucindolol	3	Exercise, symptoms
Gilbert[b] [21]	23	Bucindolol	3	LV function, symptoms, exercise
Woodley[b] [22]	50	Bucindolol	3	LV function, symptoms, exercise
Paolisso[a] [23]	10	Metoprolol	3	Metabolic and LV function, symptoms
MDC [24]	383	Metoprolol	18	Need for transplantation/mortality
Wisenbaugh [25]	29	Nebivolol	3	LV function
Fisher [26]	50	Metoprolol	6	WHF, LV function, symptoms, exercise
Bristow [27]	139	Bucindolol	3	Dose titration study
Eichhorn [28]	25	Metoprolol	3	LV function
Metra [29]	40	Carvedilol	6	LV function, symptoms, exercise
CIBIS [30]	641	Bisoprolol	23	Mortality
Olsen [31]	60	Carvedilol	4	LV function, symptoms, exercise
Krum [32]	49	Carvedilol	3.5	LV function, symptoms, exercise
ANZ [33]	415	Carvedilol	20	LV function, symptoms, exercise
US MOCHA [43]	345	Carvedilol	6.5	LV function, exercise, QOL
US PRECISE [44]	278	Carvedilol	6	LV function, exercise, QOL
US "Severe" [42]	105	Carvedilol	3.5	LV function, symptoms, exercise
US Mild [46]	366	Carvedilol	6	Disease progression
TOTAL	3141		12.9	

[a] cross-over trial; [b] 23 patients appear in both totals from these two trial reports (but are included only once in the column total); N, number of patients; IHD, ischemic heart disease; FU, follow-up (months); MDC, Metoprolol in dilated cardiomyopathy; CIBIS, Cardiac Insufficiency Bisoprolol Study; ANZ, Australia-New Zealand Heart Failure Reasearch Collaborative Group; LV, left ventricular; WHF, worsening heart failure; QOL, quality of life.

toms and improved NYHA functional class [16-29, 31,32] although others have not confirmed these findings [14, 15, 33]. The Australian-New Zealand carvedilol trial [33], in patients with chronic stable heart failure due to ischemic heart disease, has shown a trend to worsening of symptomatic status after 6 months of treatment [35], with no overall effect on symptoms after 12 months [33]. This study involved a significant proportion of patients in NYHA functional class I at entry into the study and this may partially account for the apparent slight worsening of symptoms early during treatment.

Effects of β-Blockade on Exercise Tolerance

The effects of β-blockade on exercise performance in heart failure have been variable, as with symptomatic effects. Some studies have reported improvement in maximal exercise duration [14, 19, 20, 23, 24, 26] while others have shown no effects [15, 21, 22, 25, 29, 31-33] or even a decrease in exercise performance [14, 27]. Long-term β-blockade attenuates maximum oxygen consumption [36], consequently, maximal exercise testing may not be the most appropriate method for assessing improvement in functional capacity. Submaximal exercise may better reflect limitations in regular daily physical activities in patients with heart failure [37]. Some studies have shown that six minute walk distance improves with β-blocker therapy [25,31,32] although this has not been a consistent finding [33]. It is now recognised that the central hemodynamic abnormalities that occur in heart failure are poor predictors of exercise limitation [38]. Abnormalities of skeletal muscle metabolism and function, of ventilation [39], and of the peripheral circulation [40] are more closely linked with exercise limitation in heart failure.

Effects of β-Blockade on Left Ventricular Function

A recent pooled analysis has shown that left ventricular ejection fraction is increased by about 5 absolute percentage points over 3 to 6 months with β-blocker therapy [6]. Similar effects were also shown in the recent Australian-New Zealand carvedilol trial [33], where patients with heart failure due to ischemic heart disease showed an improvement in ejection fraction of about 5.4% after six months of treatment, which was maintained at 12 months. Such improvement has recently been shown to be associated with reductions in left ventricular end diastolic and end systolic volumes [41] suggesting that β-blockade results in intrinsic improvement in left ventricular function. These beneficial effects occur in patients already on optimal standard treatment for heart failure, including ACE-inhibitor therapy.

Effects of β-Blockade on Survival and Hospitalisation

In March 1995 a trial programme in the United States [34] involving patients with heart failure of mixed etiology was terminated early by the Data and Safety Monitoring Board due to an early reduction in mortality with carvedilol. Entry to the four studies in the programme [42-45] was on the basis of the distance covered in a six minute walk test prior to randomisation. Each trial had different randomisation protocols and secondary end-points but total mortality was a pre-specified end-point for the four trials combined. There was a total of 53 deaths among 1094 patients enrolled in these four trials during an average of 6 months follow up and a 65% reduction in total mortality with carvedilol. This large mortality benefit has not been seen with any heart failure treatment before. While it is likely that β-blockade does indeed have a significant mortality benefit in patients with heart failure, it appears likely that this result was an extreme effect from analysis of a relatively small data set and that plausibly the actual effect is likely to be more moderate.

Following publication of the results from the US Carvedilol Trials [34], opinion has been expressed both for [46] and against [47] accepting the current data as sufficient to warrant widespread use of carvedilol in all patients with heart failure. While the US carvedilol trials yielded a statistically significant mortality reduction, it is possible to examine all the available data on total mortality among all the β-blocker trials. One such meta-analysis has recently been published [48]. In this systematic overview, mortality data were obtained from all of the 24 completed randomised controlled trials. There were a total of 135 deaths among the 1775 patients allocated to treatment with a β-blocker compared with 162 deaths among the 1366 patients allocated to control during an average follow-up of approximately one year. This represents a 31% reduction in total mortality (odds ratio 0.69, 95% confidence interval 0.54 to 0.89, 2 p = 0.0035), and a reduction in mean annual mortality rate from 9.7% to 7.5% [48].

Such overviews allow all the available data to be easily presented and examined but should not provide the basis for widespread treatment recommendations in the community generally. Reliable definitive data on the relative benefits and risks in all grades of heart failure should be available from appropriately powered clinical trials before such recommendations are made. Interestingly, the US Food and Drug Administration approved the use of carvedilol for patients with heart failure in March 1997 on the basis of data from the US carvedilol trial program [34] and Australian New Zealand carvedilol trial [33]. While this "labelling approval" allows carvedilol to be promoted for use in heart failure patients, it does not constitute a clear recommendation or requirement for use.

Clinical Use of β-Blockers in Patients with Heart Failure

Several factors should be considered when contemplating whether to use β-blocker therapy in an individual patient presenting with heart failure.

Overall Effect of β-Blockers in Heart Failure

As summarised above a consistent effect of β-blocker therapy in patients with heart failure appears to be toward improving left ventricular size and function with long-term treatment. This effect probably mediates in part the improvement in long-term outcomes with associated reduction in hospital admissions and improved survival. Symptomatic and exercise improvement are not a consistent effect of β-blocker treatment and these effects should not be a primary expectation with β-blocker use.

Selection of Patients for β-Blocker Treatment

The experience in clinical trials is mainly in patients with mild to moderate chronic stable heart failure (NYHA II-III). Only approximately 100 patients with NYHA class IV symptoms have been involved altogether in these trials. Consequently, if such therapy is to be used, then it should be started when the patients are clinically stable and preferably early in the course of the disease. The primary aim should be that of improving long-term outcomes rather than providing additional symptomatic benefit.

Initiation of β-Blockade

Clinical recommendations for use of β-blockers can be derived from clinical trial application and experience. Patients should be clinically stable and relatively free of signs of overt congestion. ACE-inhibitor therapy should be established in adequate dosages and diuretics optimised to control symptoms and signs of congestion. Most trials have used a 2-3 week phase prior to randomisation during which eligible patients received a low-dose of open-label β-blocker (eg metoprolol 5mg bd, carvedilol, 3.125-6.25mg bd). The aim of this phase was to identify those patients who should not tolerate even a low dose of β-blocker. In the patients who were selected for these trials the tolerability was excellent, with only about 5% of patients being intolerant, mainly due to dizziness or hypotension. This tolerability is similar to that with initiation of ACE-inhibitors, although it should be noted that these were carefully selected patients with stable heart failure who were deemed eligible for the trial after careful clinical assessment by heart failure specialists.

Following initiation of treatment, further titration can continue with the dosage increments at weekly intervals according to tolerability. Possible adverse effects include bradycardia, hypotension, worsening heart failure and atrioventricular block. Signs of increasing congestion may be controlled with adjustment of diuretic dose and do not necessarily imply long-term intolerance of the drug. However, symptomatic hypotension is more difficult and often suggests intolerance. With this graduated approach, 70%-80% of patients should be satisfactorily established on maintenance treatment with the dosages employed in the clinical trials (eg carvedilol 25 mg bd, metoprolol 50-75 mg bd).

Monitoring of β-Blocker Therapy

Generally, patients should be reviewed at 3 monthly intervals, or more often as required. Once on established β-blocker therapy, subsequent deterioration, for example with worsening heart failure, does not necessarily imply intolerance and should be controlled with an increase in standard anti-failure treatment. As is evident, for clinicians to use β-blockers in patients with heart failure safely and effectively, careful monitoring and regular review is required to ensure that the safety and tolerability, that have been demonstrated in the trials under conditions of close supervision, are reproduced.

Selection of a β-Blocker Agent

The vasodilator β-blocker carvedilol has been used in almost half of the patients in the randomised trials. Newer agents possess certain theoretical advantages, although whether these will translate into significant clinical benefits is the subject of futher ongoing comparative clinical trials.

Conclusions

The present role of β-blockers in heart failure treatment appears to be as an addition to standard treatment in patients with chronic stable heart failure, carefully selected and monitored. The aims of treatment are to provide long-term improvement in left ventricular function and in the natural history of the condition, with improved survival and reduced hospital admissions. β-blockers are however not as easy to use as ACE-inhibitors and clinical trial experience is still relatively limited in patients with more severe symptoms and also in the elderly, who represent a large part of the heart failure population.

As more clinical trial data are provided during the next few years from studies now in progress, it is likely that β-blockade will become a more standard component of combination therapy in heart failure.

References

1. Doughty R, Yee T, Sharpe N, MacMahon S (1995) Hospital admissions and deaths due to congestive heart failure in New Zealand 1988-91. NZ Med J 108:473-475
2. McMurray J, Hart W, Rhodes G (1993) An evaluation of the cost of heart failure to the National Health Service in the UK. Br J Med Econ 6:99-110
3. The CONSENSUS Trial Study Group (1987) Effects of enalapril on mortality in severe congestive heart failure. Results of the Cooperative North Scandinavian Enalapril Survival Study (CONSENSUS). N Engl J Med 316:1429-1435
4. The SOLVD Investigators (1991) Effect of enalapril on survival in patients with reduced left ventricular ejection fraction and congestive heart failure. N Engl J Med 325:293-302
5. Packer M, Carver JR, Rodeheffer RJ, Ivanhoe RJ, Di Bianco R, Zeldis SM, et al for the PROMISE Study Research Group (1991) Effect of oral milrinone on mortality in severe heart failure. N Engl J Med 325:1468-1475
6. Doughty RN, MacMahon S, Sharpe N (1994) β-blockers in heart failure: promising or proved? J Am Coll Cardiol 23:814-821
7. Packer M (1992) The neurohormonal hypothesis: a theory to explain the mechanism of disease progression in heart failure. J Am Coll Cardiol 20:248-254.
8. Szakacs JE, Cannon A (1958) Norepinephrine myocarditis. Am J Clin Pathol 30:425-435
9. Bigger JT. (1987) Why patients with congestive heart failure die: arrhythmias and sudden cardiac death. Circulation 75 [Suppl IV] IV-28-IV-35

10. Mancia G (1990) Sympathetic activation in congestive heart failure. Eur Heart J 11 [Suppl A]:3-11
11. Waagstein F, Hjalmarson A, Varnauskas E, Wallentin I (1975) Effect of chronic β-adrenergic receptor blockade in congestive cardiomyopathy. Br Heart J 37:1022-1036
12. Swedberg K, Hjalmarson A, Waagstein F, Wallentin I (1980) Beneficial effects of long-term β-blockade in congestive cardiomyopathy. Br Heart J 44:117-133
13. Swedberg K, Hjalmarson A, Waagstein F, Wallentin I (1979) Prolongation of survival in congestive cardiomyopathy by β-receptor blockade. Lancet 1:1374-1376
14. Ikram H, Fitzpatrick D (1981) Double-blind trial of chronic oral β-blockade in congestive cardiomyopathy. Lancet 2:490-492
15. Currie PJ, Kelly MJ, McKenzie A, Harper RN, Lim YL, Federman J et al (1984) Oral β-adrenergic blockade with metoprolol in chronic severe dilated cardiomyopathy. J Am Coll Cardiol 3:203-209
16. Anderson JL, Lutz JR, Gilbert EM, Sorensen SG, Yanowitz FG, Menlove RL et al (1985) A randomised trial of low-dose β-blockade therapy for idiopathic dilated cardiomyopathy. Am J Cardiol 55:471-475
17. Engelmeier RS, O'Connell JB, Walsh R, Rand N, Scanlon PJ, Gunnar RM (1985) Improvement in symptoms and exercise tolerance by metoprolol in patients with dilated cardiomyopathy: a double-blind, randomised, placebo-controlled trial. Circulation 72:536-546
18. Sano H, Kawabata N, Yonezawa K, Hirayama H, Sakuma I, Yasuda H (1989) Metoprolol was more effective than captopril for dilated cardiomyopathy in Japanese patients Circulation 80 [Suppl II]:II-118 (abstr)
19. Leung WH, Lau CP, Wong CK, Chen CH, Tai YT, Lim SP (1990) Improvement in exercise performance and haemodynamics by labetalol in patients with idiopathic dilated cardiomyopathy. Am Heart J 119:884-890
20. Pollock SG, Lystash J, Tedesco C, Craddock G, Smucker ML (1990) Usefulness of bucindolol in congestive heart failure. Am J Cardiol 66:603-607
21. Gilbert EM, Anderson JL, Deitchman D, Yanowitz FG, O'Connell JB, Renlund DG et al. (1990) Long-term β-blocker vasodilator therapy improves cardiac function in idiopathic dilated cardiomyopathy: a double-blind, randomized study of bucindolol versus placebo. Am J Med 88:223-229
22. Woodley SL, Gilbert EM, Anderson JL, O'Connell JB, Deitchman D, Yanowitz FG, et al. (1991) β-blocker with bucindolol in heart failure caused by ischaemic versus idiopathic dilated cardiomyopathy. Circulation 84:2426-2441
23. Paolisso G, Gambardella, Marrazzo G, Varza M, Teasuro P, Varricchio M, et al. (1992) Metabolic and cardiovascular benefits deriving from β-adrenergic blockade in chronic congestive heart failure. Am Heart J 123:103-110
24. Waagstein F, Bristow MR, Swedberg K, Camerini F, Fowler MB, Silver MA et al. for the Metoprolol in Dilated Cardiomyopathy (MDC) Trial Study Group (1993) Beneficial effects of metoprolol in idiopathic dilated cardiomyopathy. Lancet 342:1441-1446
25. Wisenbaugh T, Katz I, Davis J, Essop R, Skulargis J, Middlemost S et al. (1993) Long-term (3 month) effects of a new β-blocker (nebivolol) on cardiac performance in dilated cardiomyopathy. J Am Coll Cardiol 21:1094-1100
26. Fisher ML, Gottlieb SS Plotnick GD, Greenberg NL, Patten RD, Bennett SK, et al. (1994) Beneficial effects of metoprolol in heart failure associated with coronary artery disease: a randomised trial. J Am Coll Cardiol 23:943-950
27. Bristow MR, O'Connell JB, Gilbert EM, French WJ, Leatherman G, Kantrowitz NE, et al. for the Bucindolol Investigators (1994) Dose-response of chronic β-blocker treatment in heart failure from either idiopathic dilated cardiomyopathy or ischemic cardiomyopathy. Circulation 89:1632-1642
28. Eichorn EJ, Heesch CM, Barnett JH, Alvarez LG, Fass SM, Grayburn PA et al. (1994) Effect of metoprolol on myocardial function and energetics in patients with non-ischemic dilated cardiomyopathy: a randomised, double-blind, placebo-controlled study. J Am Coll Cardiol 24:1314-1320
29. Metra M, Nardi M, Giubbini R, Dei Cas L.(1994) Effects of short- and long-term carvedilol administration on rest and exercise hemodynamic variables, exercise capacity and clinical conditions in patients with idiopathic dilated cardiomyopathy. J Am Coll Cardiol 24:1678-1687

30. CIBIS Investigators and Committees (1994) A Randomized Trial of β-Blockade in Heart Failure. The Cardiac Insufficiency Bisoprolol Study (CIBIS). Circulation 90:1765-1773.
31. Olsen SL, Gilbert EM, Renlund DG, Taylor EO, Yanowitz FD, Bristow MR (1995) Carvedilol improves left ventricular function and symptoms in chronic heart failure: a double-blind randomised study. J Am Coll Cardiol 25:1225-1231
32. Krum H, Sackner-Bernstein JD, Goldsmith RL, et al. (1995) Double-blind, placebo controlled study of the long-term efficacy of carvedilol in patients with severe chronic heart failure. Circulation 92:1499-1506
33. Australia New Zealand Heart Failure Research Collaborative Group (1997) Effects of carvedilol in patients with congestive heart failure due to ischemic heart disease: final results from the Australia New Zealand Heart Failure Research Collaborative Group trial. Lancet 349:375-380
34. Packer M, Bristow MR, Cohn JN, Colucci WS, Fowler MB, Shusterman NH, for the US Carvedilol Heart Failure Study Group (1996) The effect of carvedilol on morbidity and mortality in patients with chronic heart failure. N Engl J Med 334:1349-1355.
35. Australia New Zealand Heart Failure Research Collaborative Group (1995) Effects of carvedilol, a vasodilator β-blocker in patients with congestive heart failure due to ischemic heart disease. Circulation 92:212-218
36. Sweeney ME, Fletcher BJ, Fletcher GF (1989) Exercise testing and training with β-adrenergic blockade: role of drug washout period in "unmasking" a training effect. Am Heart J 118:941-948
37. Lipkin DP, Scriven AJ, Crake T (1986) Six minute walk test for assessing exercise capacity in chronic heart failure. Br Med J 92:653-655
38. Franciosa JA, Park M, Levine TB (1981) Lack of correlation between exercise capacity and indexes of resting left ventricular performance in heart failure. Am J Cardiol 47:33-39
39. Clark A, Coats A (1994) Mechanisms of exercise intolerance in cardiac failure: abnormalities of skeletal muscle and pulmonary function. Curr Opin Cardiol 9:305-314
40. Drexler H (1995) Changes in the peripheral circulation in heart failure. Curr Opin Cardiol 10:268-273
41. Doughty RN, Whalley GA, Gamble G, MacManon S, Sharpe N on behalf of Australia New Zealand Heart Failure Research Collaborative Group (1997) Left ventricular remodeling with carvedilol in patients with congestive heart failure due to ischemic heart disease. J Am Coll Cardiol 29:1060-1066
42. Cohn JN, Fowler MB, Bristow MR, Colucci WS, Gilbert EM, Kinal V et al. for the Carvedilol Study Group (1996) Effect of carvedilol in severe chronic heart failure J Am Coll Cardiol 27 [Suppl A]:169A (abstr)
43. Bristow MR, Gilbert EM, Abraham W, Adams KF, Fowler MB, Hershberger RE et al. for the MOCHA Investigators (1996) Carvedilol produces dose-related improvements in left ventricular function and survival in subjects with chronic heart failure. Circulation 94:2807-2816
44. Packer M, Colucci WS, Sackner-Bernstein O, Liang CS, Goldscher DA, Freeman I et al. for the PRECISE Study Group (1996) Double-blind placebo-controlled study of the effects of carvedilol in patients with moderate to severe heart failure. The PRECISE Trial. Circulation 94:2793-2799
45. Colucci WS, Packer M, BristowMR, Gilbert EM, Cohn JN, Fowler MB et al. (1996) Carvedilol inhibits clinical progression in patients with mild symptoms of heart failure. Circulation 94:2800-2806
46. Cleland JGF, Swedberg K (1996) Carvedilol for heart failure, with care. Lancet 347:1199-1200
47. Pfeffer MA, Stevenson LW (1996) β-adrenergic blockers and survival in heart failure. N Engl J Med 334:1396-1397
48. Doughty RN, Rodgers A, Sharpe N, MacManon S (1997) Effects of β-blocker therapy on mortality in patients with heart failure. A systematic overview of randomised controlled trials. Eur Heart J 18:560-565

Controversial Issues on β-Blocker Treatment: Has Metoprolol an Additive Effect to Conventional Medical Treatment in Heart Failure Due to Dilated Cardiomyopathy?

G. Sinagra, D. Gregori, A. Perkan, A. Di Lenarda, B. Pinamonti, F. Longaro, A. Poletti, D. Chersevani, S. Klugmann and F. Camerini

Introduction

Despite the introduction of ACE-inhibitors and the consequent improvement in prognosis, mortality rates in patients with heart failure remain high, ranging from 10% to 40% depending on severity [1, 2]. Thus additional therapies are required to reduce the morbidity and mortality associated with heart failure.

Both experimental and clinical evidence suggest that activation of the sympathetic nervous system contributes importantly to the progression of left ventricular dysfunction to end stage heart failure [3]. This belief has lead to the evaluation of β-adrenergic blocking drugs in patients with heart failure, in an attempt to interfere with the deleterious effects of prolonged sympathetic stimulation.

Controlled trials have shown that long-term administration of metoprolol, bucindilol, nebivolol, bisoprolol and carvedilol can improve ventricular function and clinical status in patients with heart failure [4-8]. Pooled evidence [9] from randomized clinical trials suggests that β-blockade reduces mortality in patients with heart failure of different etiology. However, many aspects of the clinical use of β-blockers and of the evaluation of trial results still remain controversial or undefined (Table 1).

All the observed beneficial effects of β-blockers in heart failure were obtained in patients already on standard drug therapy for heart failure, that included ACE-inhibitors in more than 80% of patients. This aspect, in absence

Table 1. Controversial or unsolved issues on beta-blockers in heart failure

Which patients should (or should not) be treated?
Can we predict improvement on beta-blockers?
Which compound to choose and which are the optimal doses of beta-blockers?
Should the results of trials be extrapolated to elderly patients?
Do beta-blockers improve diastolic function?
Do beta-blockers improve exercise performance?
Do beta-blockers reduce sudden death in heart failure?
Are we ready for an extensive although cautious use of beta-blockers in heart failure?
Have beta-blockers an independent and additive effect to ACE-inhibitors in heart failure?

of standardized criteria on dosage and time of assumption makes it difficult to extrapolate the beneficial effects due to β-blockers from the effects due to long term treatment with ACE-inhibitors.

The participation in the MDC trial [5] gave us the opportunity to analyze the effect of beta-blockade as additional treatment in patients randomized to placebo and maximal medical therapy, who were crossed to metoprolol at the end of the study.

Methods

Twenty-nine patients with idiopathic dilated cardiomiopathy were enrolled at our center as part of the Multicenter International Trial MDC (Metoprolol in Dilated Cardiomiopathy) between 1987 and 1991 [5]. The trial was a randomized, placebo-controlled, parallel group study of metoprolol on mortality and need for heart transplantation. Patients eligible for enrollment had to be symptomatic for heart failure with a left ventricular ejection fraction $< 40\%$ and were subsequently followed for 12-18 months. The protocol recommended that, if vasodilator therapy was necessary, it should have been started more than two weeks before enrollment. At the beginning of our study, 26 patients were still alive. Eleven out of the 26 patients had been randomized to treatment for one year with placebo and a standard optimal conventional therapy, which included ACE-inhibitors (Group 1). The remaining patients had metoprolol added to their treatment. After one year, at the end of the randomized study, all patients continued the treatment with β-blockers, and were followed for a second year. Therefore the study had an incomplete cross-over design (Fig.1), where the metoprolol group (Group 2) continued to be treated, because of the results of ongoing randomized clinical trials and the clinical evidence of treatment efficacy. The MDC trial proved, in fact, a beneficial effect of metoprolol on the main clinical and instrumental parameters [5].

The statistical model is based on the general methodology for analyzing cross-over designs, but for some restrictions in the parameters. The approach we used in estimating the model is based on the use of the Generalized Esti-

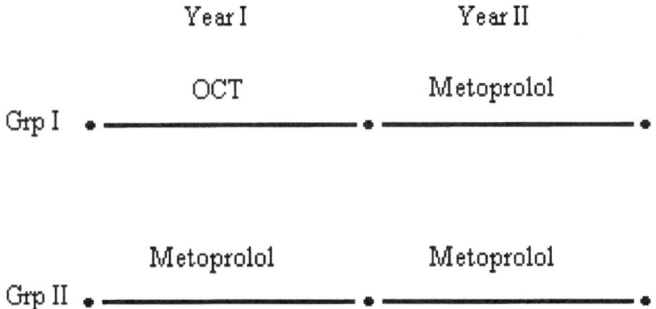

Fig 1. - Design of the study. OCT, optimal conventional treatment

mating Equations [10,11], applied to a continuous response model [12]. The linear predictor is modeled using non-orthogonal contrasts, set up in such a way as to give an answer to some issues of practical interest.

Results

The design is biased with respect to length of the disease at diagnosis (median value 43 months in Group 2 versus 5 months in Group 1), age of patients (Group 1 is younger by about 10 years; median 42 vs 52 years) and NYHA class (class III more frequently represented in Group 2 than in Group 1: 47% vs 27%).

In Group 1 the absolute effect of optimal conventional treatment, with ACE-inhibitors and digitalis being administered to all patients, during the first year period is markedly high, in terms of improvement in overall clinical conditions, right ventricular diastolic function and left ventricular geometry and function. A strong indication of the efficacy of both strategies, in terms of treatment, is given by the fact that patients were classified in lower NYHA classes at the end of the two years. The improvement was further confirmed by the decrease of the congestive heart failure score (Table 2). Group 1 gained

Table 2. Distribution of the parameters for Group 1 (PLACEBO → METOPROLOL) with respect to time and treatment. Numbers indicates median absolute values in patients crossed to metoprolol (first and third quartile are in pedix)

	First Year		Second Year (metoprolol)	
	Base	End	Base	End
Age	$_{33}42_{55}$			
History of hypertension	100% (11)			
Symptoms duration (months)	$_{3}5_{24}$			
New York Heart Association Class 1	0% (0)	73% (8)	64% (7)	73% (8)
New York Heart Association Class 2	73% (8)	9% (1)	18% (2)	18% (2)
New York Heart Association Class 3	27% (3)	18% (2)	18% (2)	9% (1)
Clinical heart failure score	$_{1.0}2.0_{3.5}$	$_{0.0}0.0_{0.5}$	$_{0.0}0.0_{1.5}$	$_{0.0}0.0_{0.5}$
Cardiac thoracic ratio (X-ray)	$_{0.50}0.52_{0.55}$	$_{0.46}0.50_{0.54}$	$_{0.46}0.47_{0.54}$	$_{0.46}0.49_{0.51}$
Mean heart rate (b/min) at Holter	$_{73}86_{93}$	$_{76}79_{83}$	$_{69}78_{84}$	$_{61}67_{75}$
LV end diastolic diameter (cm/m^2)	$_{3.7}4.0_{4.1}$	$_{3.1}3.4_{4.3}$	$_{3.1}3.4_{4.0}$	$_{3.1}3.2_{3.6}$
LV shortening fraction (%)	$_{10}13_{14}$	$_{12}14_{17}$	$_{12}14_{16}$	$_{16}19_{26}$
RV end diastolic area (cm^2)	$_{14}21_{22}$	$_{14}16_{18}$	$_{12}16_{18}$	$_{10}12_{19}$
RV shortening fraction (%)	$_{40}41_{50}$	$_{50}53_{59}$	$_{50}56_{62}$	$_{45}55_{64}$
LV end systolic volume (ml/m^2)	$_{99}129_{143}$	$_{52}79_{129}$	$_{64}71_{93}$	$_{62}74_{94}$
LV ejection fraction (%)	$_{23}24_{27}$	$_{25}33_{44}$	$_{26}33_{44}$	$_{26}37_{54}$
E deceleration time* (msec)	$_{128}136_{145}$	$_{160}200_{209}$	$_{175}200_{212}$	$_{220}230_{255}$
Exercise duration (min)	$_{480}540_{720}$	$_{600}660_{750}$	$_{570}660_{750}$	$_{456}686_{810}$
Minimum heart rate (b/min) at Holter	$_{84}100_{108}$	$_{78}85_{102}$	$_{72}92_{105}$	$_{60}67_{75}$
Serum sodium (mEq/l)	$_{136}141_{142}$	$_{139}140_{141}$	$_{138}140_{141}$	$_{137}141_{142}$
Dosage of beta blocker (mg/day)	$_{0}0_{0}$	$_{0}0_{0}$	$_{0}0_{0}$	$_{138}150_{150}$

LV, left ventricular; RV, right ventricular.
* echo-doppler mitral flow

Table 3. Distribution of the parameters for Group 2 (METOPROLOL → METOPRO-LOL) with respect to time and treatment. Numbers indicates median absolute values in patients continued to be treated with metoprolol (first and third quartile are in pedix)

	First Year		Second Year (metoprolol)	
	Base	End	Base	End
Age	$_{43}52_{59}$			
History of hypertension	40% (6)			
Symptoms duration (months)	$_{12}43_{52}$			
New York Heart Association Class 1	0% (0)	40% (6)	40% (6)	47% (7)
New York Heart Association Class 2	53% (8)	40% (6)	40% (6)	40% (6)
New York Heart Association Class 3	47% (7)	20% (3)	20% (3)	13% (2)
Clinical heart failure score	$_{2}3_{4}$	$_{0}1_{2}$	$_{0}1_{2}$	$_{0}1_{1}$
Cardiac thoracic ratio (X-ray)	$_{0.50}0.53_{0.59}$	$_{0.48}0.50_{0.55}$	$_{0.48}0.50_{0.55}$	$_{0.47}0.50_{0.51}$
Mean heart rate (b/min) at Holter	$_{71}76_{82}$	$_{64}73_{86}$	$_{64}73_{86}$	$_{65}77_{84}$
LV end diastolic diameter (cm/m^2)	$_{3.9}4.1_{4.3}$	$_{3.2}3.8_{3.9}$	$_{3.2}3.6_{3.9}$	$_{3.1}3.4_{3.5}$
LV shortening fraction (%)	$_{8.4}11.4_{13.5}$	$_{12.3}16.5_{23.6}$	$_{12.3}16.7_{23.6}$	$_{10.0}19.4_{25.4}$
RV end diastolic area (cm^2)	$_{16}21_{24}$	$_{12}15_{19}$	$_{12}15_{19}$	$_{16}18_{24}$
RV shortening fraction (%)	$_{24}41_{53}$	$_{48}53_{59}$	$_{48}54_{59}$	$_{49}54_{60}$
LV end systolic volume (ml/m^2)	$_{90}126_{174}$	$_{67}96_{131}$	$_{76}94_{102}$	$_{65}91_{98}$
LV ejection fraction (%)	$_{21}27_{28}$	$_{29}33_{43}$	$_{29}33_{43}$	$_{35}39_{43}$
E deceleration time* (msec)	$_{100}140_{175}$	$_{209}210_{240}$	$_{210}212_{240}$	$_{205}232_{250}$
Exercise duration (min)	$_{450}540_{780}$	$_{600}720_{840}$	$_{600}720_{840}$	$_{510}720_{810}$
Minimum heart rate (b/min) at Holter	$_{79}100_{109}$	$_{75}100_{110}$	$_{75}100_{110}$	$_{68}80_{90}$
Serum sodium (mEq/l)	$_{136}139_{142}$	$_{138}141_{144}$	$_{138}141_{144}$	$_{140}142_{144}$

LV, left ventricular; RV, right ventricular.
* echo-doppler mitral flow

during conventional medical treatment 9 left ventricular ejection fraction points in the first year, and another 4 in the second, when metoprolol was added (from 24% at baseline to 37% after two-years). Also remarkable was the improvement of left ventricular diastolic parameters and the reduction of left ventricular volumes after the two-year period of treatment (Tables 2, 4). The average β-blocker dosage in the second year for Group 1 was 150 mg. In Group 2 (Table 3), a number of patients almost double those of Group 1 was at baseline in functional class NYHA III; however, after two years, the low percentage of patients in NYHA III was the same in both groups. Interestingly, the gradual gain in left ventricular ejection fraction in Group 2, although slightly smaller than in Group 1, continued during the two-year period of observation. The same finding was observed for left ventricular volumes.

The median changes for Group 1 (Table 4 and Figure 2) show that, although most of the improvement was achieved in the first year, during optimal conventional treatment, switching to metoprolol gave an additional gain for left ventricular shortening fraction, ejection fraction and diastolic function. After adjustment, the additive effect of metoprolol appears evident for NYHA class, left ventricular shortening fraction, ejection fraction and right ventricular end diastolic area ($p < 0.05$). These changes reproduce, at least partially, the effect observed in Group 2 during the first year of combined therapy with metoprolol and ACE-inhibitors.

As expected, exercise duration increased significantly after long-term opti-

Table 4. Distribution of the two groups of patients with respect to time and treatment. Numbers indicate median absolute changes between first and second year (first and third quartile are in pedix)

	GR 1 - OCT (n = 11)	GR 2 - Metropolol (n = 15)	GR 1 Crossed (n = 11)	GR 2 - Unchanged (n = 15)
New York Heart Association Class	$_1$ -1 $_1$	$_{-1}$ -1 $_0$	$_0$ 0 $_0$	$_0$ 0 $_0$
Clinical heart failure score	$_{-2.0}$ -1.0 $_{-1.0}$	$_{-3.0}$ -1.0 $_{-0.5}$	$_{1.0}$ 0.0 $_{0.0}$	$_{-1.0}$ 0.0 $_{0.0}$
Cardiac thoracic ratio (X-ray)	$_{-0.047}$ -0.030 $_{-0.015}$	$_{-0.080}$ -0.050 $_{0.005}$	$_{-0.060}$ 0.000 $_{-0.035}$	$_{-0.025}$ 0.000 $_{0.015}$
Mean heart rate (b/min) at Holter	$_{-14.5}$ -9.0 $_{-6.5}$	$_{-8.5}$ -6.0 $_{6.5}$	$_{-21.5}$ -6.0 $_{-2.5}$	$_{-14.0}$ -3.0 $_{9.0}$
LV end diastolic diameter (cm/m^2)	$_{-0.553}$ -0.206 $_{-0.062}$	$_{-0.939}$ -0.300 $_{-0.162}$	$_{-0.333}$ -0.252 $_{-0.079}$	$_{-0.363}$ -0.121 $_{0.117}$
LV shortening fraction (%)	$_{-4.848}$ 0.604 $_{7.180}$	$_{-0.033}$ 5.071 $_{12.808}$	$_{1.408}$ 8.474 $_{10.657}$	$_{-3.127}$ 0.644 $_{3.778}$
RV end diastolic area (cm^2)	$_{-6.0}$ -3.0 $_{0.5}$	$_{-8.0}$ -5.0 $_{-3.0}$	$_{-5.5}$ 0.0 $_{2.0}$	$_{1.4}$ 3.0 $_{5.9}$
RV shortening fraction (%)	$_{-0.43}$ 11.54 $_{20.26}$	$_{3.77}$ 10.00 $_{21.32}$	$_{-10.00}$ -6.49 $_{6.43}$	$_{-4.50}$ 0.42 $_{11.21}$
LV end systolic volume (ml/m^2)	$_{-60.92}$ -18.10 $_{4.63}$	$_{-41.41}$ -20.18 $_{-9.09}$	$_{-22.16}$ -3.71 $_{0.92}$	$_{-27.33}$ -2.11 $_{2.13}$
LV ejection fraction (%)	$_{1.10}$ 8.68 $_{18.18}$	$_{4.08}$ 10.81 $_{18.85}$	$_{2.71}$ 5.60 $_{10.18}$	$_{-0.44}$ 3.49 $_{6.86}$
E deceleration time* (msec)	$_{26.1}$ 60.0 $_{86.1}$	$_{34.3}$ 68.6 $_{115.0}$	$_{-1.9}$ 60.0 $_{75.0}$	$_{-25.9}$ 0.0 $_{25.0}$
Exercise duration (min)	$_{-120}$ 120 $_{150}$	$_0$ 60 $_{190}$	$_{-60}$ 0 $_{36}$	$_{-60}$ -60 $_{20}$
Minimum heart rate (b/min) at Holter	$_{19.0}$ -12.0 $_{8.0}$	$_{-9.5}$ 2.0 $_{15.0}$	$_{-34.5}$ -25.0 $_{-15.0}$	$_{-21.5}$ -10.0 $_{-7.5}$
Serum sodium (mEq/l)	$_{-2.5}$ 1.0 $_{4.5}$	$_{1.0}$ 2.0 $_{4.0}$	$_{-2.0}$ -2.0 $_{3.5}$	$_{-1.5}$ 2.0 $_{5.5}$

LV, left ventricular; RV, right ventricular.
* echo-doppler mitral flow

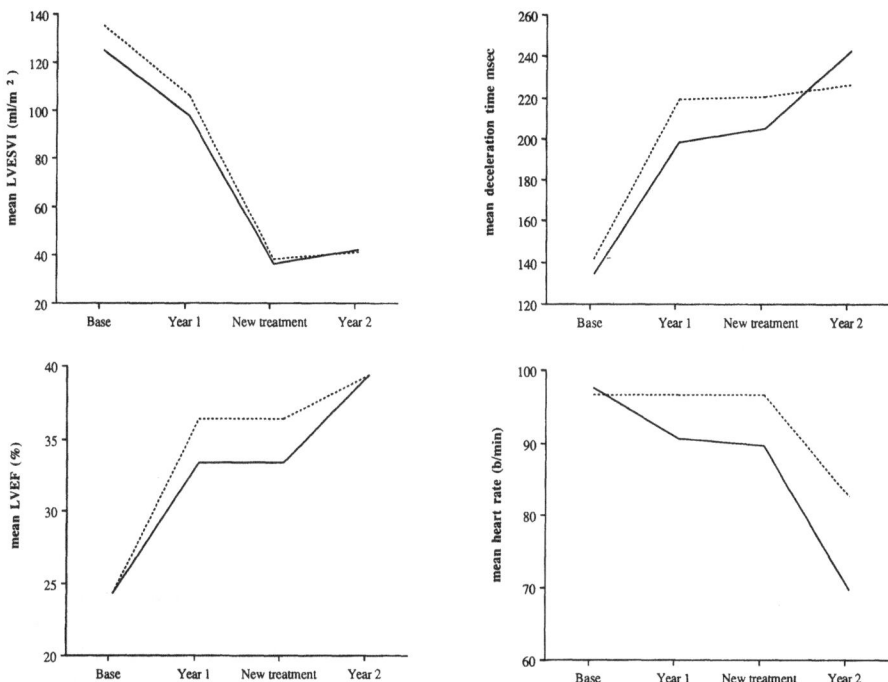

Fig 2. Behaviour of left ventricular end-systolic volume (LVESVI), left ventricular ejection fraction (LVEF), deceleration time and heart rate in Groups 1 (*continuous line*) and 2 (*hatched line*) at each observation time

mal conventional treatment, but not during the different phases of metoprolol treatment, because of the impairment in chronotropic response after β-blockade.

Discussion

Our understanding of the pathophysiology of heart failure has changed greatly in the past few years. It is becoming increasingly clear that abnormal cell growth and gene expression may be more important in the development and progression of heart failure than impaired hemodynamics.

In the latter part of the 1980s and early 1990s, evidence began to appear that certain types of medical therapy might have a beneficial effect on the natural history of left ventricular dysfunction, despite having initial hemodynamic effects that where either unimpressive or even adverse.

Treatment for congestive heart failure with β-blockers has been controversial since Waagstein [3] first reported their beneficial effects in 1975. Randomized clinical trials have shown that β-blockers improve hemodynamics, ejection fraction, ventricular remodelling and myocardial energetics [4,13].

Despite the impressive results of the US carvedilol program [6] data on improvement of survival are still incomplete. A recent meta-analysis [9] of 17 randomized clinical trials is consistent with a beneficial effect on total and cardiovascular mortality. The overall decrease in the odds of death was 31%, with one death prevented per 35 patients treated. The reduction in the odds of non sudden cardiac death (− 42%) was more marked than for sudden death (− 16%). The carvedilol trials were associated with a greater sudden death survival benefit (odds ratio 0.51) compared with the non carvedilol trials (odds ratio 1.03; $p = 0.04$). However, the summary odds ratio of 0.84 (95% confidence intervals 0.59-1.2) did not reach statistical significance and the scientific community should wait for more data on a large number of sudden death events before reaching definitive conclusions.

Previous studies have suggested that patients with ischemic and non-ischemic cardiomyopathies may respond differently to β-blocker therapy [8]. The results of the US carvedilol program [6] and of the meta-analysis by Heidenreich et al [9] found that the etiology of heart failure did not necessarily affect the response to β-blocker therapy.

The identification of predictors of acute response to β-blockers in heart failure still remains a further, unsolved issue. In the prospective and comprehensive study of Di Lenarda et al. [14], according to a logit model, a higher probability of a good response to metoprolol (sensitivity 75%, specificity 81%) was estimated for patients with dilated cardiomyopathy, history of mild hypertension, high resting heart rate, associated with stabilized heart failure or moderate to severe left ventricular dysfunction (ejection fraction 0.20-0.33).

In clinical practice, patients are usually treated with β-blockers after a short period of conventional therapy, which includes digitalis, ACE-inhibitors and diuretics. Therefore the evaluation of the role of the single therapeutic intervention is difficult. The present incomplete cross-over study was designed at the end of the MDC trial [5] to assess whether β-blockers had an additive, independent effect on those variables significant for prognosis. There is an evident limitation to the study, mostly due to the bias in baseline conditions of the patients. This bias however came from the MDC trial, which did not adjust enrollment by time before diagnosis and age. The model-based adjustment helped in reducing the effect, but at a high price in terms of degrees of freedom [15].

On the basis of this analysis, two main conclusions can be drawn. First, as shown in the experience of Hall et al. [16] improvement on β-blockers takes place after a long-term treatment. Our data confirm that the gain attributed to metoprolol continues after 12-18 months. Second, the addition of β-blockers in patients who had been treated for a long time with optimal conventional therapy, including ACE-inhibitors, digitalis and diuretics, allowed a further, significant and independent improvement of all the indexes of well being, and of prognostically relevant parameters, such as left and right geometry and function, and left ventricular diastolic properties [13]. This last conclusion does not authorize clinicians to prescribe β-blockers without concomitant ACE-inhibition, but suggests that in selected patients, such as those intolerant to ACE-inhibitors or those with asymptomatic left ventricular dysfunction and indicators of marked sympathetic activation, β-blockers can be used and beneficial effects should be observed.

In summary, evidence accumulated from our experience and from several large trials strongly suggests that it is appropriate to add β-blockers to conventional therapy. Beta-blockers are much better tolerated and effective when used accurately in selected patients. To confirm the improvement in survival we need further large prospective trials on patients in NYHA class III-IV, using different beta-blockers.

References

1. The CONSENSUS Trial Study Group (1987) Effects of enalapril on mortality in severe congestive heart failure: results of the Cooperative North Scandinavian Enalapril Survival Study (CONSENSUS). New Engl J Med 316:1429-1435
2. The SOLVD Investigators (1991) Effect of enalapril on survival in patients with reduced left ventricular ejection fraction and congestive heart failure. New Engl J Med 325:293-302
3. Waagstein F, Hjalmarson A, Varnauskas E, Wallentin I (1975) Effect of chronic beta-adrenergic receptor blockade in congestive cardiomyopathy. Br Heart J 37:1022-1036
4. Slatton ML, Eichhorn EJ (1996) Beta-blocker therapy for heart failure. Curr Op Cardiol 11:263-268
5. Waagstein F, Bristow MR, Camerini F, Fowler MB, Silver MA, Gilbert EM, Johnson MR, Goss FG, Hjalmarson A (1993) Beneficial effect of metoprolol in idiopathic dilated cardiomyopathy. Lancet 342:1441-1446
6. Packer M, Bristow MR, Cohn JN, Colucci WS, Fowler MB, Gilbert EM, Shusterman NH (1996) The effect of carvedilol on morbidity and mortality in patients with chronic heart failure. New Engl J Med 334:1349-1357
7. Australia New Zealand Heart Failure Research Collaborative Group (1997) Randomized, placebo-controlled trial of carvedilol in patients with congestive heart failure due to ischaemic heart disease. Lancet 349:375-380
8. CIBIS Investigators and Committees (1994) A randomized trial of β-blockade in heart failure. The Cardiac Insufficiency Bisoprolol Study. Circulation 90:1765-1773
9. Heidenreich PA, Lee TT, Massie BM (1997) Effect of beta-blockade on mortality in patients with heart failure: a meta-analysis of randomized clinical trials. J Am Coll Cardiol 30:27-34
10. Liang KY, Zeger SL (1986) Longitudinal data analysis using generalized linear models. Biometrika 73:13-22
11. Zeger SL, Liang KY (1986) Longitudinal data analysis for discrete and continous outcomes. Biometrics 42:121-130
12. Taesung Park (1993) A comparison of the generalized estimating equation approach with the maximum likelihood approach for repeated measurement. Statistics in Medicine 12:1723-1732
13. Eichhorn EJ, Bristow MR (1996) Medical therapy can improve the biological properties of the chronically failing heart. A new era in the treatment of heart failure. Circulation 94:2285-2296
14. Di Lenarda A, Gregori D, Sinagra G, Lardieri G, Perkan A, Pinamonti B, Salvatore L, Secoli G, Zecchin M, Camerini F (1996) Metoprolol in dilated cardiomyopathy: is it possible to identify factors predictive of improvement? J Cardiac Failure 2:87-102
15. Fitzmaurice GM, Laird NM, Rotnizky AG (1993) Regression models for discrete longitudinal responses. Statistical Science 8: 284-309
16. Hall SA, Cigarroa CG, Marcoux L, Risser RC, Grayburn PA, Eichhorn EJ (1995) Time course of improvement in left ventricular function, mass and geometry in patients with congestive heart failure treated with β-adrenergic blockade. J Am Coll Cardiol 25:1154-1161

β-Blockers for Heart Failure: Practical Issues

J.G.F. Cleland

Introduction

Carvedilol, and possibly other β-blockers, are rapidly becoming established as part of the routine treatment for chronic heart failure [1,2]. In clinical trials chronic β-blocker therapy slows progression of left ventricular dysfunction and heart failure symptoms, postpones the need for transplantation, reduces the frequency of hospitalisations and reduces the risk of death. In these trials, β-blockers have been well tolerated, with withdrawal rates similar to that observed in trials of angiotensin converting enzyme (ACE) inhibitors.

However, the results of clinical trials must be implemented in clinical practice in order that patients can benefit [2]. This paper deals with issues such as which patients to target and which to avoid, when to start treatment and how to avoid or manage problems at the time of initiation.

Selection of Patients with Heart Failure for β-Blocker Therapy

Indications: Chronic Heart Failure

β-blockers are indicated for chronic stable heart failure secondary to left ventricular systolic dysfunction. This implies that patients must be investigated by an imaging technique, usually echocardiography, for the cause of their heart failure and that it is inappropriate to treat patients on the basis of a clinical diagnosis alone [3].

Over 90% of patients in the large trials of β-blockers have also been receiving ACE-inhibitors. It is important to emphasise that the benefits of β-blockade are in addition to those of ACE-inhibition. There are theoretical reasons to support a synergistic action of these 2 classes of agent in heart failure. β-blockers suppress plasma renin [1] and therefore may thereby enhance the ability of ACE-inhibitors to suppress angiotensin II long-term. However, it is likely that β-blockers are also effective in patients who cannot tolerate an ACE-inhibitor.

Recent Onset Heart Failure

Studies with β-blockers after myocardial infarction indicate that patients with evidence of heart failure have a high mortality and the greatest absolute benefit from β-blocker therapy [4,5] (Figures 1-2). Patients after myocardial infarction with a tachycardia or third heart sound or with marked but asymptomatic left ventricular dysfunction are appropriately treated with a β-blocker. Patients with cardiogenic shock or pulmonary oedema should have these problems treated first before institution of a β-blocker.

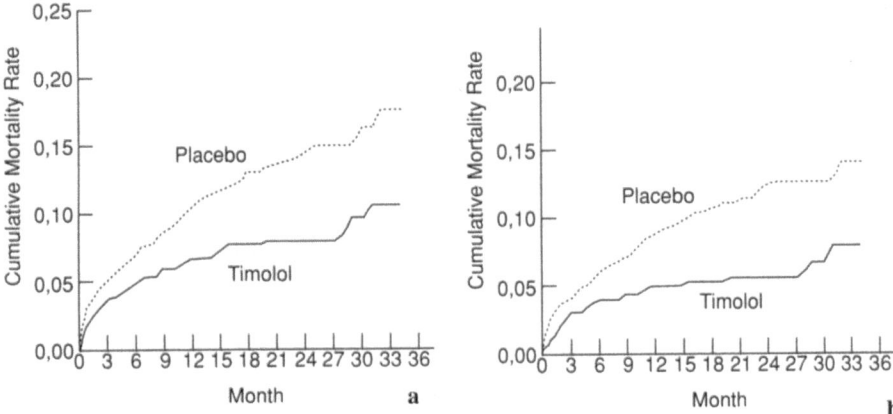

Fig. 1. a. Life-table cumulated rates of death from all causes. These deaths occurred while patients were taking the test medication or within 28 days of administration of last dose. **b.** Life-table cumulated rates of sudden cardiac death during administration of medication or within 28 days of the last dose (reproduced with permission from [25])

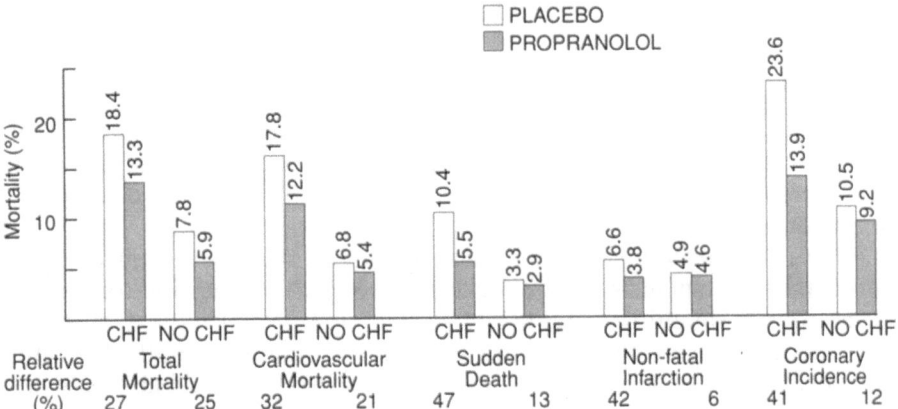

Fig. 2. Effect of propanolol on morbidity and mortality related on the presence or absence of congestive heart failure (CHF) (reproduced with permission from [5])

Table 1. Mortality and mode of death in patients with asymptomatic left ventricular dysfunction

Study [7]	No. of Deaths and (%) Mortality	
	Patients not developing CHF	Patients Developing CHF
SOLVD (Prevention) (2,117 on placebo) [23]	178 deaths in 1477 without CHF (12% of those at risk)	156 deaths in 640 developing CHF (24% of those at risk)
SAVE (active and placebo combined) [24]	248 deaths in 1755 without CHF (14% of those at risk)	174 deaths in 456 developing CHF (34% of those at risk)

Asymptomatic Left Ventricular Dysfunction

The most common cause of asymptomatic left ventricular (LV) dysfunction is myocardial infarction, a condition that clearly benefits from β-blockade [6]. Asymptomatic LV dysfunction indicates a high risk of sudden death and progression to heart failure (Table 1) [7] and β-blockers have been shown to be effective treatments for both conditions. It is difficult to think of a reason not to prescribe a β-blocker for most patients with this problem.

Absolute Contraindications

Asthma

There is only one absolute contraindication to treatment with β-blockers and that is asthma. Many patients with heart failure have chronic obstructive airways disease, but unless marked bronchodilatation is observed with β-agonist inhalation then such patients usually tolerate the introduction of a β-blocker.

Verapamil & Diltiazem

Some patients with dilated cardiomyopathy are treated with verapamil or diltiazem [8] while patients with heart failure and angina may be receiving such therapy. This treatment should be withdrawn for 24 hours prior to the first dose of β-blocker.

There is no specific contraindication to the combination of dihydropyridine calcium antagonists and β-blockers, although the indication for the use of the former should be carefully reviewed. However, if the patient has a low arterial pressure then calcium antagonists should generally be withdrawn [7]. Other unnecessary hypotensive medications should also be withdrawn (eg: nitrates [7]).

In trials, amiodarone patients taking β-blockers appeared to do rather well [9,10] but few patients in the β-blocker trials were receiving amiodarone.

Amiodarone does not constitute a contraindication but does suggest that increased care is required.

Other Relative Contra-indications

Recent Exacerbation of Chronic Heart Failure

Probably the most important common contraindication to a β-blocker is a recent exacerbation of heart failure. It is vital to remember that, unlike diuretics, nitrates, digoxin or ACE inhibitors, beta-blockers are not usually effective as short-term rescue therapy for worsening *chronic* heart failure. β-blockers should not be used in the same way as these other therapies, but should be used when the patient is clinically stable.

In selected patients with severe heart failure requiring prolonged hospitalisation, β-blockers may be utilised but this is a highly specialised use of these agents and β-blockers should only be employed in this way by doctors with expert knowledge.

β-blockers have been given widely to patients developing new onset heart failure after a myocardial infarction and shown to reduce mortality in this setting [5]. It is important to note that patients with incipient cardiogenic shock or acute pulmonary oedema were excluded from these studies, at least until the patient had improved and stabilised with conventional treatment for heart failure. Thus β-blockers should be used, albeit with care, for new onset post-infarction heart failure.

Currently it is not clear how β-blockers should be used for patients with pre-existing chronic heart failure and recurrent myocardial infarction and the balance of their risks and benefits in this setting should be weighed carefully.

Bradycardia and A-V Block

Complete heart block requires pacing and hence the contraindication to β-blockade is removed. Patients with lesser degrees of A-V block are at risk of progressing to more severe degrees and the risks and benefits of β-blockade should be weighed carefully.

Even small doses of β-blockers (eg: carvedilol 6.25mg bd) appear to exert some benefit. A trial of low dose therapy is often appropriate in patients with bradycardia or lesser degrees of heart block. Patients may be titrated to higher doses depending on the effect on A-V conduction.

Recently dual chamber pacing with a short A-V delay has been advocated for the management of heart failure in order to reduce diastolic mitral regurgitation and increase left ventricular filling times [11-14]. The efficacy of pacing in this setting is disputed [12], but PR prolongation has been reported to predict the benefit of short A-V delay pacing. If these studies prove correct, then pacing combined with β-blockade could become common place for patients with PR prolongation requiring a β-blocker.

In patients with bradycardia, consideration should be given to stopping drugs that slow heart rate such as digoxin, diltiazem and verapamil.

Hypotension

A low arterial pressure indicates that additional care needs to be taken with the introduction of a β-blocker to prevent syncope. In addition, as renal function is highly dependent on perfusion pressure in patients with heart failure, it should be monitored. Hypotension is most frequently a problem related to initiation of therapy. As ventricular function improves during chronic β-blockade, an effect that may take 2-3 months to appear, arterial pressure often increases and may actually rise above pre-therapy values in the long term.

Renal or Hepatic Dysfunction

Patients with a serum creatinine greater than about 200 μmol/L were generally excluded from the clinical trials. Patients with renal dysfunction should be carefully monitored during initiation of a β-blocker, especially for hypotension that may exacerbate their renal dysfunction. The β-blockers currently being considered for the treatment of heart failure are excreted predominantly by the hepatic route. Lower doses should be used in patients with severe liver dysfunction, but renal dysfunction generally has little impact on the plasma concentrations of the β-blockers considered for heart failure.

Generally Inappropriate Contraindications

Diabetes

Diabetes has long been considered, like heart failure, to be a relative contraindication to β-blockers. β-blockers can mask symptoms of hypoglycaemia and have adverse metabolic effects including increasing triglycerides. However, studies of β-blockers postinfarction suggest that diabetes identifies a group of patients who benefit particularly well from β-blockers [15]. The landmark studies of heart failure confirm that diabetics obtain marked benefit with the use of a β-blocker.

Peripheral Vascular Disease

Peripheral vascular disease is another traditional contraindication to β-blockers. However, several studies have shown that β-blockers have little impact on claudication distance. β-blockers can be used safely except, perhaps, in those patients in whom the viability of the appendage is in doubt. These patients have a high cardiac mortality and as such even severe peripheral ischaemia cannot be considered an absolute contraindication to β-blockade.

Peripheral vascular disease is a good marker of renal artery stenosis [16]. Any treatment that reduces arterial pressure may precipitate renal failure in this setting, especially if the patient is receiving an ACE inhibitor [7].

Unexplored Indications

Currently there is little data on patients > 75 years of age, patients with NYHA IV heart failure, patients with normal systolic function (eg: possible 'diastolic' heart failure) and the benefits and risks of treatment should be weighed on a case by case basis in these groups.

When to Start Treatment

As stated above, patients with heart failure should be stable for 3-4 weeks before initiating a β-blocker. Beta-blockers should rarely be used in patients with severe heart failure requiring hospitalisation and then only under expert guidance. This does cause some problems as stable patients may not wish to have additional treatment. This is an attitudinal problem (for doctors and patients) that must be overcome. Introducing the β-blocker early in the course of heart failure, when the patient has a less activated sympathetic nervous system and is at lower risk of exacerbation of heart failure or hypotension during the initiation of the β-blocker, reduces the risk of adverse reactions [17-19]. It is also logical to start the β-blocker early, as one of the principal effects of β-blockers is to slow the progression of heart failure.

There is one possible exception to the above rule about initiating in stable patients. Acute onset of heart failure after myocardial infarction indicates a high early mortality and this group of patients, providing they are free of pulmonary oedema or incipient shock, appear to benefit from early treatment with a β-blocker.

Which β-blocker

Bisoprolol and carvedilol have both been shown to reduce mortality in patients with dilated cardiomyopathy [1]. Carvedilol is the only β-blocker that has been shown to reduce mortality in patients with chronic heart failure and ischaemic heart disease. A large mortality trial (COMET) is underway to compare the effects of metoprolol and carvedilol on mortality.

Initiation and Titration (Tables 2-5)

The motto is 'start low and go slow'. β-blockers should be started at low doses (Table 2) and titrated up at intervals of 2-4 weeks. Few hospitals have the luxury, or patients the desire to stay in hospital, for the entire initiation phase nor is it generally necessary. β-blockers are best started in out-patients. Patients should be kept under observation for 2-3 hours after initiation or increase in the dose of a β-blocker, at least until sufficient experience in their use has been gathered by the prescribing doctor. In those rare instances when beta-blockers are started in hospital, the temptation to increase the speed of titration should be resisted.

Even with such a cautious approach 3%-8% of patients may not tolerate the introduction of a β-blocker. The greatest reported experience has been with the initiation of carvedilol. In general few adverse effects are observed

Table 2. Initiation and titration of beta-blocker therapy in heart failure

Agent	Initial dose	Target dose	Titration schedule
Metoprolol	5 mg bd	50 mg tid	Increase at weekly intervals to 5mg tid, 10mg tid, 25mg tid and 50mg bd and then 50mg tid over 7 weeks.
Bisoprolol	1.25 mg/day	5 mg/day	Increase to 2.5mg/day after 2 days Increase to 5mg/day after 1 month
Carvedilol	3.125 mg bd	25 mg bd	Increase to 6.25mg bd after 2 weeks then to 12.5mg bd after 2 weeks then to 25mg bd after 2 weeks (If >85Kg Increase to 50mg bd after 2 weeks)

Table 3. Suggested routine checklist before and after initiating a beta-blocker

Before
• Heart rate, blood pressure and weight
• Urea and electrolytes and blood or urine glucose
• 12 lead ECG
• Echocardiogram (if not done recently)
After
• Check heart rate, blood pressure and weight at every visit
• Check renal function and blood or urine glucose at monthly intervals for 3 months
• If on digoxin: check serum digoxin in older patients, patients on large doses of digoxin and in patients with impaired renal function
• 12 lead ECG once on maintenance dose

Table 4. Practical tips to initiating therapy in selected patients with chronic heart failure

• Exclude patients with contraindications to beta-blockers
• Avoid treating in-patients with recent exacerbation of heart failure
• Initiate treatment in stable out-patients
• Initiate beta-blockers in mild heart failure to reduce problems with initiation
• Educate patients about possible side effects, and to contact medical personnel *at onset* of problems. Tell them that they may feel worse, temporarily, during the titration phase.
• Initiate at the minimum dose. Give after food.
• Wait for 2 weeks before up-titration, longer if side effects
• Adjust other medications as indicated throughout initiation phase to maintain beta-blocker therapy
• Titrate to maximum tolerated dose

Table 5. Outcomes after the initiation of carvedilol

Outcome	Adverse Events: Incidence	Leading to Withdrawal	Action to be taken (initial action + subsequent actions as required)
No Adverse Events	70%-80%	not applicable	Routine Checks see Table 3
Dizziness and Hypotension	13% (33%[a])	~ 0.5%	Wait and see. Give after food Stagger medication Withdraw non-essential vasodilators Temporarily reduce dose of ACE-inhibitor Reduce or do not increase beta-blocker
Worsening of Heart Failure	0.1-2.0% depending on initial severity of heart failure	0.1%-2%	Do not withdraw beta-blocker Do not increase the dose of beta-blocker Increase the dose of diuretic temporarily Reduce dose of beta-blocker
Bradycardia	8% (9%[a])	~ 1.0%	Withdraw other rate lowering drugs Withdraw digoxin with care in some cases Reduce dose of beta-blocker
Worsening Renal Function	2% (7%[a])	< 0.3%	Withdraw non-essential vasodilators Reduce dose of diuretic if possible Reduce dose of ACE-inhibitor Reduce or do not increase dose of beta-blocker
Hyperglycaemia	4% (13%[a])	~ 0%	Manage as for diabetes

[a] percentage with this problem without correction for placebo (ie: 33% of patient may report dizziness going onto carvedilol but 20% would report this symptom on placebo).

with 3.125 mg bd of carvedilol; problems are more likely to be observed with up-titration to 6.25 mg bd. It is not yet clear if a protracted period of treatment (eg: 4-6 weeks) with 3.125 mg bd can overcome this problem or whether use of an intermediate 3.125 mg t.i.d. or q.i.d. dose can help, but these strategies should be explored in a patient who has difficulty tolerating introduction of higher doses.

Target doses of β-blockers were set (Table 2) in the landmark studies and largely achieved. However, it appears that relatively low doses of β-blockers may exert considerable effects and it is not entirely clear that 25 mg bd of carvedilol is clinically superior to 6.25 mg bd. It is also not clear whether higher doses than used in the clinical trials might not be even more effective.

Management of Hypotension

Asymptomatic and symptomatic hypotension are not infrequent during titration and may be more common with carvedilol due to its vasodilator properties. Blood pressure reaches its nadir 2-3 hours after dosing with carvedilol and it is appropriate to monitor the patient for some hours after the first dose at each level of titration.

If hypotension is asymptomatic and has not led to a decline in renal function it requires no specific management other than to perhaps delay up-titration. With time blood pressure will often rise, either due to tolerance to the alpha-blocking properties of carvedilol or due to improvement in left ventricular function.

In patients who have minor symptoms due to hypotension, reassurance and a delay in further titration will often result in spontaneous resolution of symptoms. Administration after food will slow absorption and may improve symptoms. Staggering the dose of β-blocker, diuretic and ACE-inhibitor may also get round this problem. For instance, giving captopril and carvedilol at the same time means that both agents will exert a maximum hypotensive effect at a similar time. If carvedilol is given 2 hours before the ACE-inhibitor their maximum hypotensive effects will not coincide. Similarly patients who have just had a vigorous diuresis may be more susceptible to the hypotensive effects of carvedilol. In patients with troublesome symptoms carvedilol may be given at 8 a.m. and in the evening before going to bed. Diuretics and ACE-inhibitors could then be given later in the morning (10-11 a.m.) with further dosing later in the day if required. Switching to a long-acting ACE-inhibitor (eg: enalapril, quinapril or ramipril bd, or lisinopril, trandolapril once daily) will smooth out the peak and trough hypotensive effects of ACE inhibition and may improve the tolerability of the β-blocker. Such manipulation of therapy is often required only temporarily, and once maintenance doses have been achieved dosing at standard times can usually be resumed.

In patients with more severe hypotensive symptoms vasodilators such as calcium antagonists and nitrates should be withdrawn. If such manipulation fails, then it is appropriate to either accept a lower dose of β-blocker (although doses of carvedilol below 6.25 mg bd have not been shown to have any effect) or to reduce the doses of ACE-inhibitors or diuretics. Although target doses of ACE-inhibitors as achieved in the landmark trials (eg: enalapril 10-20 mg bd) are currently recommended for heart failure, it is possible that lower doses are equally effective. Similarly clear evidence of superiority of low versus high dose β-blockade does not exist, although doctors should strive to titrate patients to the doses achieved in the clinical trials.

Management of Bradycardia

Asymptomatic bradycardia should be managed by reassurance alone, always recognising that excessive bradycardia could manifest itself as increased fatigue or breathlessness. If bradycardia is symptomatic, the need for other rate limiting medications (eg: amiodarone, digoxin, diltiazem etc.) should be reviewed. In patients with mild heart failure digoxin may be stopped; in patients with more advanced heart failure withdrawal of digoxin in the titration phase may expose the patient to the risk of worsening heart failure. If bradycardia develops as a problem in the maintenance phase, then digoxin withdrawal should be considered. If the above are not options, then the dose of carvedilol should be reduced to relieve symptoms. As long as the patient has no symptoms attributable to the bradycardia, then heart rates of 50 bpm or less are acceptable.

Management of Worsening Heart Failure

Increased fluid retention should be sought for by weighing the patient daily. The patient should be instructed to increase the dose of diuretic, temporarily, if they gain more than 2 kg in weight.

For patients with a mild exacerbation of symptoms simple reassurance, control of fluid retention with diuretics and waiting for the benefits of β-blockade to appear usually suffice. The patient should not receive an increase in β-blocker dose until symptoms have re-stabilised. More marked worsening may require a reduction in β-blocker dose and further adjustment of the ACE-inhibitor or the introduction of digoxin.

In extreme cases hospitalisation for diuresis and the use of intravenous low renal-dose dopamine or a phosphodiesterase inhibitor may be required. In patients on full doses of β-blocker the dose should be cut to 25%-50% of target. Withdrawing the β-blocker altogether should be avoided if at all possible, as these patients may then be at high risk of sudden death. Any improvement due to β-blocker withdrawal is often only temporary.

Other Side Effects

Hyperglycaemia

Both selective [20,21] and non-selective β-blockers may impair insulin sensitivity and although carvedilol, by virtue of its alpha-blocking qualities, has been reported not to impair insulin sensitivity [20] more hyperglycaemia was observed with its use compared to placebo in the US carvedilol trials [22]. Patients should have urine or blood glucose checked monthly for the first 3 months. Hyperglycaemia should be managed as for patients not receiving β-blockers. It is not appropriate to withdraw the β-blocker.

Diarrhoea

This is a not uncommon side effect of carvedilol and may improve with time. If marked, it may require reduction in the dose of carvedilol. Other causes of diarrhoea should be excluded.

Renal Dysfunction

Renal dysfunction is usually a manifestation of hypotension in a patient who is already receiving a diuretic and an ACE-inhibitor [7]. If there are no signs of fluid overload (eg: oedema, weight gain) then the dose of diuretic should be reduced cautiously. If this is not effective then reduction of the dose of carvedilol or the ACE-inhibitor, or both, may be required. Serum creatinine should be checked monthly for the first 3 months.

Increased Serum Digoxin Levels

A small increase in serum digoxin occurred in the trials of carvedilol, possibly reflecting a small decline in glomerular filtration rate. In patients at risk of digoxin toxicity serum digoxin levels should be checked monthly for the first 3 months.

Conclusions

Physicians and patients need to understand the time course of the effects of β-blocker therapy. The initial effects are neutral or adverse, and the beneficial effects occur gradually over a period of weeks to months. For patients with moderately severe heart failure only with patience, perseverance and education can patients hope to reap the full benefits of β-blocker therapy. However, in milder heart failure β-blockers can usually be introduced with little difficulty. Early treatment maximises the effectiveness and acceptance of therapy.

References

1. Cleland JGF, Bristow M, Erdmann E, Remme WJ, Swedberg K, Waggstein F (1996) β-blocking agents in heart failure. Should they be used and how? Eur Heart J 17:1629-1639
2. Cleland JGF, Swedberg K (1996) Carvedilol for heart failure, with care. Lancet 347:1199-1201
3. Cleland JGF, Erdmann E, Ferrari R, Hess OM, Poole Wilson PA, Remme WJ, Riegger G, Soler Soler J, Swedberg KB, Tavazzi L, Waagstein F, Dargie HJ, Kjekshus OM, Pouleur H (1995) Guidelines for the diagnosis of heart failure. Eur Heart J 16:741-751
4. Yusuf S, Peto R, Lewis J, Collins R, Sleight P (1985) β blockade during and after myocardial infarction: an overview of the randomized trials. Prog Cardiovasc Dis 27:335-371
5. Chadda K, Goldstein S, Byington R, Curb JD (1986) Effect of propranolol after acute myocardial infarction in patients with congestive heart failure. Circulation 73:503-510
6. Cleland JGF, Ray SG, McMurray JJV (1994) Prevention strategies after myocardial Infarction. London: Science Press
7. Cleland JGF, JJF McMurray, PJ Cowburn (1997) Heart failure: A systematic approach for clinical practice. London, Science Press, pp 1-123
8. Figulla HR, Gietzen F, Zeymer U, Raiber M, Hegselmann J, Soballa R, Hilgers R (1996) Diltiazem improves cardiac function and exercise capacity in patients with idiopathic dilated cardiomyopathy: results of the diltiazem in dilated cardiomyopathy trial. Circulation 94:346-352
9. Singh SN, Fletcher RD, Fisher SG, Singh BN, Lewis HD, Deedwania PC, Massie BM, Colling C, Lazzeri D (1995) Amiodarone in patients with congestive heart failure and asymptomatic ventricular arrhythmia. N Engl J Med 333:77-82
10. Massie BM, Fisher SG, Deedwania PC, Singh BN, Fletcher RD, Singh SN, for the CHF-STAT group (1996) Effect of amiodarone on clinical status and left ventricular function in patients with congestive heart failure. Circulation 93:2128-2134

11. Innes D, Leitch JW, Fletcher PJ (1994) DDD pacing at short atrioventricular intervals does not improve cardiac output in patients with dilated heart failure. PACE 17:959-965
12. Gold MR, Feliciano Z, Gottlieb SS, Fisher ML (1995) Dual-chamber pacing with a short atrioventricular delay in congestive heart failure: A randomized study. J Am Coll Cardiol 26:967-973
13. Linde C, Gadler F, Edner M, Nordlander R, Rosenqvist M, Ryden L (1995) Results of atrioventricular synchronous pacing with optimized delay in patients with severe congestive heart failure. Am J Cardiol 75:919-923
14. Brecker SJD, Xiao HB, Sparrow J, Gibson DG (1992) Effects of dual-chamber pacing with short atrioventricular delay in dilated cardiomyopathy. Lancet 340:1308-1312
15. Jonas M, Reicherreis H, Boyko V, Shoton A, Mondelzweig L, Goldbourt V, Behar S (1996) Usefulness of β-blocker therapy in patients with non-insulin-dependent diabetes mellitus and coronary artery disease. Am J Cardiol 77:1273-1277
16. Choudhri AH, Cleland JGF, Rowlands PC, Tran TL, McCarty M, Al Kutoubi MAO (1990) Unsuspected renal artery stenosis in peripheral vascular disease. Br Med J 301:1197-1198
17. Packer M, Colucci WS, Sackner-Bernstein J, Lang C, Goldschef DA, Freeman I, Kukin ML, Kinhal V, Udelson JE, Klapholz M (1995) Prospective Randomized Evaluation of Carvedilol on Symptoms and Exercise Tolerance in Chronic Heart Failure: Results of the PRECISE Trial. Circulation 92 [Suppl I]:1-143
18. Bristow MR, Gilbert EM, Abraham WT, Adams KF, Fowler MB, Hershenberger R, Kubo SH, Narahara KA, Ingersoll N (1995) Multicenter Oral Carvedilol Heart Failure Assessment (MOCHA): a six-month dose-response evaluation in class II-IV patients, Circulation 92 [Suppl I]:I-142 (abstr)
19. Colucci WS, Packer M, Bristow MR, Cohn JN, Fowler MB, Gilbert EM, Krueger SK, Adams KF, Hershenberger R, Uretzky BF (1995) Carvedilol inhibits clinical progression in patients with mild heart failure. Circulation 92 [Suppl I]:1-395 (abstr)
20. Jacob S, Rett K, Wicklmayr M, Agrawal B, Augustin HJ, Dietze GJ (1996) Differential effect of chronic treatment with two β blocking agents on insulin sensitivity: the carvedilol-metoprolol study. J Hyper 14:489-494
21. Pollare T, Lithell HO, Selinus I, Berne C (1989) Sensitivity to insulin during treatment with atenolol and metoprolol: a randomised, double-blind study of effects on carbohydrate and lipoprotein metabolism in hypertensive patients. Br Med J 298:1152-1157
22. Packer M, Bristow MR, Cohn JN, Colucci WS, Fowler MB, Gilbert EM, Shusterman NH, for the US carvedilol study group (1996) The effect of carvedilol on morbidity and mortality in patients with chronic heart failure. N Engl J Med 334:1349-1355
23. Yusuf S, Nicklas JM, Timmis G, Breneman G, Jafri SM, Duvernoy WFC, Davis SW, Goldberg MJ, Blair J, Mancini GBJ, Johnson T, Luckoff C, Henry G, Wlodkowski MB, Czajka M, Reinstein D, Richards J, Lewis R, Davey DE, et al (1992) Effect of enalapril on mortality and the development of heart failure in asymptomatic patients with reduced left ventricular ejection fractions. N Engl J Med 327:685-691
24. Rutherford JD, Pfeffer MA, Moye LA, Davis BR, Flaker GC, Kowey PR, Lamas GA, Miller HS, Packer M, Rouleau JL, Braunwald E, on behalf of the SAVE investigators (1994) Effects of captopril on ischemic events after myocardial infarction. Results of the Survival And Ventricular Enlargement trial. Circulation 90:1731-1738
25. The Norvegian Multicenter Study Group (1981) Timolol-induced reduction in mortality and reinfarction in patients surviving acute myocardial infarction. N Engl J Med 304:801-807

DDD Pacing in Dilated Cardiomyopathy

D. Gibson

It is well recognised that pacing from a right ventricular site leads to abnormal left ventricular activation, and thus loss of the normal physiological contraction pattern. When a DDD pacemaker is inserted for abnormal atrioventricular conduction, left ventricular contraction is not impaired, so that any deterioration caused by abnormal activation is of no physiological consequence. DDD pacing has been proposed, however, in patients with dilated cardiomyopathy in whom left ventricular function may be profoundly impaired [1]. At first sight, this would seem paradoxical; if benefit were to occur, it is likely to be seen in patients in whom ventricular activation is so abnormal under control conditions that it is actually contributing significantly to the overall impairment of ventricular function.

Disturbances of Activation in Dilated Cardiomyopathy

It has long been known that abnormal activation directly affects ventricular contraction, [2] but such effects have been little studied in patients with dilated cardiomyopathy. Activation can readily be assessed from QRS duration on the 12 lead ECG, which is now automatically determined by inbuilt software in most modern ECG machines. Figure 1 shows a normal frequency plot of QRS duration in 60 patients with dilated cardiomyopathy. Values extend from 75 to 190 ms, but more significantly, the plot is linear, and does not differ significantly from a single normal frequency distribution [3]. There is no evidence of any discontinuity at 120 ms, which would correspond to "complete left bundle branch block", a term probably best avoided in the setting of the complex activation disturbances seen in patients with dilated cardiomyopathy. A second ECG disturbance frequently noted in these patients is the presence of a prolonged PR interval, which is often assumed to be due to concomitant disease of the conducting system.

Mechanical Effects of Disturbed Activation

The overall duration of left ventricular systole, equivalent to the time period over which the left ventricular myocardium develops pressure, is measured

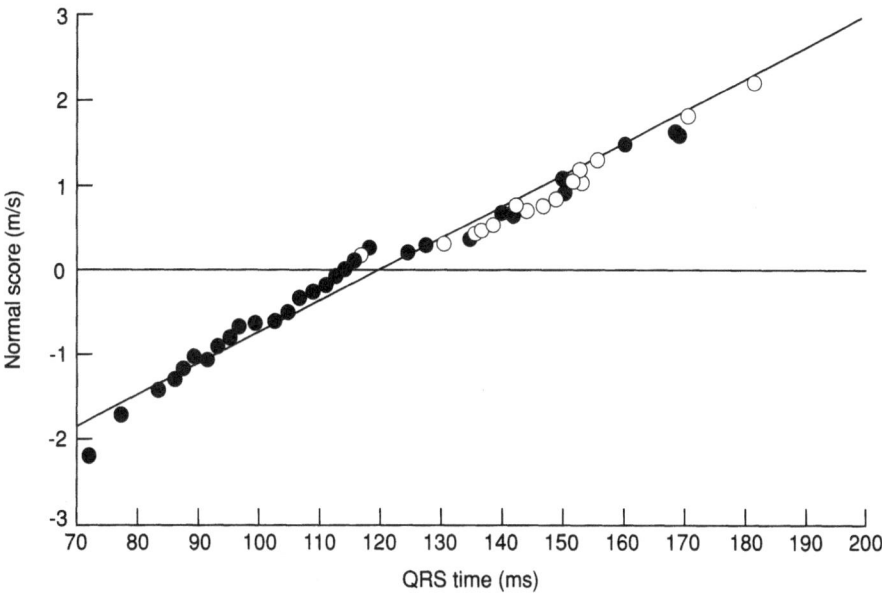

Fig. 1. Normal frequency plot of QRS duration in 50 patients with dilated cardiomyopathy. Note that values are normally distributed as a single population. There is no evidence of any discontinuity at 120 ms, which would correspond to orthodox definitions of complete left bundle branch block

from the high fidelity left ventricular pressure pulse [4]. It has recently been demonstrated that the time course of pressure development is reflected to within 5 ms by the continuous wave Doppler trace of functional mitral regurgitation (MR). Since the latter is frequently present in patients with DCM, it can be used as a simple noninvasive measure of left ventricular contraction time. Disturbances of ventricular activation greatly prolong the MR signal, as shown in Figure 2. Furthermore, while ejection time is unaffected, contraction and relaxation times are strikingly prolonged. This prolongation is little affected by tachycardia during exercise, so that as heart rate increases, left ventricular filling time, the interval between the pulses of mitral regurgitation, is selectively shortened, and may fall to 200 ms or less at rest [5]. On transmitral pulsed Doppler, this leads to the normal E and A waves being lost and replaced by a single pulse (Fig. 3). In order for the whole stroke volume to enter the ventricle in such a short period, blood velocity and thus acceleration must be high, implying a high atrioventricular pressure drop. It was our hypothesis that it was this short filling period rather than systolic function that limited stroke volume. If filling period could be lengthened by modifying ventricular activation, then the time for filling would increase, so that stroke volume would increase and AV pressure gradient fall.

Further electromechanical abnormalities are apparent when the timing of the onset of mitral regurgitation is correlated with the onset of the Q wave in patients with abnormal activation. In a substantial number of such patients, electromechanical delay (EMD), rather than being prolonged, is abnormally

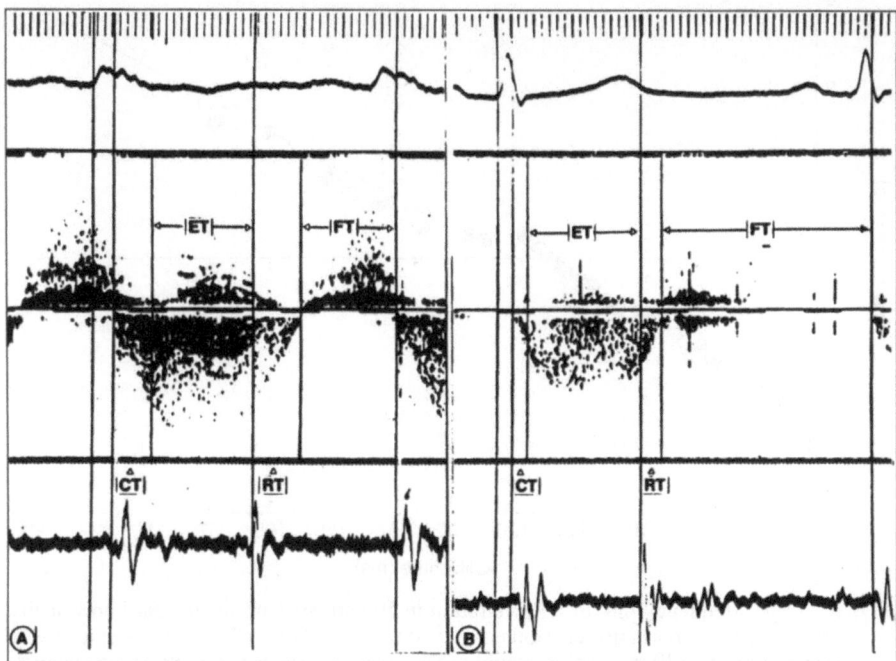

Fig. 2. Effect of ventricular activation on the duration of mitral regurgitation, as recorded by continuous wave Doppler. On the left is the record from a patient with a broad QRS complex, while that on the right is normal. Note that the duration of mitral regurgitation is greatly prolonged in the former. Ejection time is the same in both, but with an activation delay, contraction and relaxation times are more than doubled. Filling time, the interval between the pulses of mitral regurgitation is correspondingly shortened, though heart rate is the same. CT, contraction time; RT, relaxation time; ET, ejection time; FT, filling time

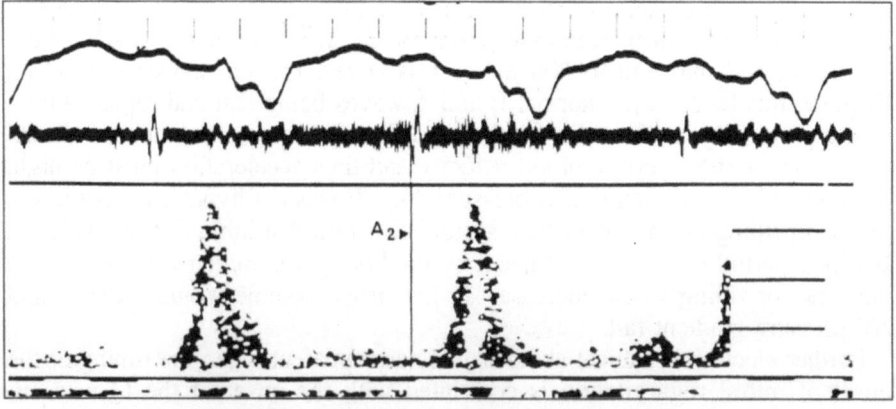

Fig. 3. Transmitral flow pulse from a patient with DCM and a very short filling time (130 ms) due to abnormal ventricular activation

short [6]. Furthermore a short EMD is characteristically correlated with a long PR interval. This combination suggested that the onset of the QRS complex did not represent the true onset of ventricular activation, but that low potentials were present, below the threshold of the 12 lead ECG. This finding was confirmed by signal averaged ECG. Furthermore, detailed electromechanical mapping demonstrated that this early regurgitation arose from contraction in the upper part of the septum. The onset of left and right ventricular free wall contraction were both delayed, suggesting bilateral complete bundle branch block with activation of the whole ventricular mass from fibres close to the AV node. This mechanism is quite different from the assumed activation pathway in isolated left bundle branch block, with left ventricle activated from the right. The ultimate proof of these ideas is to pace such patients from the right ventricle: if the generally accepted idea applies, then there should be no change, but if bilateral complete block is present, then the overall duration of contraction should be shortened. The results are consistent. An example is shown in Figure 4, where it is quite clear that the duration of MR is significantly shortened by pacing. These findings form the basis of our approach to DDD pacing in DCM.

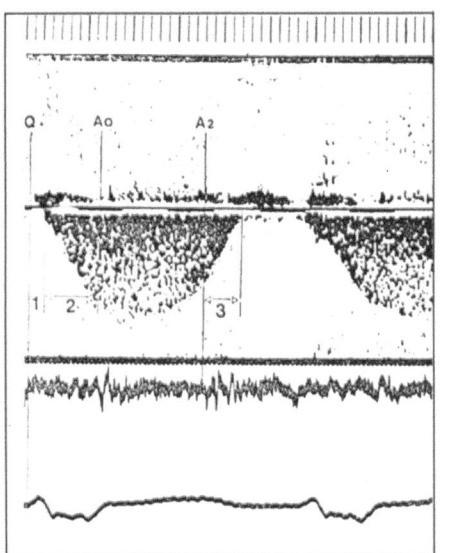 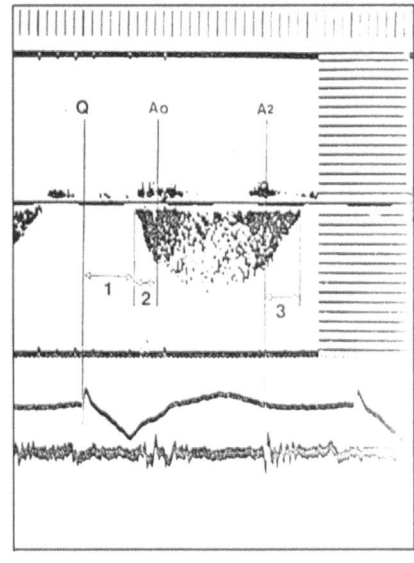

Fig. 4. Effect of RV pacing on ventricular contraction pattern: *left panel* before pacing, and *right panel* after pacing

Criteria for Selection

Patients considered for pacing must be in sinus rhythm, and symptomatic in spite of established treatment with diuretics and ACE-inhibitors. The 12 lead ECG is likely to show a QRS duration of more than 140 ms, a normal axis, and a prolonged PR interval. The ultimate selection criteria, however, are echocardiographic, with MR duration of more than 450 ms, a total left ventricular filling time (i.e. the interval between the pulses of MR) of less than 200 ms and a monophasic transmitral inflow pulse. It is important that this condition be distinguished from simple restrictive filling, when the duration of the E wave may be short, but the interval between the MR pulses is more than 200 ms. We usually set the AV delay on the pacemaker to 70 ms. This abolishes any presystolic MR, and leads to more coordinated activation of the ventricular mass.

Assessment of the Results of Pacing

The immediate effects of pacemaker insertion are judged from MR duration and ventricular filling time. However, the aim of pacing is to improve exercise tolerance, so we do not depend on resting haemodynamics. This proved unreliable in identifying drugs for treating patients with heart failure, and there seems no reason to repeat the mistake with pacemakers. We have therefore formally assessed exercise tolerance in terms of maximal oxygen consumption (MVO_2), and exercise time.

In all patients, the pattern of MR and filling time was modified, with a reduction in the former and an increase in the latter of 90 ms each [7]. This effect becomes apparent within 2-3 beats of turning the pacemaker on, and persists unchanged thereafter, at any rate up to 1 year after insertion. In those patients capable of exercise before treatment, there is an acute increase in exercise time and MVO_2 of 30%, which gradually increases to just under 50% over the succeeding year [8]. At the end of this time, there is also a fall in cavity size. More recently, we have been interested in using the technique in patients who are very disabled at rest, including those with cardiogenic shock.

Future Developments

These are likely. It is possible that multisite pacing might further improve results. It is also conceivable that patients exist in whom activation becomes abnormal only with exercise; they would be identified by pharmacological stress testing, and pacemaker settings varied accordingly. Optimal AV delay has not been settled. We have always used a short one (75 ms) when instituting pacing, since this has an optimum effect on MR duration, and since ventricular filling is restrictive with no blood entering the ventricle with atrial systole.

On occasion, though, a very short AV delay aggravates functional MR, so this should be checked by colour flow Doppler. In addition, as the patients improve clinically over the months after insertion, the potential value of atrial systole increases, as occurs with administration of an ACE-inhibitor. It may well be, therefore, that AV delay should be prolonged in these circumstances.

Summary

DDD pacing is not applicable in the large majority of patients with DCM, and, not surprisingly, inappropriate use causes haemodynamic deterioration [9,10]. However, in a clearly defined minority, who can be identified noninvasively, its effects are beneficial, as well as being prompt and reproducible to a degree not seen with pharmacological therapy. We believe, therefore, that DDD pacing has a significant place in the overall treatment of these patients, both as a primary means of therapy and as a bridge to transplantation.

References

1. Hochleitner M, Hortnagl H, Fridrich I, Geschnitzer F (1992) Long term efficacy of physiological dual chamber pacing in the treatment of end-stage dilated cardiomyopathy. Am J Cardiol 70:1320-1325
2. Wiggers CJ (1922) The interpretation of the intraventricular pressure curve on the basis of rapidly summated fractionate contraction. Am J Physiol 80:1-11
3. Xiao HB, Brecker SJD, Gibson DG (1992) Effects of abnormal activation on the time course of the left ventricular pressure pulse in dilated cardiomyopathy. Br Heart J 68:403-407
4. Xiao HB, Jin XY, Gibson DG (1995) Doppler reconstruction of left ventricular pressure from functional mitral regurgitation: potential importance of varying orifice geometry. Br Heart J 73:53-60
5. Ng KSK, Gibson DG (1990) Relation of filling pattern to diastolic function in severe left ventricular disease. Br Heart J 45:209-214
6. Xiao HB, Roy C, Gibson DG (1994) Nature of ventricular activation in patients with dilated cardiomyopathy: evidence for bilateral bundle branch block. Br Heart J 72:167-174
7. Brecker SJD, Xiao HB, Sparrow J, Gibson DG (1993) Effects of dual-chamber pacing with short atrioventricular delay in dilated cardiomyopathy. Lancet 340:1308-1312
8. Brecker SJ, Kelly PA, Chua TP, Gibson DG (1995) Effects of permanent dual chamber pacing in endstage dilated cardiomyopathy (abstract). Circulation 92 [Suppl. I]:I-724 (abstr.)
9. Gold MR, Feliciano Z, Gottlieb SS, Fisher ML (1995) Dual chamber pacing with a short atrioventricular delay in congestive heart failure: a randomized study. J Am Coll Cardiol 26:967-973
10. Nishimura RA, Hayes DL, Holmes DR JF, Tajik AJ (1995) Mechanism of hemodynamic improvement by dual-chamber pacing for severe left ventricular dysfunction: an acute Doppler and catheterization study. J Am Coll Cardiol 25:281-288

End-Stage Heart Failure and Timing of Heart Transplantation

M.F. Leonen and J.B. O'Connell

During the 30 years since the first successful operation, cardiac transplantation has evolved to a procedure of choice in heart failure patients who have otherwise dismal short term prognosis. Refinements in surgical approach, tissue preservation, immunology and infectious disease control have produced survival rates up to 85% at one year and 70% at five years [1]. By operational definition, patients with refractory symptoms whose prognoses are estimated to be worse than transplantation should be considered in end-stage heart failure.

Because of the aging population and the advances in management of coronary artery disease, the number of patients deemed to be "end-stage" has logarithmically increased. This is reflected by the growth of the patients on the transplant waiting list and subsequently, the transplant waiting times [2]. Unfortunately, the availability of donor hearts has not kept up with the demand, limiting the number of procedures to less than 3500 per year worldwide [1]. Because of the critical donor shortage, there is an increasing need to better identify the patients who are likely to exhibit the most pronounced improvement in functional capacity and life expectancy after transplantation [3,4]. Current priorities in organ allocation limit this procedure to those who are hospital-dependent or ambulatory patients who have waited the longest. It has been shown, however, that patients who have already survived six months on the list have a one-year mortality comparable with patients who have been transplanted [5]. Thus, the selection must be a dynamic process, with periodic listing and "de-listing" of patients, as necessary. Management schemes that have improved heart failure treatment must be optimized, while support for active clinical research for alternative options is emphasized. As the current advances in medical and surgical nontransplant strategies provide sufficient stabilization in a majority of patients, transplantation will only be utilized for those with limited options.

With periodic re-evaluation, the optimized approach in determining the timing of surgery involves three general processes: (1) delineation of the etiology and *alternative treatment strategies*, (2) evaluation of *comorbid conditions* that may affect post-transplantation prognosis, and (3) *prognostication* by quantification of the degree of cardiovascular dysfunction.

Alternative Treatment Strategies

Defining the etiology

An important first step in the evaluation of potential heart transplant candidates is ascertaining the etiology of the heart failure. This will not only outline a rational treatment strategy, but also would provide prognostic information. In some patients, symptoms and objective assessment of cardiac function have been noted to ameliorate with time. Spontaneous improvement of cardiomyopathy has been demonstrated, especially in those with a shorter duration of symptoms [6-7]. Significant increase in ejection fraction occurs in about 27% of patients referred for cardiac transplantation, mostly in those with the least hemodynamic compromise and least degree of mitral regurgitation at the time of referral [8]. Specific etiologies - like peripartal [9], alcohol [10], obesity [11], and tachycardia-related [12] cardiomyopathies have shown spontaneous improvement, especially after removal of the corresponding inciting factor.

Medical Treatment

The medical approach to managing patients with severe congestive heart failure has shown considerable improvement over the past two decades (Fig. 1). Angiotensin-converting enzyme (ACE)-inhibition has revolutionized pharmacologic therapy, but still produces inferior short and medium-term survival results as compared to the transplantation experience. The first controlled trial that looked at comparably sick patients is the CONSENSUS trial in the 1980s has shown a greater than 40% one year mortality in NYHA Class IV patients treated with digoxin, diuretics and enalapril [13]. In a more recent trial of patients with severe heart failure and ejection fraction less than 30 percent (PRAISE), the one year mortality in both the placebo and amlodipine group appeared to be better, with a one year mortality of around 30% [14]. This still contrasts with current results with transplantation, with approximately 15%-20% mortality within the first year.

Optimization of medical treatment is imperative prior to any consideration for transplantation. In a study describing the outcome of alternative therapies in patients with end-stage heart failure, a group of patients, who were denied heart transplantation because of a positive response to intensified medical therapy, had similar survival within the first two to three years as those who were accepted for transplantation [15]. Despite preponderance of evidence from large scale trials of survival benefit, ACE-inhibitors are still being underutilized [16]. In patients who have absolute contraindication to ACE-inhibitors, the combination of hydralazine and nitrates at doses used in the VHEFT trials [17] must be prescribed prior to any consideration of transplantation listing. Agents that have shown probable survival benefit in patients with NYHA Class III-IV CHF patients like carvedilol [18] and amiodarone [19] must also be considered.

Undoubtedly, there is a pressing need to further evaluate pharmacologic

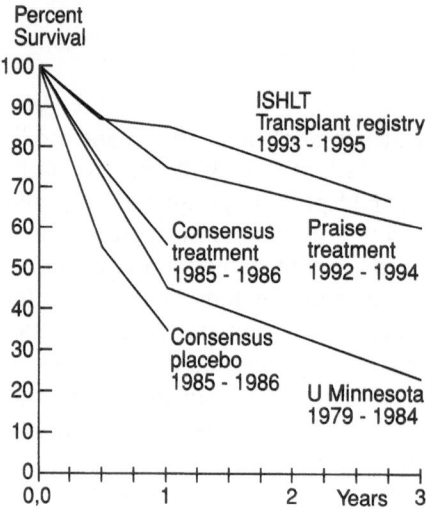

Fig. 1. Medical treatment vs transplantation in severe congestive heart failure

agents that may improve current survival rates in medical therapy on a background of ACE-inhibition. Clinical trials with beta-blockers have variously suggested clinical benefit, although the question of mortality reduction would be best answered by the ongoing BEST (β-blocker Evaluation of Survival trial) utilizing bucindolol in about 2800 patients. Efforts are underway to find an inotropic agent with a favorable mortality benefit after recently published trials have shown no mortality reduction with digoxin [20] and a dose-related deleterious outcome with vesnarinone [21]. Intermittent dobutamine therapy has produced symptomatic benefit in previously moribund patients, but its effect on mortality is unsettled [22].

Surgical Treatment

Aggressive surgical approach to the management of the heart failure patient who is deemed "end-stage" must be carefully examined as an alternative to transplantation listing. Cardiac transplantation in patients who have undergone previous nontransplant cardiac operations has been carried out without compromising immediate or long-term outcome [23]. Novel and aggressive surgical treatment to heart failure may therefore be used to preserve functional status and survival, thus deferring listing for transplantation.

Coronary Revascularization

Ischemic cardiomyopathy is the major indication for cardiac transplantation, accounting for more than 40% of patients who eventually are allocated donor hearts. With improved surgical techniques, myocardial preservation, and postoperative intensive care, the outcome of patients with severe heart failure who undergo coronary artery bypass grafting has improved. Early experience with bypass surgery from the CASS database [24] has demonstrated that although perioperative risk is high, the greatest increment in both symptomatic and survival benefit with surgical revascularization is observed in the patients who have the lowest left ventricular (LV) ejection fraction. Predictors of adverse outcome include increasing age [25] and LV dimension [26]. Latest experience with aggressive coronary revascularization in patients with angina and poor left ventricular function have provided results comparable to heart transplantation, with one year survival rates of up to 90% [27,28]. In patients who have no angina, the use of PET-scanning has enabled identification of the presence of viable myocardium and has predicted improved functional status after revascularization [29]. It is therefore important that before listing for transplantation, aggressive revascularization surgery should be considered in patients with ischemic cardiomyopathy and presence of viable myocardium, adequate targets, and LV end diastolic dimension of less than 75 mm.

Valvular Heart Disease Surgery

Although transplantation for "end-stage" valvular heart disease has produced results comparable to those transplanted for other underlying etiologies of heart failure, the important strategy for managing these patients is the optimal timing of valve replacement to prevent the higher perioperative morbidity and mortality once LV dysfunction evolves. There is hardly any need to consider transplantation for patients with *mitral stenosis*, as patients with Class IV symptoms and severe pulmonary hypertension may still have excellent surgical outcomes [30]. In patients with severe LV dysfunction secondary to critical *aortic stenosis*, aortic valve replacement is indicated because relief of "afterload mismatch" produces remission of functional symptoms and improvement in ventricular performance [31]. Although the operative mortality may be as high as 10% [32], patients with *aortic regurgitation* and significant ventricular dysfunction must be evaluated for aortic valve replacement, since the natural history of these patients indicates a poor outcome without surgery. The functional improvement is dependent on the severity and duration of symptoms and the impairment in LV systolic function [33].

Because replacing the mitral valve increases LV afterload and consequently further decreases LV function, patients with severe *mitral regurgitation* and low LV ejection fraction were previously considered formidable risks to surgical management. In the past decade, increasing experience with reparative techniques has shown that preservation of the subvalvular apparatus with mitral valve repair or in conjunction with mitral valve replacement have improved overall mortality and morbidity [34]. Experience at the University of Michigan with mitral valve reconstruction with end stage cardiomyopathy has shown no operative or hospital deaths and a 75% one year actuarial survival [35]. Nonetheless, LV dysfunction remains a major cause of mortality and morbidity following mitral valve surgery [36]. Therefore, early surgery before the development of severe symptoms and demonstrable LV impairment is the cornerstone of management for patients with severe mitral regurgitation [37].

Newer Surgical Approaches

Research efforts are underway to further define optimal patient selection for novel surgical approaches to refractory heart failure. In preliminary analysis, *dynamic cardiomyoplasty* has been shown to improve ventricular systolic function and functional status in patients with congestive heart failure [38], although operative risk may limit its use to patients with NYHA Class III symptoms [39]. Initial experience with ventriculotomy in association with mitral valve reconstruction (*Batista procedure*) in 120 patients with refractory heart failure produced 30% in hospital and 60% 1-year mortality [40]. *Left ventricular assist device* support has intensified the transplant donor shortage by allowing temporary stabilization of patients who would otherwise not have survived awaiting transplantation [41]. The low 30-day mortality [42], demonstrable improvement in function, and possible cost savings [43] in the care of these patients have stimulated the development and research of devices intended for long-term use.

Comorbid conditions

Although the traditional secondary exclusions have been narrowed with the improvement in transplantation techniques, the basic tenet remains that patients should not be listed if they have limited post-transplant potential for rehabilitation.

Systemic Diseases

Experience in patients with systemic illnesses such as amyloidosis [44], sarcoidosis [45], Chagas disease [46], and myocarditis [47] has shown recurrence post-transplantation. Active rheumatologic disease such as systemic lupus erythematosus, severe rheumatoid arthritis and scleroderma have been considered by themselves contraindications because of poor prognosis apart from the underlying cardiovascular disease [48]. On the other hand, isolated cases of successful outcome have been reported in patients with muscular dystrophy [49], pre-existing malignancies [50] and endocarditis [51,52]. Insulin-dependent diabetes mellitus is no longer a contraindication in patients without end-organ damage [53]. The majority of responders at a recent consensus conference believe that positive testing for the human immunodeficiency virus is an absolute contraindication to transplantation [48].

Age, Gender, Body Habitus

At the current time, most transplant centers accept 55 as their age limit for cardiac transplantation. Cardiac transplantation in the patient over 60 years of age may be successfully undertaken with acceptable mortality and survival [54], although age-related comorbidities may limit functional rehabilitation post-transplantation [55]. The number of females undergoing heart transplantation is significantly lower than the number of males, which has been explained to result partly from a sex difference in disease prevalence and possibly treatment preference [56]. Interestingly, women seem to experience allograft rejection more than their male counterparts [57], and may be at-risk for reduced actuarial survival up to three years after transplantation [58]. Although there is a paucity of data on risks of obesity in transplant recipients, it is generally believed that weight more than 50% greater than ideal body weight is an absolute contraindication to transplantation [48].

Pulmonary Hypertension

Pulmonary vascular disease is one of the most important comorbid conditions that has had a significant impact on transplantation outcomes. Early post operative right ventricular failure and death have been associated with elevated pulmonary vascular resistance of greater than 6 Wood units or a transpulmonary gradient greater than 15 mm Hg [59]. Lack of significant hemodynamic response of pulmonary pressures to vasodilators has been shown to be a stronger predictor of morbidity and mortality than baseline pulmonary hemodynamics [60]. Excessive pulmonary vascular resistance that is unresponsive to maneuvers such as nitroprusside [60], prostaglandin E-1 [61] or adenosine infusion [62] is therefore a contraindication to heart transplantation. Serial right heart catheterization in thus essential in the proper selection and timing of transplant surgery in potential candidates.

Other Organ Dysfunction

During the pre-transplantation evaluation, objective measurement of the lung, liver and kidney function must be performed after optimal medical therapy for heart failure has been ensured. Patients with pulmonary function tests showing less than 50% of predicted forced expiratory velocity in 1 second (FEV_1) or FEV_1 over forced vital capacity (FVC) ratios [63], creatinine clearance less than 50 ml/min for an average square area, and liver transaminase levels twice their normal values in association with coagulation abnormalities irreversible by inotropic therapy may be poor transplantation candidates. Although anecdotal reports of successful combined-organ transplantation seem promising [64-66], allocation of limited donor organs must at present be prioritized to those who would have the most benefit from conventional procedures.

Psychosocial Factors

Transplantation is a lifelong commitment to intensive monitoring, drug therapy and rehabilitation. It is of utmost importance that issues such as psychological stability, alcohol and tobacco abuse, and social support be addressed, as noncompliance remain a major factor in adverse post-transplant outcomes [67]. The potential for rehabilitation is the point of emphasis in considering the comorbidities in the cardiac transplantation candidate, physiologic and nonphysiologic issues are of equal importance.

Prognostication

After optimization of medical and surgical therapy and exclusion of limiting co-morbid conditions, an important, yet complex step in listing patients for heart transplantation is assessing the patient's short term prognosis. In patients with congestive heart failure, four variables have been useful in assessing risk for mortality: (1) functional capacity, (2) hemodynamic measures of cardiac performance, (3) Indices of neurohormonal stimulation, and (4) spontaneous arrhythmias.

Functional Capacity

Most patients who should be considered for transplantation have limiting symptoms at rest and with any physical activity – that is, Class IV by NYHA criterion. Most studies have in fact shown that these are the patients with the worst prognosis – with annual mortality exceeding 50% [68]. In patients with Class III symptoms, exercise duration may provide incremental prognostic value [69]. Unfortunately, exercise duration is influenced by factors such as patient motivation. In the heart transplant candidate, an objective measure of exercise tolerance with anaerobic threshold and peak O_2 consumption (VO_2 max) must be measured. In a group of ambulatory patients awaiting transplantation, Mancini et al [70] have demonstrated that a VO_2 max greater than 14ml/kg/min predicts good one-year survival approaching 94%. In these patients, transplantation can be safely deferred despite severe hemodynamic impairment at rest. It is important, however, to prove maximal exercise tolerance by documenting achievement of anaerobic threshold at 50%-70% of VO_2 max. In addition, although 14 ml/kg/min is the accepted criteria threshold for most transplant centers, this level of exercise tolerance may not be acceptable for an active young person and thus age must be taken into consideration. In a study of Class II - IV patients, mean peak age- and gender-adjusted percent predicted oxygen consumption ($\%VO_2$) rather than VO_2 was found to be an independent predictor of overall survival [71].

Measures of Cardiac Performance

The LV ejection fraction (LVEF) has traditionally been accepted as a measure of systolic dysfunction which can be quantified by echocardiography or nuclear techniques. Although there is a direct relationship of LVEF to mortality, studies of patients with refractory heart failure have shown that this measure of cardiac systolic performance looses its prognostic value at the time a patient is sick enough to consider transplantation [72]. In these patients, right ventricular ejection fraction greater or equal to 0.35 may be a more potent predictor of favorable outcomes [71].

Like the LVEF, hemodynamic parameters lose their prognostic value in patients with refractory heart failure. Wilson et al [73], for example, found no hemodynamic measure that distinguished survivors from nonsurvivors in patients with NYHA Class III-IV symptoms. A more recent study [74] suggests that right atrial pressure alone (< 12 mm Hg) is a significant predictor of survival in patients awaiting heart transplantation. In another study, identification of poor responders to isoproterenol infusion has been suggested as a means to establish priorities on the waiting list for heart transplantation [75].

Neurohormone Levels

The use of indices of neurohormonal activation to further stratify patients awaiting heart transplantation has not been fully determined. However, studies have shown that plasma norepinephrine [76], plasma renin activity and atrial natriuretic peptide [77] were all independent survival predictors using a multivariate model.

Spontaneous Arrhythmias

The weight of evidence suggests that frequency and complexity and occurrence of ventricular arrhythmias are associated with poorer outcome in patients with varying degrees of ventricular failure. In a study that has focused on patients with severe heart failure, however, ventricular premature beat frequency did not contribute independent prognostic information [72]. To date, evidence has not justified the use of Holter monitoring or programmed electric stimulation to further stratify patients with end stage heart disease in the absence of hemodynamic compromise or symptoms attributable to spontaneous arrhythmias. In those transplant candidates who develop symptomatic ventricular arrhythmias, drug therapy with amiodarone, or implantable cardioverter-defibrillator placement as appropriate, may help extend survival. However, prophylaxis is not justified.

Timing of Transplantation

There is no question regarding the benefit of transplantation in patients who have refractory symptoms despite optimal medical and surgical therapy. This general indication includes patients with NYHA class IV symptoms, refractory angina after aggressive efforts of percutaneous, surgical or medical management, and hemodynamically-compromising arrhythmias despite drug or device-related therapy.

For the ambulatory patient, the timing of heart transplantation is not as dependent on its potential benefits to the heart recipient as it is on the critical donor shortage. As the number of co-morbidities that contraindicate transplantation continue to shrink with the improvement in transplantation experience and technology, the donor shortage problem will continue to intensify. Use of older donors [78] and liberalization of donor-recipient weight match criteria [79] to expand the donor pool have not increased transplantation volume [1]. Efforts should thus be directed to optimizing available medical and surgical approaches, while intensifying research on alternative strategies of managing refractory heart failure.

The growing transplant list and longer waiting times have enabled analyses demonstrating that the survival benefit of transplantation decreases as patients wait longer than six months for a donor heart [80]. Moreover, in some patients on the transplant list, re-examination of exercise capacity has documented improvement in peak oxygen uptake accompanied by stable clinical symptoms [81]. This has led to the concept of a dynamic transplant listing strategy (Fig. 2), where intensified medical and aggressive surgical therapy is combined with periodic re-evaluation that allows active listing and "de-listing" of patients. By adapting this approach to determine the timing of transplantation, we recognize that although stringent criteria must be applied, the selection is a time-dependent process as a result of our limited ability to prognosticate.

Optimization of conventional medical therapy and consideration of unconventional approaches to the care of these patients with already limited options must involve heart failure specialists. In order for this to be effective, the establishment of regional comprehensive heart failure centers is desirable [82]. An integrated scheme emphasizes the best alternative approach, at the same

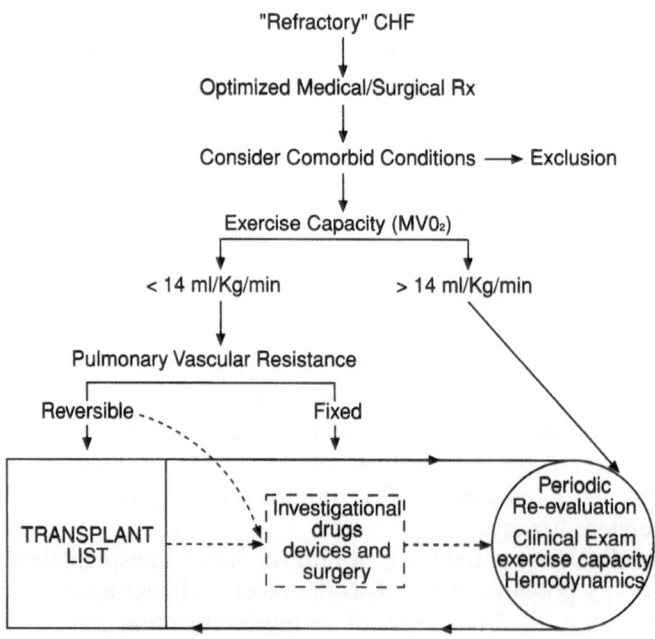

Fig. 2. Dynamic listing for heart transplantation

time providing an arena of active research that would facilitate efforts to decrease the medical and economic burden of end stage heart disease.

Conclusion

Heart failure must not be deemed "end-stage" until conventional medical and aggressive surgical therapy have been optimized. The timing of heart transplantation is a dynamic process, with periodic prognostication and re-evaluation of comorbid conditions. The critical donor shortage mandates a listing program that integrates specialists' care and consideration of investigational drugs, devices, and surgery that may later produce more favorable outcomes for the growing heart failure population.

References

1. Hosenpud JD, Novick RJ, Bennett L Keck BN, Fiol B, Dair OP (1996) The Registry of the International Society for Heart and Lung Transplantation: Thirteenth Official Report-1996. J Heart and Lung Transplant 15:655-675
2. Stevenson LW (1994) Selection and management of patients for cardiac transplantation. Curr Opin Cardiol 9:315-325
3. O'Connell J, Bourge R, Costanzo-Nordin M, Driscoll DJ, Morgan JP, Rose EA, Uretsky BF (1992) Cardiac transplantation: Recipient selection, donor procurement and medical follow-up. Circulation 86:1061-1079
4. Costanzo M, Augustine S, Bourge R, Bristow M, O'Connell JB, Driscoll D, Rose E (1995) Selection and treatment of candidates for heart transplantation. Circulation 92:3593-3612
5. Stevenson LW, Wamer SL, Steimle AE, Fonarow GC, Hamilton MA, Moriguchi JD, Kobashigawa JA, Tillisch JH, Drinkwater DC, Laks H (1994) The impending crisis awaiting cardiac transplantation-Modeling a solution based on selection. Circulation 89:450-457
6. Stevenson LW, Fowler MB, Schroeder SS, Stevenson WG, Dracup KA, Fond V (1987) Poor survival of patients with idiopathic cardiomyopathy considered too well for transplantation. Am J Med 83:871-976
7. Keogh AM, Baron DW, Hieckie JB (1990) Prognostic guides in patients with idiopathic or ischemic dilated cardiomyopathy assessed for cardiac transplantation. Am J Cardiol. 65:903-908
8. Steimle AE, Stevenson LW, Fonarow GC, Hamilton MA, Moriguchi JD (1994) Prediction of improvement in recent-onset cardiomyopathy after referral for heart transplantation. J Am Cardiol 23:553-559
9. O'Connell J, Constanzo-Nordin MR, Subramanian R, Robinson JA, Wallis DE, Scanlow PJ, Gunnar RM (1986) Peripartum cardiomyopathy. Clinical, hemodynamic, histologic, and prognostic characteristics. J Am Coll Cardiol 8:52-56
10. Regan TJ (1991) Alcohol and the cardiovascular system. A review. JAMA 264:377-381
11. Alexander JK (1895) The cardiomyopathy of obesity. Prog Cardiovasc Dis 27:325-334
12. Middlekauff HR, Stevenson WG, Saxon LA, Stevenson LW (1992) Low dose amiodarone for atrial fibrillation in advanced heart failure restores sinus rhythm and improves functional capacity. Circulation [Suppl I] 86:I-808 (abstr)
13. The CONSENSUS Trial Study Group (1987) Effects of enalapril on mortality in severe congestive heart failure: results of the Cooperative North Scandinavian Enalapril Survival Study (CONSENSUS). N Engl J Med 316:1429-1435
14. Packer M, O'Connor C, Ghali J, Pressler ML, Carson PE, Belkin RN, Miller AB, Neuberg GW, Frid D, Wertheimer JH, Cropp AB, DeMets DL for the Prospective Randomized Amlodipine Survival Evaluation Study Group (1996) Effect of amlodipi-

ne on morbidity and mortality in severe chronic heart failure. N Engl J Med 335:1107-1114

15. Lindelow B, Andersson B, Waagstein F and Bergh CH (1995) Prognosis of alternative therapies in patients with heart failure not accepted for heart transplantation. J Heart Lung Transplant 14:1204-1211

16. Rajfer SI (1993) Perspective of the pharmaceutical industry on the development of new drugs for heart failure. J Am Coll Cardiol 22[Suppl A]:198-200

17. Cohn JN, Johnson G, Ziesche S, Cobb F, Francis G, Tristani F, Smith R, Dunkman WB, Loeb H, Wong M (1991) A comparison of enalapril with hydralazine-isosorbide dinitrate in the treatment of chronic congestive heart failure. N Engl J Med 325:303-310

18. Packer M, Bristow M, Cohn J, Colucci WS, Fowler MB, Gilbert EM, Shusterman NH (1996) The effect of Carvedilol on morbidity and mortality in patients with chronic heart failure. N Engl J Med 334:1349-1355

19. Doval H, Nul D, Grancelli H, Perrone SV, Bortman GR, Curiel R (1994) Randomized trial of low-dose amiodarone on severe congestive heart failure. Lancet 344:493-498

20. The Digitalis Investigation Group (1997) The effect of digoxin on mortality and morbidity in patients with heart failure. N Engl J Med 336:525-533

21. Feldman AM, Young J, Bourge R et al (1997) Mechanism of increased mortality from vesnarinone un the severe heart failure trial (VesT). Circulation 29[SupplA]:64A

22. Dies F, Krell MJ, Whitlow P et al (1986) Intermittent dobutamine in ambulatory outpatients with chronic heart failure. Circulation 74[Suppl II]:11-38

23. Ott GY, Norman D, Hosenpud J, Hersaberger RE, Ratkovec RM, Cobanoglu AM (1994) Heart transplantation patients with previous cardiac operations: excellent clinical results. J Thorac Cardiovasc Surg 107:203-209

24. Alderman EL, Fisher LD, Litwin P, Kaiser GC, Myers WO, Maynard C, Levine F, Schloss M (1983) Results of coronary artery surgery in patients with poor left ventricular function (CASS). Circulation 68:785-795

25. Langenburg SE, Buchanan SA, Blackbourne LH, Scheri RP, Sinclair KN, Martinez J, Spotnitz WD, Trible CC, Kron IL (1995) Predicting survival after coronary revascularization for ischemic cardiomyopathy. Ann Thorac Surg 60:1193-1197

26. Louie H, Laks H, Milgalter E, Drinkwater DC Jr, Hamilton MA, Brunken RC, Stevenson LW (1991) Ischemic cardiomyopathy: Criteria for coronary revascularization and cardiac transplantation. Circulation 84[Suppl III]:290-295

27. Elefteriades J, Tolis G, Levi E, Mills K, Zaret B (1993) Coronary artery bypass grafting in severe left ventricular dysfunction: excellent survival with improved ejection fraction and functional state. J Am Coll Cardiol 22:1411-1417

28. Hausmann H, Ennker J, Topp H, Schuler S, Schiessler A, Hempel B, Friedel N, Hofmeister S, Hetzer R (1994) Coronary bypass grafting and heart transplantation in end stage coronary artery disease: A comparison of hemodynamic improvement and ventricular function. J Card Surg 9:77-84

29. Di Carli MF, Asgarzadie F, Schelbert HR, Brunken RC, Laks H, Phelps ME, Naddahi J (1995) Quantitative relation between myocardial viability and improvement in heart failure symptoms after revascularization in patients with ischemic cardiomyopathy. Circulation 92:3436-3444

30. Carabello B (1991) Timing of surgery in mitral and aortic stenosis. Cardiology Clinics 9:229-238

31. Carabello BA, Green LH, Grossman W, Cohn LH, Koster JK, Collins SS (1980) Hemodynamic determinants of prognosis of aortic valve replacement in critical aortic stenosis and advanced congestive heart failure. Circulation 62:42

32. Bonow R, Picone A, McIntosh C, Jones M, Rosing DR, Maron BS, Lakatos E, Clark RE, Epstein SE (1985) Survival and functional results after valve replacement for aortic regurgitation from 1976-1983: Impact of preoperative left ventricular function. Circulation 72:1244-1256

33. Bonow R, Dodd J, Maron B, O'Gara PT, White CC, McIntosh CC, Clark RE, Epstein ST(1988) Long term serial changes in left ventricular function and reversal of ventricular dilatation after valve replacement for chronic aortic regurgitation. Circulation 78:1108-1120

34. Lee EM, Shapiro LM, Wells FC (1996) Importance of subvalvular preservation and early operation in mitral valve surgery. Circulation 94:2117-2123
35. Bolling SF, Deeb GM, Brunsting LA, Bach DS (1995) Early outcome of mitral valve reconstruction in patients with end-stage cardiomyopathy. J Thorac Cardio Surg 109:676-682
36. Lee EM, Shapiro LM, Wels FC (1995) Mortality and morbidity after mitral valve repair: the importance of left ventricular dysfunction. J Heart Valve Dis 4:460-468
37. Sousa Uva M, Dreyfus G, Rescigno G, Al Aile N, Mascagni R, La Marra M, Povillart F, Parkaoncar S, Palsky E, Raffoul R, Scorsin M, Noera G, Lessana A (1996) Surgical treatment of asymptomatic and mildly symptomatic mitral regurgitation. J Thorac Cardio Surg 112:1240-1248
38. Furnary AP, Jessup FM, Moreira LP (1996) Multicenter trial of dynamic cardiomyoplasty for chronic heart failure. The American Cardiomyoplasty Group. J Am Coll Cardiol 28:1175-1180
39. Furnary AP, Chachques JC, Moreira LF, Grunkemeier GL, Swanson JS, Stolf N, Haydars S, Acar C, Starr A, Jatene AD, Carpentier AF (1996) Long term outcome, survival analysis, and risk stratification of dynamic cardiomyoplasty. J Thorac Cardio Surg 112:1640-1649
40. Communication, American College of Cardiology 46th Annual Scientific Session, Anaheim, USA, March 1997
41. Massad MG, McCarthy PM, Smedira NG, Miller CA, Pierce WS (1996) Does successful bridging with the implantable left ventricular device affect cardiac transplantation outcome? J Thorac Cardio Surg 112:1275-1281
42. Mehta SM, Aufiero TX, Pae WE, Miller CA, Pierce WS (1995) Combined registry for the clinical use of mechanical ventricular assist pumps and the total artificial heart in conjunction with heart transplantation: sixth official report 1994. J Heart Lung Transplant 14:585-593
43. Mehta SM, Aufiero TX, Pae WE, Miller CA, Pierce WS (1995) Mechanical ventricular assistance: an economical and effective means of treating end stage heart disease. Ann Thorac Surg 60:284-290
44. Hosenpud JD, De Marco T, Frazier H, Griffith BP, Uretsky BF, Mekisah H, O'Connell JB, Olivari MT, Valantine HA (1991) Progression of systemic disease and reduced long term survival in patients with cardiac amyloidosis undergoing heart transplantation. Circulation [Suppl III] 84:338-343
45. Oni AA, Hershberger RE, Norman DJ, Ray J, Hovaguinian N, Cobanoglu AM, Hosenpud JD (1991) Recurrence of sarcoidosis in a cardiac allograft: Control with augmented corticosteroids. J Heart Transplant 11:367-369
46. Stolf NAG, Higushi L, Bocchi E, Bellotti O, Auler JO, Vip D, Amatoneto V, Pileggi F, Jatenz AD (1987) Heart transplantation in patients with Chagas disease cardiomyopathy. J Heart Transplant 6:307-312
47. Loria K, Jessurun J, Shumway S, Kubo S (1994) Early recurrence of chronic active myocarditis after heart transplantation. Hum Pathol 25:323-326
48. Miller L, Kubo S, Young J, Stevenson LW, Loh E, Costanzo MR (1995) Report of the consensus conference on candidate selection for heart transplantation-1993. J Heart Lung Transplant 14:562-571
49. Rees W, Schuler S, Hummel M, Hetzer R (1993) Heart transplantation in patients with muscular dystrophy associated with end stage cardiomyopathy. J Heart Lung Transplant 12:804-807
50. Dillon T, Sullivan M, Ladowski J, Schatzlein MH, Peterson AC, Scheeringa RA, Clark WR Jr, Ladowski JS (1991) Cardiac transplantation in patients with preexisting malignancies. Transplantation 52:82-85
51. Pulpon LA, Crespo MG, Sobrino M, Segovia J, Ortigosa J, Burgos R, Silva L, Serrano S, Artzara M, Tellel G (1994) Recalcitrant endocarditis successfully treated by heart transplantation. Am Heart J 127:958-960
52. Park S, Sullivan H, Lonchyna v et al (1993) Heart transplantation for complicated and recurrent early prosthetic valve endocarditis. J Heart Lung Transplant 12:802-203
53. Munoz E, Lonquist J, Frazier O, Radovancevic B, Baldwin RT, Ford S, Duncan JM,

Frazieroa (1992) Long term results in diabetic patients undergoing heart transplantation. J Heart Lung Transplant 11:943-949

54. Bergin P, Rabinov M, Esmore D (1995) Cardiac transplantation in patients over 60 years. Transplant Proc 27:2150-2151
55. Heroux A, Costanzo-Nordin MR, O'Sullivan J, Kao WG, Liao Y, Mullen GM, Johnson MR (1993) Heart transplantation as a treatment option for end stage heart disease in patients older than 65 years of age. J Heart Lung Transplant 12:573-579
56. Aaronson K, Schwartz S, Goin J, Mancini D (1995) Sex differences in patient acceptance of cardiac transplant candidacy. Circulation 91:2753-2761
57. Crandall B, Renlund D, O'Connell J, Burton NA, Jones KW, Gay WA Jr, Doty DB, Karwande SV, Lee HR, Holland C (1988) Increased cardiac allograft rejection in female heart transplant recipients. J Heart Transplant 7:419-423
58. Wechler M, Giardina E, Sciacca R, Rose E, Barr M (1995) Increased mortality in women undergoing cardiac transplantation. Circulation 91:1029-1035
59. Kirklin JK, Naftel DC, Kirklin JW, Blackstone EH, White-Williams C, Bourge RC, (1988) Pulmonary vascular resistance and the risk of heart transplantation. J Heart Transplant 7:331-336
60. Costard-Jale A, Fowler MB (1992) Influence of preoperative pulmonary artery pressure on mortality after heart transplantation. Testing of potential reversibility of pulmonary hypertension with nitroprusside is useful in defining a high risk group. J Am Coll Cardiol 19:48-54
61. Murali S, Uretsky BF, Armitage JA, Tokarczyk TR, Betschart AR, Kormos RL, Stein KL, Reddy PS, Hardesty RL, Griffith P (1992) Utility of prostaglandin E1 in the pretransplantation evaluation of heart failure patients with significant pulmonary hypertension. J Heart Lung Transplant 11:716-723
62. Haywood G, Sneddon B, Bashir Y, Jennison SH, Gray HH, McKenna WS (1992) Adenosine infusion for the reversal of pulmonary vasoconstriction in biventricular failure - a good test but a poor therapy. Circulation 86:892-902
63. Light RW, George RB (1983) Serial pulmonary function in patients with acute heart failure. Arch Intern Med 143:429-433
64. Levy R, Guerraty A, Yacub M, Loertscher R (1993) Prolonged survival after heart-lung transplantation in systemic lupus erythematosus. Chest 104:1903-1905
65. Gonwa T, Husberg B, Klintmakn G (1992) Simultaneous heart and kidney transplantation: a report of three cases and review of literature. J Heart Lung Transplant 11:152-155
66. Olivieri N, Liu PP, Shern G, Olivieri MF, Lio PP, Osherm CD, Daly PA, Greig PD, McCusker PJ, Collins AF, Fracombe WH, Templeton DM, Butany J (1994) Brief report: combined liver and heart transplantation for end-stage iron-induced organ failure in an adult with homozygous beta-thalassemia. N Engl J Med 330:1125-1127
67. Rodriguez MD, Colon A, Santiago-Delphin EA (1991) Psychosocial profile of noncompliant patients. Transplant Proc 23:1807-1909
68. Massie BM, Conway M (1987) Survival of patients with congestive heart failure: Past, present, and future prospects. Circulation 75 [suppl IV]:IV-11
69. Griffin BP, Shah PK, Ferguson J, Rubin SA (1991) Incremental prognostic value of exercise hemodynamic variables in chronic congestive heart failure secondary to coronary artery disease or to dilated cardiomyopathy. Am J Cardiol 67:848-853
70. Mancini DM, Eisen H, Kussmaul W, Mull R, Edmunds LH Jr, Wilson Jr (1991) Value of peak exercise oxygen consumption for optimal timing of cardiac transplantation in ambulatory patients with heart failure. Circulation 83:778-786
71. Di Salvo T, Mathier M, Semigran MJ, Dec W (1995) Preserved right ventricular ejection fraction predicts exercise capacity and survival in advanced heart failure. J Am Coll Cardiol 25:1143-1153
72. Dec GW, Fifer MA, Hermann HC, Cocca-Spofford D, Semigran MJ (1993) Long term outcome of enoximone therapy in patients with refractory heart failure. Am Heart J 125:423-429
73. Wilson JR, Schwartz JS, Sutton JSJ, Ferraro N, Horowitz LN, Reicher N, Josephson MG (1983) Prognosis in severe heart failure: Relation to hemodynamic measurements and ventricular ectopic activity. J Am Coll Cardiol 2: 403-410

74. Morley D, Brozena SC (1994) Assessing risk by hemodynamic profile in patients awaiting cardiac transplantation. Am J Cardiol 75:379-383
75. Kopelev B, Chestukhin V, Mironov B, Golovchiwer GN, Mogilevsky GN, Shumacov VI (1992) Heart transplantation: Additional criteria for patient selection. Trans Proc 24:2006
76. Cohn JN, Levine TB, Olivari MT (1984) Plasma norepinephrine as a guide to prognosis in patients with chronic congestive heart failure. N Engl J Med 311:819-823
77. Nicklas JM, Benedict C, Johnstone DE, Kay R, Kirklin PC, Weiner D, Bourassa MG, Yusuf S (1991) Relationship between neurohormonal profile and one year mortality in patients with CHF and/or LV dysfunction. Circulation (suppl II) II-468
78. Luciani G, Livi U, Faggian G, Mazzucco A (1992) Clinical results of heart transplantation in recipients over 55 years of age with donors over 40 years of age. J Heart Lung Transplant 11:1177-1183
79. Sethi G, Lanauze P, Rosado L et al (1993) Clinical significance of weight difference between donor and recipient in heart transplantation. J Thorac Cardiovasc Surg 108:444-448
80. Kao W, Mc Gee D, Liao Y, Heroux AL, Mullen GM, Johnson MR, Costanzo MR (1994) Does heart transplantation confer additional benefit over medical therapy to patients who have waited > 6 months for heart transplantation? J Am Coll Cardiol 24:1547-1551
81. Stevenson L, Steimle A, Fonarow G, Kermani M, Kermani D, Hamilton MA, Moriguchi SD, Walden S, Tillisch JA, Drinkwater DC, Laks H (1995) Improvement in exercise capacity of candidates awaiting heart transplantation. J Am Coll Cardiol 25:163-170
82. O'Connell J, Bristow M (1993) Economic impact of heart failure in the United States: time for a different approach. J Heart Lung Transplant 13:S107-112

Cardiomyoplasty: Surgical Therapy for Ischemic and Idiopathic Dilated Cardiomyopathies

J.C. Chachques and A. Carpentier

Introduction

The discovery of an adequate substitute for cardiac muscle to treat loss of muscle mass or functional cardiac insufficiency, has long been one of man's great dreams. Rather than approaching the problem with heart transplantation or artificial heart-assist devices, the ideal would be to have a substitute contractile tissue [1, 2].

Dynamic cardiomyoplasty is a surgical procedure that combines cardiac and plastic surgery with electrophysiology and biomedical engineering. This procedure was conceived to enhance cardiac performance by assisting myocardial contraction. The surgical technique consists of placing a pedicled Latissimus Dorsi muscle (LDM) around the heart via a partial resection of the 2nd rib and suturing it around the ventricles (Fig. 1). Postoperatively the LDM is stimulated by a CardioMyostimulator (pulse train generator) in synchrony with ventricular systole. The goal of this technique is the support of hypokinetic, akinetic or dyskinetic myocardial areas secondary to ischemic, dysplastic or idiopathic dilated cardiomyopathies. The LDM was chosen for use in cardiomyoplasty due to the anatomy of its neurovascular supply, facility of transposition into the thoracic cavity, and its relatively large surface area allowing placement around the heart [3, 4].

Physiological, histological, metabolic and biochemical properties of skeletal muscle alter in response to chronic electrical stimulation. Histochemical and electrophysiological studies of conditioned LDM show that muscle fatigue resistance can be greatly improved after training.

The cardiomyoplasty postoperative muscle electrostimulation protocol provided a full fiber conversion from glycolytic to oxidative fatigue-resistant type, with similar histochemical characteristics to myocardium. This adaptative response of skeletal muscle to working demands, as those required for myocardial assistance, is the basic principle to a cardiac support function [5, 6].

History

Three stages mark the evolution of techniques involving use of skeletal muscle in cardiac surgery [7, 8]:

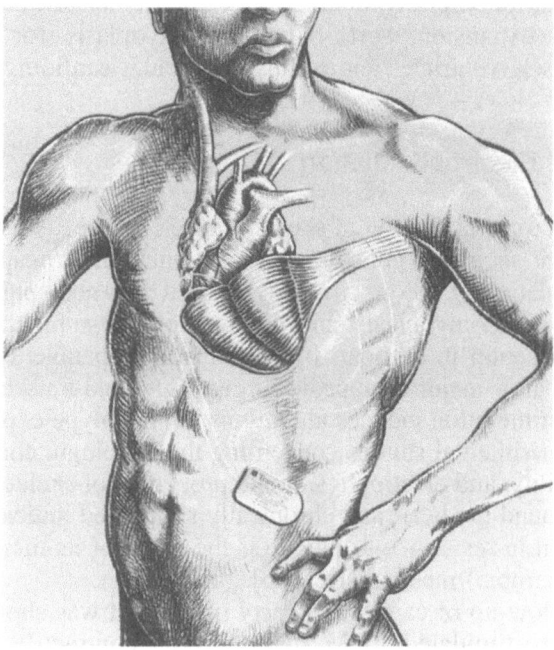

Fig. 1. Surgical technique of cardiomyoplasty. The pedicled left latissimus dorsi muscle is placed into the chest and wrapped around both ventricles. A specific pulse train generator (Cardio-Myostimulator) is used for long term systolic LDM pacing

– Use of non-stimulated skeletal muscle. These techniques were proposed experimentally and clinically. The aim was to reinforce the ventricular wall and to improve myocardial perfusion.

– Experimental use of electrostimulated skeletal muscle over a short time period. Several groups working in heart and aortic myoplasties demonstrated a rapid fatigue of skeletal muscle, with development of a partial and diminished contraction [9].

– Use of the electrostimulated Latissimus Dorsi muscle on a chronic basis. Experimental use of the LDM technique of dynamic cardiomyoplasty originated in 1980 by our group in Paris. The conception and development of new electrodes for skeletal muscle stimulation, an implantable Cardio-Myostimulator, as well as a protocol of progressive and sequential electrostimulation of the LDM, allowed development of a hemodynamically efficacious muscle contraction on a chronic basis, in synchrony with cardiac activity. Simultaneously, the surgical technique of cardiomyoplasty was conceived and developed. The first world clinical case using this technique was then performed by our group in January 1985. Over 1000 patients worldwide to date have undergone the cardiomyoplasty procedure and the long-term clinical effectiveness of this approach has been demonstrated by several groups [10-13].

Simultaneously with the clinical application of cardiomyoplasty, new myoplasty techniques for circulatory support have been developed (4): aortomyoplasty, atriomyoplasty, double flap cardiomyoplasty, balloon for preoperative LDM expansion, aorto-pulmonary myoplasty for counterpulsation, skeletal muscle ventricles and cellular-molecular cardiomyoplasties.

Functional Electrostimulation

Chronic electrical activation of skeletal muscle is already used in various clinical situations such as: 1) diaphragmatic stimulation for respiratory support, 2) electrostimulation of the gracilis muscle used as a neo-sphincter in colorectal surgery, 3) vesicomyoplasty and creation of neo-sphincters in urology, 4) postural correction in scoliosis by stimulation of paravertebral muscles, and, 5) recovery after major orthopedic surgery (to avoid muscle disuse atrophy).

Chronic stimulation induces alterations in phenotype expression of skeletal muscle. Experimental studies concerning the histologic changes, histochemical adaptability, and electrophysiologic properties of skeletal muscle which is wrapped around the heart and chronically stimulated indicate that the marked enhancement in resistance to fatigue is the result of its increased capacity for oxidative (aerobic) metabolism [5, 6].

In the follow-up of cardiomyoplasty patients, it was shown that the chronically electrostimulated LDM maintains its contractile force and shows fatigue resistance when a "systolic activity" is imposed. These properties are directly related to the careful preservation of the LDM neurovascular pedicle during surgery [4] and with the postoperative electrostimulation protocol, which must avoid muscle overstimulation.

Electronic Device and Stimulation Protocol

Preclinical studies of cardiomyoplasty led to the design and development of new devices required for cardiomyostimulation (12). Previous stimulators and electrodes were not capable of producing a chronic and diffuse muscle contraction in synchrony with the cardiac cycle.

The pulse generator developed for cardiomyoplasty (CardioMyostimulator) is a double chamber device, including two channels: a sensing channel, which functions to detect cardiac activity, and a pacing channel, which stimulates muscle contraction based on the detection of QRS complexes. An electronic circuit synchronizes stimulation of muscle contraction with cardiac activity and determines the heart:muscle synchronization ratio (i.e., 1:1, 2:1, 3:1) and the synchronization delay. In the event of atrio-ventricular block, the sensing channel automatically acts as a cardiac pacemaker.

The LDM is chronically stimulated using pulse trains (bursts) to produce a fused skeletal muscle contraction. Single impulses entrain a moderate muscle contraction. A diffuse and vigorous muscle contraction is obtained by multiple, spaced impulses. The train of impulses results in a temporal summation with recruitment of all muscle fibers. The duration of contraction is physiologically adapted to ventricular systole.

The device (Transform System, Medtronic) possesses the particularity of delivering an adaptative cycle for chronic electromyostimulation, with the possibility of programming a 28% of the RR' interval for LDM stimulation, allowing enough time for muscle relaxation, delay in which the LDM is mainly irrigated [14].

Indications for Cardiomyoplasty

Patient selection constitutes the most important factor determining early and late outcome following cardiomyoplasty. Cardiomyoplasty must be considered prior to development of extreme end-stage cardiac insufficiency. As the hemodynamic benefits of cardiomyoplasty are not achieved until after a delay of several weeks necessary for the postoperative muscle stimulation protocol, the selection of patients to undergo this procedure must take into account their residual myocardial function [4, 15].

Indications for cardiomyoplasty include heart failure due to ischemic or idiopathic cardiomyopathies, without significant mitral valve regurgitation and preferently in sinus rhythm. Candidates must present an intact latissimus dorsi muscle (Table 1).

Contraindications are: hypertrophic and restrictive cardiomyopathies, intractable NYHA IV status, preoperative dependence on intravenous inotropes or intra-aortic balloon pump (IABP) and cardiac cachexia.

Concerning the ischemic etiology, cardiomyoplasty might be considered when myocardial revascularization is impossible or without anticipated significant functional benefit. Inoperable coronary artery disease, diffuse ventricular hypokinesis not improved with myocardial revascularization and large ventricular ischemic aneurysms with hypokinesis of the remaining myocardium are indications for dynamic cardiomyoplasty.

After 12 years of clinical experience, it was demonstrated that cardiomyoplasty has an important role for patients who are severely symptomatic and do not respond adequately to medication but have not reached the end-stage

Table 1. Patient selection for cardiomyopathy

Indications
- Heart failure that is symptomatic but not yet end stage; i.e., patient has some cardiac reserve (peak VO_2 > 10 ml/kg/min, radioisotopic LV ejection fraction > 15%)
- Dilated or ischemic cardiomyopathy without significant mitral regurgitation
- Intact Latissimus Dorsi muscle
- Adult (full grown)
- Adequate pulmonary function (forced vital capacity > 55%)
- Stable cardiac rhythm

Contraindications
- Intractable NYHA IV status
- Preoperative dependence on IV inotropes or IABP
- Primary hypertrophic or restrictive cardiomyopathy
- LDM has previous surgical damage or neuromuscular disease

of heart failure. For this subset of patients (with LV ejection fraction between 15% and 30% of normal), cardiomyoplasty play an important role in slowing the cardiac deterioration and postponing or eliminating the need of heart transplantation.

Mechanism of Action

Despite a widely varying and diverse etiology of congestive heart failure, the pathophysiology is, to a great extent, constant. The predominant factor is the alteration of myocardial contractility. This contractility defect causes an elevation of the ventricular wall tension resulting in a progressive decline in the contractile state of myocardial fibers. In ischemic and idiopathic dilated cardiomyopathies, contractility and distensibility are both impaired. These changes lead to a decrease in stroke volume and an increase in left ventricular diastolic pressure.

From the physiologic standpoint cardiomyoplasty works principally due to a combination of mechanisms [16]: 1) systolic assist, 2) limitation of ventricular dilatation, 3) reduction of ventricular wall stress (sparing effect), 4) ventricular remodeling with an active girdling effect, 5) angiogenesis, and 6) a neurohumoral effect.

Studies involving left ventricular pressure-volume curves assessed by conductance catheters, demonstrate improved systolic and diastolic functions after cardiomyoplasty. The stimulated LDM provides a "dynamic elastic girdle" which contributes to decreased *myocardial* stress and improved myocardial energetics as well as reverse remodeling of the heart itself [17, 18].

Postoperative Management

The early postoperative period in cardiomyoplasty patients is characterized by the absence of improvement in ventricular function, for LDM electrostimulation is started only two weeks following surgery. This delay is necessary for LDM flap vascular recovery and to facilitate the development of adhesions between the LDM and the heart. During this critical period, patients are generally assisted by intravenous inotropic drugs or by ABP. In our experience the early introduction of an IABP has proved very important in patients presenting perioperative hemodynamic instability. IABP avoids high doses of inotropic support that can be potentially deleterious to the LDM. Most of these drugs are vasoconstrictors and potentially dangerous for muscle fiber viability.

Clinical Experience

This surgical procedure is intended for use in patients *with chronic* low cardiac output refractory to pharmacological support, due to myocardial deficiencies of ischemic, neoplastic, dysplastic or idiopathic etiologies. before the end-stage period when the only possibility is heart transplantation or mechanical assist devices.

Following the first clinical case, performed at the Broussais Hospital in January 1985, more than 1000 patients have undergone this operation worldwide. At our institution, 95 patients (aged 15 to 72, mean 50 years) were operated upon. Patients presented with severe chronic heart failure, refractory to maximal medical treatment. The etiology of heart failure was ischemic 55%, idiopathic cardiomyopathy 34%, ventricular tumor 6%, other 5%. The mean follow-up period was 44 months (range: 3 months to 12 years). The mean NYHA functional class improved postoperatively from 3.2 to 1.8. Average radioisotopic left ventricular ejection fraction increased from $17 \pm 5\%$ to $27 \pm 4\%$ ($p < 0.05$), and remained stable in the long term. Stroke-volume index increased from 32 ± 7 to 43 ± 8 ml/beat/m^2 ($p < 0.05$). The heart size also remained stable at long term. Electron beam CT scans showed at long-term a preserved LDM structure in 82% of patients. No tendency of the LDM to compress or constrict the heart was observed at long-term.

Improvement of physical activity and work performance was observed at long-term in most of the patients operated on. Following cardiomyoplasty the number of rehospitalizations due to congestive heart failure was reduced to 0.4 hospitalizations/patient/year (preoperative: 2.5, $p < 0.05$). In 63% of patients the need for pharmacological therapy was reduced after surgery.

Survival probability at 7 years is 54% for the entire group of patients, and 70% for patients operated in NYHA functional class 3. No significant difference has been found in the survival rates of patients with ischemic cardiomyopathy vs idiopathic cardiomyopathy. The preoperative predictive factors for late mortality were severe biventricular cardiac failure, LV ejection fraction (isotopic) < 15%, and permanent functional class IV (NYHA).

Six patients (6%) underwent heart transplantion after cardiomyoplasty after a mean delay of 25 months, due principally to the natural evolution of the underlying heart disease, without major technical difficulties. Ten years of rigorous clinical evaluation have resulted in improved patient selection and management to increase survival [19, 20].

Discussion

Despite recent technical advances in cardiac surgery, profound refractory heart failure remains a significant cause of mortality. Although there has been a relative decrease in cardiovascular deaths in the past few years, the problem of heart failure continues to be a major one with an estimated 2 300 000 patients, and 400 000 new cases each year in the United States alone. Cardiac transplantation and externally powered cardiac prostheses used as bridge to transplant have given satisfactory and promising results but the problem of donors and procurement limits the widespread application of these techniques.

Cardiac transplantation is limited in some regions by legal, cultural and religious issues and particularly where socio-economic or geographic conditions prevent development of a transplantation program. Furthermore, the procedure is costly, the follow-up of patients is difficult and there is risk involved with immunosuppressive therapy.

Cardiomyoplasty can be considered indicated in patients with chronic cardiac insufficiency refractory to appropriate medical therapy, with progressive and irreversible loss of ventricular contractility. The aim of adapting the work capacity of skeletal muscle for use in a cardiac assist role, as applied in the cardiomyoplasty procedure, is to prolong and improve the quality of life of patients with severe and irreversible chronic cardiac insufficiency by improving ventricular contraction and limiting cardiac dilatation. Increased ventricular volume is one of the most powerful predictors of reduced survival in patients with heart disease. Cardiomyoplasty brings an elastic limitation of ventricular dilatation without restriction of compliance, useful to prevent intrinsic arrhythmias and mitral or tricuspid regurgitation due to cardiac dilatation.

What is evident studying the relative risks of recent pharmacological placebo-controlled trials is that, although most vasodilator trials show a survival benefit, there is substantial residual mortality in the treatment groups. Also, although important gains have been achieved by cardiac transplantation, continuing problems with rejection, heart failure, sepsis, accelerated atherosclerosis, supply of donors, and psychosocial adjustement remain a concern and pose opportunities for creative solutions. While comparative reviews are still awaited, there is an evident need for further progress in the treatment of heart failure.

Dynamic cardiomyoplasty deals with two of the most important scientific advances in recent years in the fields of electrophysiology and cardiac surgery. The first is the recent advance in muscle physiology resulting in the capability of transformation of skeletal muscle fibers to a fatigue resistant state. The second is the development of pacemaker technology as applied to synchronization of skeletal muscle contraction with ventricular systole to produce a new concept of cardiac bio-assist [4].

The optimal harnessing of skeletal muscle power, which can produce four times the strength of contraction of cardiac muscle and which we have seen continue to function for more than ten years, remains the objective of our continued studies and a challenge. In the development of cardiomyoplasty many further doors of investigation have been opened which hopefully will in the future lead to improved results and a wider application of the procedure. The results of cardiomyoplasty have improved with increased technical experience, with rigorous selection of patients, and with improved protocols of intensive care management and long-term care post-operation [21].

A few alternatives exist for chronic heart failure that is refractory to medical therapy. Long-term clinical results are showing that cardiomyoplasty is for the great majority of patients a definitive alternative. It may apply to the same population as heart transplantation, but there are some specific points that make patient selection different. Indications include patients with severe heart failure and without valvular disease, stabilized in NYHA functional class III at the time of surgery. Dilated cardiomyopathies either of ischemic or idiopathic etiologies are concerned.

A multicentric international clinical investigation in conjunction with surgical centres from fifteen countries was initiated to evaluate the results of cardiomyoplasty. An international committee for evaluation of results of cardiomyoplasty was set up in 1993. In the United States, dynamic cardiomyoplasty is currently being evaluated by a Food and Drug Administration mandated randomized trial which includes 400 patients in 20 centers. These 400 patients will be randomized to receive either dynamic cardiomyoplasty or remain on standard medical therapy. Enrollment continues at this time. Also in Europe, a randomized trial was organized.

A new tendency to associate cardiomyoplasty with electrophysiological therapies is emerging. These therapies include: 1) the implantation of ventricular defibrillators, 2) multisite cardiac pacing, and, 3) permanent cardiac pacing following the induction of a complete AV block in cardiomyoplasty patients presenting with atrial fibrillation. Clinical experience from many centers demonstrates the feasibility of these combined therapies and promising short-term results [22, 23].

Conclusion

Patients with advanced heart failure need evaluation for the full spectrum of care that modern cardiology offers, ranging from advanced medical therapy to skeletal myoplasty, left ventricular assist devices, and heart transplantation.

Congestive heart failure is a common and costly health issue. Dynamic cardiomyoplasty is a relatively inexpensive option for many patients who are not responsive to medical therapy. Data to date continue to support functional capacity improvements in patients following cardiomyoplasty. Recent studies have indicated that several mechanisms of action contribute to clinical improvements [24-27].

Our 12 year clinical experience demonstrates that cardiomyoplasty increases ejection fraction, improves functional class and ameliorates quality of life. Ventricular volumes and diameters remain stable at long-term. LDM structure is maintained at long-term if electrostimulation is performed avoiding excessive myostimulation. Patient selection is the most important determinant for early and late outcome. Cardiomyoplasty may delay or prevent end-stage heart failure and the need for heart transplantation.

References

1. McManus R, O'Hair D, Beitzinger J et al (1993) Patients who die awaiting heart transplantation. J Heart Lung Transplant 12:159-171
2. Packer M (1996) Do angiotensin-converting enzyme inhibitors prolong life in patients with heart failure treated in clinical practice? J Am Coll Cardiol 28:1323-1327
3. Chachques JC, Grandjean PA, Schwartz K, et al. (1988) Effect of latissimus dorsi dynamic cardiomyoplasty on ventricular function. Circulation 78 [Suppl 3]:203-216
4. Carpentier A, Chachques JC, Grandjean P (eds) (1997) Cardiac Bioassist. Futura Publishing, New York
5. Pette D, Smith ME, Staudte HW et al (1973) Effects of long-term electrical stimulation

on some contractile and metabolic characteristics of fast rabbit muscles. Pfluegers Arch 338:257-272

6. Salmons S, Streter FA (1976) Significance of impulse activity in the transformation of skeletal muscle type. Nature 263:30-34

7. Chiu RCJ (Ed) (1986) Biomechanical Cardiac Assist. Futura Publishing, New York

8. Carpentier A, Chachques JC, Grandjean PA (eds) (1991) Cardiomyoplasty. Futura Publishing, New York

9. Termet H, Chalencon JL, Estour E, Gaillard P, Favre JP (1966) Transplantation sur le myocarde d'un muscle strié excité par pacemaker. Ann Chir Thorac Cardio 5:568-571

10. Chachques JC, Mitz V, Hero M, et al (1985) Experimental cardioplasty using the Latissimus Dorsi muscle flap. J Cardiovasc Surg 26:457-462

11. Carpentier A, Chachques JC, Grandjean PA, Perier P, Mitz V, Bourgeois I (1985) Transformation d'un muscle squelettique par stimulation séquentielle progressive en vue de son utilisation comme substitut myocardique. C R Acad Sc Paris 301:581-586

12. Chachques JC, Grandjean PA, Smits K. Method and apparatus including a sliding insulation lead for cardiac assistance. U.S. Patent 4,735,205, 1988. European Patent 0,234,457, 1987

13. Carpentier A, Chachques JC (1985) Myocardial substitution with a stimulated skeletal muscle: first successful clinical case. Lancet 1:1267

14. Grandjean PA, Leinders R (1997) A new stimulation system for cardiomyoplasty. In: Carpentier A, Chachques JC, Grandjean P (eds) Cardiac Bioassist. Futura Publishing, New York 277-284

15. Chachques JC, Grandjean PA, Carpentier A (1989) Latissimus Dorsi Dynamic Cardiomyoplasty. Ann Thorac Surg 47:600-604

16. Hwan J, Badhwar V, Chiu RCJ (1996) Mechanisms of dynamic cardiomyoplasty: current concepts. J Card Surg 11:194-199

17. Schreuder JJ, Van der Veen FH, Van der Velde ET, et al (1995) Beat-to-beat analysis of left ventricular pressure-volume relation and stroke volume by conductance catheter and aortic model flow in cardiomyoplasty patients. Circulation 91:2010-2017

18. Kass DA, Baughman KL, Pak PH, et al (1995) Reverse remodeling from cardiomyoplasty in human heart failure. Circulation 91:2314-2318

19. Carpentier A, Chachques JC, Acar C, et al (1993) Dynamic cardiomyoplasty at seven years. J Thorac Cardiovasc Surg 106:42-54

20. Chachques JC, Berrebi A, Hernigou A, et al (1997) Study of muscular and ventricular function in dynamic cardiomyoplasty: a ten year follow up. J Heart Lung Transplant 16:854-868

21. Carraro U, Chachques JC, Desnos M, Hagège A, Fontaliran F, Carpentier A (1996) Eight-year human dynamic cardiomyoplasty: preserved structure of myofibres and vessels of the latissimus dorsi. Basic Appl Myol 6:333-336

22. Francischelli D, Peterson D, Stein PM, Gealow KK, Grandjean PA (1997) Cardiomyoplasty and defibrillator: a combined treatment for heart failure. In: Carpentier A, Chachques JC, Grandjean PA (Eds): Cardiac Bioassist. Futura Publishing, New York, pp 417-428

23. Cabrera Fischer EI, Chachques JC, Christen AI, Risk MR, Carpentier A (1996) Hemodynamic effects of cardiomyoplasty in an experimental model of acute heart failure and atrial fibrillation. Artif Organs 20:1215-1219

24. Furnary AP, Chachques JC, Moreira LFP, et al (1996) Long term outcome, survival analysis and risk stratification of dynamic cardiomyoplasty. J Thorac Cardiovasc Surg 112:1640-1650

25. Magovern GJ, Simpson KA (1996) Clinical cardiomyoplasty: review of the ten-year United States experience. Ann Thorac Surg 61:413-419

26. Moreira LFP, Stolf NAG, Braile DM, Jatene AD (1996) Dynamic cardiomyoplasty in South America. Ann Thorac Surg 61:408-412

27. Lorusso R, Milan E, Volterrani M, et al (1997) Cardiomyoplasty as an isolated procedure to treat refractory heart failure. Eur J Cardio-Thoracic Surg 11:363-372

Left Ventricular Assist Device as Bridge to Transplantation

M. Viganò, M. Rinaldi, F. Pagani, G. Minzioni, A.M. D'Armini and E. Ardemagni

Introduction

The shortage of donors is responsible for the majority of patients dying while waiting for transplantation. To rescue these critically ill patients, a wide variety of devices have been proposed for circulatory assistance as bridge to heart transplantation [1,2]. Prolonged bridging is often necessary, because of donor scarcity and because of the need to allow complete patient recovery before transplantation.

This attitude has led to the consolidation of electrically powered left ventricular assist devices (LVAD) [3]. The wearable system of the Novacor device is the result of the effort in miniaturizing the previous large external consolle. It can now be worn on a belt, allowing a high degree of mobility and a good quality of life during the waiting period [4]. For this reason its use has been spreading to a large number of transplantation centers and the duration of the assistance periods has been increasing significantly over time. In some centers patients under assistance have been discharged and followed up as outpatients, decreasing the financial impact of circulatory assistance on health care resources.

The aim of this presentation is to discuss the experience in Novacor implantation at the Cardiac Surgery Department of I.R.C.C.S Policlinico S. Matteo - University of Pavia with particular attention to the risk factors for thromboembolism, and the incidence of other complications. The issues of outpatient care while on assistance and permanent application of the device are also addressed.

Despite the immediate good results of heart transplantation in the aging population, a wider application of this surgical technique in the elderly is in reality prevented by the scarcity of donor organs. Moreover, in this subgroup of patients, a higher incidence of late complications related to chronic immunosuppression has been reported. Therefore the impact of LVAD implantation in the elderly and the suitability of a permanent application of these devices as an alternative to cardiac transplantation in the older population are also discussed.

Patients and Methods

From November 1992 to May 1996, 23 patients underwent implantation of a Novacor N100 LVAS (Novacor Division - Baxter Healthcare, Oakland - California) for end-stage cardiac failure as bridge to transplant. Demographic data are illustrated in Table 1. There were 21 males and 2 females. The mean age was 50 years (range 29 - 68). Twenty patients were on the waiting list for cardiac transplantation at our Center: thirteen of them had dilated cardiomyopathy and seven had ischemic cardiomyopathy, three of whom had previously undergone coronary artery bypass grafting. The remaining three patients were put on the list soon after the assistance was implanted: one patient had dilated cardiomyopathy, was referred to us from a peripheral hospital and underwent the same day emergency application of the device; two patients had post-cardiotomy failures after coronary artery bypass grafting and massive perioperative myocardial infarction.

Twenty-two patients were in advanced NYHA class IV on infusion of inotropes and/or vasodilators. The single patient in NYHA class III had

Table 1. Demographic data

N. pat.	Age	Sex	BSA (m²)	Diagnosis	IABP	Device	Length of assistance	Follow-up
1	37	M	1.78	DCM	yes	Consolle	16	Dead pre-tx
2	57	M	1.68	DCM	no	Consolle	13	Tx, alive
3	50	M	2.05	ICM	no	Wearable	17	Tx, alive
4	47	M	1.7	DCM	no	Wearable	47	Tx, alive
5	54	M	1.99	DCM	yes	Wearable	69	Tx, dead
6	58	M	2.03	DCM	no	Wearable	427	Tx, alive
7	38	M	1.90	DCM	no	Wearable	142	Tx, alive
8	62	F	1.74	DCM	no	Wearable	431	On assistance
9	54	M	1.52	DCM	no	Wearable	88	Tx, dead
10	44	M	2.05	DCM	no	Wearable	336	On assistance
11	57	M	1.90	ICM	no	Wearable	295	Tx alive
12	29	M	1.65	DCM	no	Wearable	39	Tx, dead
13	57	M	1.87	ICM	no	Wearable	141	Dead pre tx
14	56	F	1.50	DCM	yes	Wearable	28	Tx, dead
15	47	M	1.83	DCM	no	Wearable	241	Dead pre tx
16	64	M	1.74	ICM	no	Wearable	242	On assistance
17	67	M	1.74	ICM	no	Wearable	111	Dead pre tx
18	34	M	1.68	DCM	yes	Wearable	30	Tx, alive
19	46	M	1.92	PHF	yes*	Wearable	109	On assistance
20	39	M	1.83	PHF	no	Wearable	91	On assistance
21	68	M	1.70	ICM	no	Wearable	15	Dead pre tx
22	33	M	1.89	ICM	no	Wearable	66	On assistance
23	49	M	1.85	DCM	no	Wearable	40	On assistance

BSA, Body surface area; IABP, Intra aortic baloon pump; DCM, Dilated cardiomyopathy; ICM, Ischemic cardiomyopathy; PHF, Postcardiotomy heart failure.
* ECMO, extracorporal membrane oxygenation.

ischemic cardiomyopathy and malignant arrhythmias. Four patients were bridged to LVAD with intra-aortic balloon pump and one with extracorporeal membrane oxygenation. In the first two patients the consolle-driven model was implanted, while in the subsequent cases the wearable model was used.

Surgical Technique

In all cases we adopted a modified "ortho-dromic" technique using aortic cross-clamping and hypothermic cardioplegic arrest of the heart [5]. After sternotomy, the pocket was tailored dividing the insertion of the diaphragm to the lower ribs, to ease bleeding control. On cardiopulmonary bypass, the aorta was cross-clamped and cardioplegia administered. Apical cannulation was performed first on a dry, still field. The device was then easily deaired, with blood flowing in the physiologic direction. The aorta was declamped and the outflow conduit anastomosed. Before tying the suture, final deairing was obtained. This technique allows extreme precision in apical cannulation, easier control of bleeding and accurate deairing of the pump. The ischemic time is short (around 30 minutes). In the three patients previously operated on for coronary artery bypass grafting, the only technical problem was an accidental section of a patent graft on the right coronary artery, which caused right ventricular failure during the weaning from cardiopulmonary bypass. The reanastomose of the graft to the outflow conduit of the pump allowed the recovery of right ventricular function and the weaning from cardiopulmonary bypass.

Peri-operative prophylaxis for infection included vancomicin, norfloxacin and amphotericin B.

Anticoagulation Protocol

A critical issue in mechanical assistance is the prevention of bleeding in the immediate postoperative period and of thromboembolism in the short and long term. In the first three cases we adopted the complex protocol summarized in Table 2. In the following cases anticoagulation treatment was greatly simplified by introducing either calcium heparin (7500 UI subcutaneously) or continuous heparin infusion as soon as surgical bleeding stopped, to maintain partial thromboplastin time at 1.5 times the basal value. Subsequently, patients were started on oral acenocumarole aiming at a protrombin activity of 20%-40 % (INR 2.5-4.0), and heparin was stopped. An antiplatelet agent was also added (aspirin 100 mg/day) to prevent micro-aggregation.

Out-of-hospital Management

The wearable setting of the Novacor LVAD allows a complete mobilization of the patient. Patients were discharged to the rehabilitation center as soon as the clinical situation was stable, the patient was fully mobilized and the surgical wound healed. The rehabilitation program included an individualized physical

Table 2. Protocol of anticoagulation/antiaggregation

PREOPERATIVE:
Dipyridamole: 500 mg in 12 h I.V. continuously

INTRAOPERATIVE:
Complete heparinization: 300 UI/kg
Neutralization with 60% protamine
Aprotinine according to Royston protocol
2000000 UI at start of anesthesia
2000000 UI during cardiopulmonary bypass
500000 UI/h till the end of procedure
Dipyridamole

EARLY POSTOPERATIVE :
Heparin I.V. mantaining PTT 1.5-2.0 times of normal values
Aprotinine 500000 UI every 6 hs if bleeding
Dipyridamole 1g 24 h I.V. continuously
Antithrombin III when < 75 %

LATE POSTOPERATIVE:
Oral acenocumarol maintaining 2.5 >INR < 4
Withdrawal of heparin I.V. when INR reached the range
Oral dipyridamole 800 mg/day

training program based on a 5-days/week cycle of treadmill sessions, calisthenics and stretching exercises and psychological support to allow patients to be discharged home. The stretching exercises were mainly oriented for the back muscles and aimed at avoiding or treating possible contractures due to abnormal postures caused by the weight of the device (about 4 Kg).

Results

Postoperative Course

The operative mortality was 0. Three patients required surgical re-exploration for bleeding and a fourth one underwent surgical debridement and mediastinal irrigation for sternal dehiscence, which eventually resolved. Prolonged inotropic support with dobutamine (mean 10.7 days) was needed in all cases to support the right ventricle during the postoperative period. Pulmonary vasodilatation was also obtained in all cases with sodium nipride (0.5 - 2.0 ng/kg/min) and in three cases inhaled nitric oxide (10 - 20 ppm) was needed to wean patients from cardiopulmonary bypass. Right ventricular mechanical assistance was not required in any case. The average stay in the intensive care unit for the 21 patients with the wearable device was of 13.9 days, but the median time was 8 days. The mean and median time of mechanical ventilation were 9.6 days and 2 days, respectively. The mean implant duration is at the moment 162 days (range: 7-701 days), with a significant extension of the period in the most recent cases.

Hemodynamics and Parenchymal Function

Hemodynamic data are presented in Table 3. Statistical comparisons between the main parameters, before and after the device was implanted, are summarized in Table 4. The efficacy of the device in normalizing the circulatory conditions is well evident. The extremely compromised preoperative hemodynamic situation induced an initial deterioration of parenchymal functions. Urinary output was low in all cases, with a mean creatinine level of 1.4 ± 0.3 mg/dl (range 0.9-2.1). The mean bilirubin level was 1.9 ±1.0 mg/dl (range 0.2-4.9). Renal and hepatic function improved gradually during assistance with a significant reduction in serum creatinine (from 1.4 ± 0.3 to 0.7 ± 0.5 mg/dl, p < 0.01) and bilirubine (from 1.9 ± 1.0 to 0.9 ± 0.7 mg/dl, $p < 0.01$). Severe preoperative right cardiac failure was present in 10 patients (43%) with a mean right atrial pressure of 17.1± 4.1 mmHg, a mean right ventricular ejection fraction of 8.4 ± 3.5 % and mean pulmonary vascular resistance of 460 ± 187 dyne/m^2/sec^{-5}.

Table 3. Hemodynamic data pre- and post-implantation

| N. pat. | Pre-implant | | | | | Post-implant | | | | |
	CI	MPAP	PCWP	PVR (WU)	RVEF	CI	MPAP	PCWP	PVR (WU)	RVEF
1	1.7	42	22	6.6	8	2.9	24	4	4.0	21
2	1.8	37	22	4.8	15	2.9	34	14	4.0	20
3	1.7	46	39	1.2	15	3.3	18	2	2.3	23
4	1.3	51	42	4.0	4	2.7	20	11	1.9	15
5	2.1	42	22	4.7	9	3.7	24	13	1.4	18
6	1.8	32	22	2.6	12	2.9	18	3	2.5	14
7	1.8	50	29	5.9	10	2.6	14	6	1.6	22
8	1.4	37	28	3.7	8	3.6	25	13	1.8	24
9	1.1	47	35	6.7	15	2.0	19	10	2.7	27
10	1.9	47	36	2.7	12	2.6	12	8	0.7	19
11	0.9	43	30	7.3	7	2.7	24	9	2.9	24
12	0.9	32	24	5.0	6	2.1	9	2	2.0	12
13	1.9	34	29	2.5	29	2.6	20	5	2.4	17
14	1.0	45	40	3.5	20	3.6	27	14	2.3	39
15	1.3	31	19	2.4	12	1.4	17	13	1.5	16
16	0.9	51	34	11.3		2.4	24	11	3.6	
17	1.8	46	31	4.8		2.5	10	5	5.0	
18	1.0	24	19	2.8		2.6	16	7	1.9	15
19										
20	1.7	47	32	4.7	28	3.0	13	6	1.4	
21	1.2	44	34	5.0						
22	1.3	40	32	2.9						
23	1.2	40	30	4.6	14	2.6	19	9	2	

CI, cardiac index; MPAP, mean pulmonary artery pressure; PCWP, pulmonary capillary wedge pressure; PVR, pulmonary vascular resistance in Wood Units (WU); RVEF, right ventricular ejection fraction.

Table 4. Hemodynamic variables before and after LVAD implantation

	Pre-implant	Post-implant	p
CI	1.52 ± 0.41	2.87 ± 0.52	< 0.001
MPAP	41.7 ± 6.4	20.5 ± 6.4	< 0.001
PCWP	30.0 ± 7.2	8.1 ± 4.4	< 0.001
PVR (WU)	4.37 ± 1.81	2.32 ± 0.9	< 0.001
RVEF	12.1 ± 6.5	21.0± 6.6	< 0.001

For abbreviations see Table 3

Early Complications (< 2 months)

In 3 cases (13%) surgical revision because of bleeding was necessary. There was one case of sternal dehiscence, which was surgically resolved. Early cerebrovascular events were observed in 10 patients (43.5%). In 3 patients severe and permanent neurological damage developed, which lead to patient death. A single case of hemolysis (free Hb > 30 mg/dl) was observed in coincidence with massive transfusions. Five patients (22%) had early systemic infective episodes, all successfully treated with antibiotic therapy

Late Complications (> 2 months)

Late complications were analyzed in the 15 patients who were assisted for more than 2 months. The main long-term complication was infection of the skin and the subcutaneous tissue at the site of cable exit (4/15 cases, 17.4%). This complication was generally well controlled by local medications and intermittent systemic antibiotic treatment on the basis of cultural results. One case, however, evolved in a severe Staphylococcus aureus sepsis, twelve months after LVAD application. Prolonged treatment with vancomicin and sinercid was needed to sterilize the patient and to allow transplantation. Inspection of the device after explantation revealed an endocarditis of the inflow valve with partial cusp disruption.

The incidence of late cerebrovascular accidents was 25.2% (6 cases). One transient ischemic attack occurred in a patient with severe carotid artery disease, who subsequently underwent carotid endoarteriectomy during assistance.

Another patient developed a fatal massive cerebral hemorrhage 8 months after LVAD implantation. Two patients had limb embolism, which required emergency surgical embolectomy; both cases were related to gross deviations from anticoagulation therapy

Thromboembolic Events

The majority of these events (17/21, 81%) took place during the first 2 months. Major cerebral events, i.e. those lasting more than few minutes and/or CT scan proved, followed a similar distribution: 11/12 (92%) occurred within 2 months after LVAD implantation. In 4 cases, these episodes determined a permanent serious brain damage, which led to patient death.

Outcome

Eleven patients (48%) were successfully bridged to cardiac transplantation. Five patients (21.7%) died during assistance because of multiorgan failure. Seven patients (30.5%) are presently under assistance: 2 are still in hospital, 5 have been discharged and are followed-up as outpatients. The global survival of the procedure of bridging to transplant is 78.5%. The functional status of all patients was dramatically improved during assistance with the wearable device: all moved from NYHA class IV to NYHA class I, during daily life activities. All patients attended an appropriate training in order to improve their self-sufficiency and to minimize any associated risk related to the device. As far as the psychological aspects are concerned, all patients soon became optimistic: they really felt themselves on a bridge linking heart failure with heart transplant. Improvement in their health status overcame any discomfort. The device was highly accepted and the noise did not annoy but reassured them.

Discussion

LVAD systems have reached such a degree of technological improvement, that they can be considered absolutely reliable in their life-saving function and in the normalization of the circulatory and parenchymal parameters before transplantation [6]. Their characteristics allow prolonged application with complete mobilization, rehabilitation and even discharge. For these reasons, the use of mechanical assist devices as bridges to transplantation has been spreading in many transplant centers. The great enthusiasm and expectations have recently been attenuated by some skepticism, mainly due to social costs and the scarce impact of this approach on the global mortality of patients listed for transplantation. Clearly, even a wide application of prolonged mechanical assistance does not increase the total number of transplants, which is only affected by graft availability. Some centers have already started clinical series of LVAD application as an alternative to transplant. In those series, patients with contraindication to heart transplantation, the main one being perhaps advanced age, are treated with permanent LVAD assistance.

According to the data available until the end of 1995 [7], a total number of 993 patients have been assisted with a monoventricular assist device as bridge to transplantation, either with a Novacor or a Heartmate system. This worldwide experience is summarized in Table 5. It must be said that only 49 patients (10.1%) in the Heartmate series were assisted with the recent electromechanical and wearable configuration. The transplant rate, the mean duration of assistance and the cumulative experience is basically similar in the two groups. An extremely interesting consideration, coming from the Novacor series, is presented in Table 6: from these data it appears clear how long-term bridging, with complete stabilization of patients' conditions, allows a higher transplant rate and, ultimately, a superior survival compared to those obtained with short-term assistance. These results seem to encourage the surgeons to utilize prolonged bridging.

The only real factor which seems to limit a wider application of mechanical assistance is thromboembolism, which is by far the more serious complication emerging from our and other series [4,8,9]. The prevalence of the phenomenon has globally been 43% in the first 2 months. Most episodes were transient ischemic attacks (35%) or strokes with complete recovery (64%), but in 4 cases (36%) cerebrovascular accidents led to patient death. These disturbing figures must be carefully studied and interpreted with particular attention to the risk factors for cerebral events. If the prevalence of cerebrovascular events is expressed in linearized incidence rate, there is a ten-fold difference between the early period (less than two months) and the late period (0.40 vs 0.04 episodes/patient/month; $p < 0.001$) after LVAD implantation.

The protocol of anticoagulation and antiaggregation, which was originally (in the first 5 cases) quite complex, was greatly simplified thereafter with the utilization of heparin i.v. or subcutaneous calcium-heparin in the early postoperative period and oral acenocumarol associated to aspirin, subsequently. It must be suspected that this oversimplification has negatively influenced the thromboembolic rate. Most of the thromboembolic events have been associated in our experience to sustained rhythm disturbances, namely atrial fibrillation, septic episodes, low output of the device, and errors in tuning anticoagulation. What seems to be impressive, even if the low numbers prevent any statistical comparison, is the fact that in 3 out of 4 severe cerebrovascular accidents leading to death, the patients were older than 60 years, had ischemic cardiomyopathy and documented atherosclerosis of the carotid arteries. More careful screening of elderly patients, with the possible exclusion of those with severe systemic atherosclerosis will probably be useful to reduce these complications in the future.

The risk of infection, related to the presence of prosthetic material, is out of question. In our experience however the overall number of systemic infections was low (five episodes in 23 patients). In the late follow-up the more frequent complication was the infection of the subcutaneous tissue at the site of cable exit. These episodes were managed successfully with frequent local medications and systemic antibiotic administration; in one case the infection

Table 5. World experience with Novacor and Heartmate systems

	NOVACOR	HEARTMATE
N. of patients	451	482
% of transplanted pts	62%	64%
Mean duration of assistance	68 days	72 days
Cumulative experience	83 years	96 years

Table 6. Global clinical results according to assistance duration with the Novacor system

	SHORT-TERM (< 3 months)	LONG-TERM (> 3 months)
N. of patients	306	89
Transplanted pts	163 (58%)	52 (73%)
Ongoing assistances	22	16
Mean duration of assistance	29 days	146 days

became systemic with endocarditis of the inflow valve and the patient was transplanted successfully on an emergency basis.

An adequate protocol of rehabilitation for a long period of support is of capital importance. Continuous hospitalization is no longer necessary, because once physically rehabilitated and trained to take care of the controller and the batteries, the patient can safely be discharged home. A further step towards the normalization of the quality of life consists in the complete autonomization of the patients at home. The first step is to discharge them from the rehabilitation center during the weekend; these periods can then be extended to a definitive discharge. A long distance between the patients' home and the transplant or rehabilitation center represents a limiting factor as it would preclude routine controls of the device, anticoagulation monitoring and the rapid admission in case of transplant.

In conclusion, left mechanical assistance appears to be a reliable life-saving procedure in patients dying from heart failure. The main indication remains the implantation as bridge to transplantation. As soon as the problems of thromboembolism and of the percutaneous cable are addressed by a rational and reliable method, the application of a mechanical assistance as an alternative to cardiac transplantation could be advantageous for some categories of patients. Especially elderly patients could benefit from a quite normal life without the side effects of immunosuppressive treatment. A word of caution must be pronounced in favor of a more accurate screening in this aging population, with particular regard to the conditions of the cerebral vessels and to the presence of severe atherosclerotic disease.

References

1. De Vries WC, Anderson JL, Joice LD, Anderson FL, Hammond EH, Jarvik RH, Kolff WJ (1984) Clinical use of the total artificial heart. N Engl J Med 310:273-278
2. Ferrar DJ, Thoratec Ventricular Assist Device Principal Investigators (1994) Preoperative predictors of survival in patients with Thoratec Ventricular Assist Device as a bridge to heart transplantation. J Heart Lung Transplant 13:93-100
3. Portner PM, Oyer PE, Pennington DG, Baumgartner WA, Griffith BP, Frist WR, Magilligan DJ Jr, Noon GP, Ramasamy N, Miller PJ (1989) Implantable electrical left ventricular assist system: bridge to transplantation and the future. Ann Thorac Surg 47:142-150
4. Vetter HO, Kaulbach HG, Samithz C, First A, Uberfuhr H, Kreuzer E, Pfeiffer M, Brenner P, Dewald O, Reichart B (1995) Experience with Novacor left ventricular assist system as a bridge to cardiac transplantation, including the new wearable system. J Thorac Cardiovasc Surg 109:74-80

5. Viganò M, Martinelli L, Minzioni G, Rinaldi M, Pagani F (1996) Modified method for Novacor ventricular assist device implantation. Ann Thorac Surg 61:247-249
6. McCarthy PM, Savage RM, Fraser CD, Vargo R, James KB, Goormastic CM, Hobbs RE (1995) Hemodynamic and physiologic changes during support with an implantable left ventricular assist device. J Thorac Cardiovasc Surg 109:409-418
7. Portner PM (1997) An overview on LVAD. Oral Communication. End-stage heart failure. Milan 27-29 September
8. Frazier OH, Macris MP, Myers TJ, Duncan JM, Radovancevic B, Parnis SM, Cooley DA (1994) Improved survival after extended bridge to cardiac transplantation. Ann Thorac Surg 57:1416-1422
9. Smith JA, Oyer PE (1995) Development of the Novacor left ventricular assist device. In: Shumway SJ, Shumway NE (eds) Thoracic transplantation Blackwell Science Inc Boston, pp 134-140

Subject Index